CONTEMPORARY TOPICS IN MOLECULAR IMMUNOLOGY

VOLUME 3

CONTEMPORARY TOPICS IN MOLECULAR IMMUNOLOGY

A Continuation Order Plan is available for this series. A continuation order will bring delivery of each new volume immediately upon publication. Volumes are billed only upon actual shipment. For further information please contact the publisher.

Contemporary Topics in Molecular Immunology

Volume 3

EDITED BY

G. L. Ada

Department of Microbiology
The John Curtin School of Medical Research
Australian National University
Canberra City, Australia

PLENUM PRESS • NEW YORK AND LONDON

The first volume of this series, published under a different title,
was cataloged by the Library of Congress as follows:

Contemporary topics in immunochemistry. v. 1–
New York, Plenum Press, 1972–

   v. illus. 24 cm.

Editor: v. 1–   F. P. Inman.

1. Immunochemistry—Collected works.   I. Inman, F. P., ed.

QR180.C635   574.2′9   73–186260

Library of Congress   72 [2]

Library of Congress Catalog Card Number 73-186260

ISBN-13: 978-1-4684-2840-7   e-ISBN-13: 978-1-4684-2838-4
DOI: 10.1007/978-1-4684-2838-4

CONTRIBUTORS TO THIS VOLUME

Albert A. Benedict
Department of Microbiology
University of Hawaii
Honolulu, Hawaii

J. Donald Capra
Department of Microbiology
Mount Sinai School of Medicine
City University of New York
New York, New York

A. J. Cunningham
Department of Microbiology
John Curtin School of Medical Research, A. N. U.
Canberra, Australia

Michael J. Crumpton
National Institute for Medical Research
Mill Hill
London, England

Marc Feldmann
Imperial Cancer Research Fund Tumour Immunology Unit
Department of Zoology
University College
London, England

F. P. Inman
Department of Microbiology
University of Georgia
Athens, Georgia

J. Michael Kehoe
Department of Microbiology
Mount Sinai School of Medicine
City University of New York
New York, New York

J. Mestecky
Department of Microbiology
Institute for Dental Research
University of Alabama Medical Center
Birmingham, Alabama

Ken Shortman
The Walter and Eliza Hall Institute of Medical Research
Melbourne, Australia

Malcolm J. Simons
WHO Immunology Research and Training Centre
University of Singapore
Singapore, Singapore

David Snary
National Institute for Medical Research
Mill Hill
London, England

R. H. Stevens
Division of Biochemistry
National Institute for Medical Research
Mill Hill
London, England

A. R. Williamson
Department of Microbiology and Immunology
University of California
Los Angeles, California

Preface

A series of volumes devoted to molecular immunology will contain, for the most part, articles which attempt to explain immunological phenomena in terms of the behavior and properties of particular molecules. Many of the articles in this volume do this. At the same time, there are many instances—and this is particularly so in the case of immunology—where phenomena must first be described and interpreted in terms of the properties and behavior of cells. Most of us would hope that in due course a fuller understanding will be forthcoming.

This volume starts off with such a contribution. Perhaps the most fascinating problem in immunology is how diversity is generated. There are two broad proposals: (1) that complete information exists *ab initio* (the germ-line theory), and (2) that there is initially a limited amount of information, and diversity is generated by somatic mutation. The issue is unresolved, but Cunningham has taken many of the data which have previously been used to support the germ-line theory and shows that the interpretations are not always clear-cut and can frequently be used to support another possibility—that new specificities may arise after stimulation of appropriate cells by antigens. And he has produced experimental evidence to support this notion. On the other hand, there can be little doubt that to a considerable degree the specificity of the immune response is determined by the selection by antigen of cells with receptors of appropriate specificity. This is essentially a surface phenomenon. Further, there is increasing evidence that the behavior of cells in their interactions with one another is determined in many ways by their surface antigens. It is evident that there will be increasing emphasis on the study of the cell plasma membrane, and Crumpton and Snary have provided a detailed assessment of the preparation and properties of lymphocyte membranes. It can safely be predicted that the study of the lymphocyte plasma membrane will attract more attention from immunologists. Feldman has provided a comprehensive article on the nature of immunogenicity—that feature of antigens which seems to be all-important in their reactions with B lymphocytes in determining whether antibody production, tolerance, or neither will ensue. The evidence reinforces the importance of repeating determinants on the ability of an antigen to stimulate or inactivate a cell.

If we now move inside the activated cell, one feature is the appearance in increased amount of mRNA molecules, coding for the light and heavy chains of immunoglobulin. In an elegant series of experiments, Stevens and Williamson report on the isolation and activity of mRNA for γ chains. Particularly intriguing is the demonstration of a binding site for mRNA on the Fc portion of the γ chain and the possibility that this may be involved in regulation of the production of the γ chain.

Two articles follow on the properties of antibodies, the chief products of stimulated B cells. The first, by Inman and Mestecky, is about J chains and is a comprehensive account of current information on these polypeptides, which are found associated with the polymeric immunoglobulins IgM and IgA. There is strong recent evidence that addition of J chain to the monomer is necessary for formation of the polymer to occur. IgMs, the monomer of IgM, is now generally regarded as the receptor for antigen on virgin B lymphocytes, and perhaps the addition of J chains to IgMs might be somehow connected with activation of the cell. Kehoe and Capra have compared the heavy-chain variable region ($V_H III$) sequences from several species. Their analyses focus attention on the extensive conservation of sequence preceding the first hypervariable region, and on the phylogenetically associated residues. The relationship of these observations to the theories of antibody diversification is discussed.

Progress in any discipline depends largely on the development of new techniques, and immunology is no exception. This volume concludes with two such contributions. The first, by Shortman, is a critical evaluation of techniques available for the separation of different types of cells of interest to immunologists. Undoubtedly, future progress will depend to a large extent upon the availability of purified cell populations, and the message of this article is that many suitable techniques are already available.

There are probably more papers in immunology on the reactions between antigen and antibody than on any other topic. Why have another? The reason is that the technique of radioelectrocomplexing, described by Simons and Benedict, seems to offer so many advantages, not only in academic but in clinical immunology, compared to many other procedures, that a comprehensive description seemed to be appropriate.

I believe all the articles in this volume are on topics at the growing edge of immunological research. I hope they are as useful and fascinating to other readers as they have been to me. I warmly thank the contributors and my fellow editors for their help in preparing this volume.

G. L. Ada

Contents

Immunogenicity *In Vitro:* Structural Correlation
Marc Feldmann

**mRNA for H and L Chains of Immunoglobulin: Specific Control
of H-Chain Production**
R. H. Stevens and A. R. Williamson

The Generation of Antibody Diversity: Its Dependence on Antigenic Stimulation

A. J. Cunningham

Department of Microbiology
John Curtin School of Medical Research
Australian National University
Canberra, Australia

I. INTRODUCTION

How antibody diversity arises is a central problem in immunology. Older instructionist theories have been abandoned with increasing knowledge of mechanisms of protein synthesis, and the selectionist ideas have been experimentally confirmed: each lymphocyte seems to be restricted to the synthesis of one type of antibody-combining site. This implies that a vast array of different lymphocytes exists within an animal. How these arise is not clear. The germ-line theory (Hood and Prahl, 1971) says that all genes are carried by each cell, a process of selective gene expression ensuring that only one V_L and one V_H gene product are released per cell. Somatic mutation (Cohn, 1972) or recombination (Gally and Edelman, 1972) theories say that a range of genetically different lymphocytes is produced during ontogeny by random changes in the DNA.

Is the full complement of lymphocytes bearing different receptors generated before or after contact with antigen? The germ-line theory would say "before." For somatic theories it should not matter. In fact, it would seem simpler to carry only a few types of lymphocytes and to adapt to antigen by production and selection of mutants. This possibility has often been mentioned. Makela and Cross (1970) think that such a mechanism may contribute to antibody diversity, but most other authors either consider it unimportant (e.g., Siskind and Benacerraf, 1969) or specifically reject it (Claflin and Merchant, 1973; Davie and Paul, 1972). That is, most immunologists seem to consider that the great variety of antigen-reactive cells arise spontaneously and are present before antigen, which acts only to select from the available repertoire.

1

Historically, this view arose because of a need to explain self-tolerance: the *spontaneous* generation of diversity and elimination of self-reactive clones is one of the cornerstones of Burnet's clonal selection theory (Burnet, 1959). More recently, the idea that self-tolerance is due to an early developmental purging of self-reactive clones has become undermined. Some other possible mechanisms are discussed in a later section. If an animal can use one of a variety of suppressor mechanisms to prevent self-destruction, then there is no longer any need to prohibit the random generation of new clones during an immune response. Self-reactive cells will be dealt with as they arise.

The purpose of this chapter is to present the evidence for an obligatory role of antigen in the generation of most antibody diversity. The majority of published discussions on the generation of diversity attempt to derive possible genetic mechanisms from an analysis of the amino acid sequences of myeloma proteins. Here the argument will be mainly at the level of cellular phenotype. Do new types of immunocompetent cells commonly arise *only* after antigenic stimulation? If they do, this has important implications for immunological theory and puts some constraints on possible genetic mechanisms for the generation of diversity. Antigen-generated diversity would seem to be more consistent with somatic mutation than with germ-line ideas, although it is conceivable that some members of a clone might switch randomly from the expression of one antibody gene to another. The evidence is all indirect, and it has to be admitted at the outset that there are no experiments yet which conclusively decide the issue. Nevertheless, most existing phenomena are much more simply explained by the idea that antigen generates diversity than by its opposite.

II. EXPLANATION OF THE THEORY

Figure 1 compares conventional and "antigen-generated-diversity" theories. According to this new model, an animal would need only a relatively small number (1000–10,000?) of B-cell types* with different receptors. Multiple copies of each cell type would exist. An antigen stimulates one or a few of these types to proliferate and produce antibody. The affinity of such early receptors for any antigen must usually be weak. Stimulation of the cells would be assisted by, and perhaps be dependent on, multipoint binding of antigen, possibly on the surface of macrophages or T cells, and the antibody first produced would probably be of too low affinity to be detectable by most serological tests. The large amounts of "nonspecific" Ig often found early in a primary response (e.g., Urbain-Vansanten, 1970) might represent such early low-affinity products.

---

*The same arguments probably apply to all immunocompetent cells, whether B or T (see Section IX), but only B cells have been discussed throughout this chapter, because there is much more information about the diversity of their product.

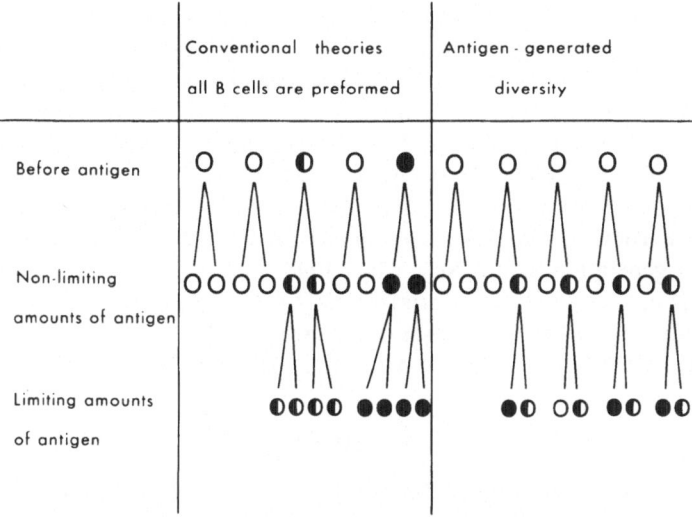

Figure 1. Changes in the patterns of B cells produced during the course
of an immune response. The highest-affinity cells are black.

Variant B-cell forms would quickly appear, the simplest idea being that
these are mutants, that is, B cells with a mutation in a structural gene for the
variable region of the light or heavy chain. Those having relatively high affinity
for the antigen would be selected by limiting concentrations of antigen, as in the
conventional scheme. That several cycles of mutation and selection occur is
compatible with the sequence data (Cohn, 1970; Jerne, 1971). Most adult
animals would have a repertoire of B cells which had been expanded considerably by contact with numerous environmental antigens. The "clonotype" would
be bigger than the "primotype," not smaller as in Gally and Edelman's (1972)
analysis.

There are echoes of the old ideas on multipotent precursor cells in this
model. The mechanism proposed is different, however. Each B cell has only one
kind of antibody receptor and will respond initially to a restricted range of
antigens. Any one B cell is able to proliferate extensively and give rise, by
mutation, to a variety of progeny which produce slightly different Ig chains.

III. CHANGES IN PATTERNS OF ANTIBODY PRODUCED
DURING THE COURSE OF AN IMMUNE RESPONSE

The primary antibody response to an antigen characteristically has the
following features: there is a lag phase of up to several days (depending on the
antigen) before any antibody is produced (see Weigle and Dixon, 1957); the

early antibody is of low affinity (Eisen and Siskind, 1964; Siskind, Dunn, and Walker, 1968), relatively homogeneous in affinity (Eisen and Siskind, 1964; Miller and Segre, 1972), and specific (Gershon and Kondo, 1972a). By contrast, in a secondary response there is little or no lag phase, the first antibody is of high affinity (Steiner and Eisen, 1967), often more heterogeneous (Miller and Segre, 1972), and less specific (Gershon and Kondo, 1972a; Eisen *et al.*, 1969). Obviously, the B-cell populations stimulated in these two cases are different in some ways. These differences are explained most simply by a theory of antigen-dependent generation of diversity, which holds that there is no rapid production of high-affinity antibody in a primary response, because the corresponding B cells do not yet exist. The conventional view requires *ad hoc* assumptions to account for the different response patterns, as discussed below.

A. Affinity

The average affinity of antibody for a simple determinant may increase at least 10^4-fold during the course of a primary immune response (Eisen and Siskind, 1964). This is probably a minimal estimate, since very-low-affinity antibody is difficult to detect (Eisen and Siskind, 1964). Large variations in affinity occur even in small animals such as the mouse (Andersson, 1972; Huchet and Feldman, 1973). By contrast, the earliest antibody released in a secondary response is typically of high affinity (Steiner and Eisen, 1967).

These serological findings have been explained in cellular terms by the antigen-selection hypothesis (Eisen, 1966; Siskind and Benacerraf, 1969). Early in an immune response when excess amounts of antigen are present, B cells bearing receptors of any affinity are stimulated, while later, as antigen becomes limiting, the clonal proliferation of high-affinity cells is favored.

The antigen-selection hypothesis is not strictly concerned with how high-affinity cells arise, but it has almost always been accepted that the full range of B cells is present before antigenic stimulation. This is the assumption which is being questioned here, because it leads to a number of difficulties.

1. Numbers of B Cells

To explain why high-affinity antibody is not found in the serum early in a response, it is usually assumed that B cells bearing low-affinity receptors for a particular antigen greatly outnumber those with high-affinity receptors. That is, moderate amounts of antigen will stimulate all B cells, but the average affinity will be low. To allow a change in the average association constant of 10^4-fold, the low-affinity cells would need to outnumber the high-affinity cells by a large factor, perhaps 100- to 1000-fold. If an animal could make 100 different kinds of high-affinity antibody, and had 100 copies of each of the corresponding B cells, it would have 10^4 "high-affinity" B cells. To allow for a substantial maturation of antibody affinity, it would need perhaps 10^6 or 10^7 low-affinity B cells.*

Clearly the two models make very different predictions about the numbers of B cells which must be present before antigen. The conventional view needs a large number, while relatively few are required if antigen generates high-affinity mutants. In fact, rather small numbers of B cells are found by functional tests on cells from unimmunized animals, as discussed in Section IV.

One way of getting around the need for large numbers of low-affinity B cells would be to assume that both high- and low-affinity cells are present in fairly small numbers, but that the high-affinity cells are selectively tolerized by high concentrations of antigen in the early stages of a response (Eisen, 1966; Siskind and Benacerraf, 1969). Under certain conditions, preferential inhibition of high-affinity antibody can be shown, especially when antigen is used in large doses or in a form which does not affect T cells (Theis and Siskind, 1968; Davie et al., 1972; Weksler et al., 1973). However, this is probably not a general mechanism; as noted by Eisen (1966), this does not usually happen in *secondary* responses, where high-affinity antibody is produced immediately, in response to doses of antigen which give low-affinity antibody in primary responses (Steiner and Eisen, 1967). Neither can it reasonably be argued that the high-affinity B cells are not tolerized in secondary responses because of other changes induced by antigen, such as increased numbers of T cells. A second injection of hapten produces antibody of equally high affinity whether it is conjugated to the same carrier as was used for priming or to a different carrier (Steiner and Eisen, 1967; Paul et al., 1967; Claflin and Merchant, 1973) while low-affinity antibody results when a hapten-protein complex is injected into an animal previously primed with the carrier only (Steiner and Eisen, 1967; Claflin and Merchant, 1973). It seems probable that when high-affinity cells are present they are normally stimulated by antigen, not selectively tolerized.

In summary, this section points out that if all B cells are present before antigen, there must be a very large number reactive against any one antigen to allow for observed changes in antibody affinity. If antigen generates new B cells, relatively small numbers of cells would be needed.

2. Dose of Antigen

Conventional theory predicts that the smaller the dose of antigen, the higher will be the affinity of antibody induced at any time. This follows from the

---

*Antigens which are relatively "thymus independent" often induce antibody responses which show very little maturation of affinity. This is presumably because these antigens for some reason (such as being polymeric) can combine with and induce B cells very readily. Variants with higher-affinity receptors would have no real selective advantage, and the affinity and heterogeneity of the antibody produced would not increase much.

antigen-selection hypothesis. By contrast, if antigen must generate high-affinity mutants, then we would expect maximum stimulation of antibody-forming cell clones to lead to the greatest number of favorable mutations. These would still require limiting amounts of antigen for their selection, but very small doses of antigen should not yield the highest-affinity antibody.

Siskind and Benacerraf (1969) have pointed out that very small doses of antigen do *not* stimulate highest-affinity antibody, either early or late in an immune response (Siskind *et al.*, 1968; Huchet and Feldman, 1973). Neither do such doses prime an animal for a very-high-affinity secondary response (Steiner and Eisen, 1967). They argue that this is because very small amounts of antigen stimulate only a small proportion of available B cells, among which, by chance, no high-affinity precursors are present. This seems unreasonable. While there is enough antigen for all B cells, affinity should not change, whereas when it is *limiting,* high-affinity precursors are said to have a selective advantage. One cannot fairly claim that when antigen is even more limiting these cells lose their advantage simply because they are less numerous.

A similar anomaly has been noted by Gershon (Gershon and Paul, 1971; Gershon and Kondo, 1972b), who also favors the idea that antigen generates new high-affinity precursor cells. Antibody induced in the relative absence of T cells was of lower affinity than that produced when T cells were plentiful. This is again the opposite of conventional predictions: where conditions for stimulating B cells are limiting, only the highest-affinity cells should be activated. It is unlikely that high-affinity cells are more readily tolerized by most antigens in the absence of T cells since several groups have shown that high-affinity antibody is preferentially stimulated when an animal is challenged with hapten coupled to a carrier protein different from that used for priming (Steiner and Eisen, 1967; Paul *et al.*, 1967; Claflin and Merchant, 1973). Siskind and Benacerraf (1969) also discuss the "coincidence" that doses of antigen giving the largest amount of antibody also give the highest affinities. This is predicted by a theory of antigen-generated diversity.

Most affinity studies are done on serum from animals injected with a depot of antigen in adjuvant, from which the antigen gradually leaks out over several months. This has led to the concept of a gradual selection of preexisting high-affinity cells which eventually come to replace their low-affinity counterparts. This picture may need some revision. There are at least four recent papers which describe an early increase in antibody affinity followed by a *decrease* as antibody production wanes (Doria *et al.*, 1972; Miller and Segre, 1972; Clem and Small, 1970; Urbain *et al.*, 1972). This is hard to explain. It seems unlikely that in the absence of antigen an animal would permanently lose its B memory cells, since high-affinity antibody is recalled immediately on challenge.

3. Heterogeneity of Antibody Affinity

The heterogeneity of the affinity (or any other property) of antibody should decrease during an immune response if certain subpopulations are being selected from an initial large array. If, on the other hand, new sequences are continually being created by mutation, antibody heterogeneity will increase, and this is commonly found (see Eisen and Siskind, 1964; Miller and Segre, 1972; Kreth and Williamson, 1973).

4. Affinity Studies with Plaque-Forming Cells

Affinity changes have recently been studied at the level of single plaque-forming cells (Andersson, 1972; Davie et al., 1972; Davie and Paul, 1972; Doria et al., 1972; Miller and Segre, 1972; Huchet and Feldman, 1973). Two studies (Davie and Paul, 1972; Claflin and Merchant, 1973) appeared to show that somatic mutational events after antigen stimulation were not crucial to generation of high-affinity antibody molecules. Davie and Paul (1972) measured the changing proportions of plaque-forming cells in different subgroups during the course of a response to DNP* in the lymph nodes of guinea pigs. They found low- and high-avidity plaque-formers both early and late: only the relative proportions were altered. The plaque inhibition method is open to some objections, however:

(a) Cells producing antibody of the highest affinity were probably not distinguished, since the affinity of serum antibody continued to rise after 30 days, while the apparent maximum avidity of plaque-forming cells did not increase after this time.

(b) Avidity of plaque-forming cells was found to drop more than 10-fold from days 6–12 after immunization. Similarly, the data show that the proportion of very-high-avidity plaque-forming cells was higher at 6 and 8 days than at 12 and 16 days. This is not in accordance with theory and suggests that the method was influenced by some property of the antibody released, other than its affinity.

(c) As a check on the method, inhibition of plaque production was tested using cells of a myeloma which were presumably all producing identical antibody. One hundred times more antigen was required to inhibit all of these plaques than to inhibit 20% of them. Two other groups, Yamada et al. (1970) and Claflin et al. (1973) found that plaques produced by the same myeloma (MOPC-315) were nearly all inhibited over a 10-fold range of antigen concentra-

---

Abbreviations: DNP, 2,4-dinitrophenyl hapten; NIP, 3-nitro-4-hydroxy-5-iodophenacetyl hapten; BSA, bovine serum albumin; HSA, human serum albumin.

tions. This last objection is the most serious. A population of cells producing antibody of identical amino acid sequence scored as having a fairly wide range of avidities. It appears that while the method gives a useful picture of the population changes involved, it is not suitable for the unequivocal detection of a small minority of high-affinity cells whose presence before antigen is debated.

To summarize this section, the conventional view is that antigen selects high-affinity B cells from among an array of preformed B cells. This number must be very large to allow for the great increases in affinity of serum antibody and the variety of different antibodies which are often observed. The view that antigen generates entirely new B cells is simpler in that it permits a much smaller initial number and diversity of B cells, and it also explains why the extent of increase in affinity is correlated with the amount of antibody produced. It is not contested that "maturation of affinity" is due in part to selection of B cells by antigen. What is being suggested is that antigen has a second role to play: in addition to selecting new B cells, it also stimulates their initial production as variants within clones whose early members are all producing antibody of relatively low affinity. This could be proved beyond doubt by a direct demonstration that such variation does occur within single clones (see Section VIII).

B. Lag Phase

After primary stimulation with some antigens, there is a period of several days or even weeks during which no measurable amounts of specific antibody are produced (see Weigle and Dixon, 1957). By contrast, antibody is formed much more quickly in a secondary response.

This difference is most simply explained as a relative lack of B cells able to produce antibody of measurable affinity in unimmunized animals. Stated in its most extreme form, the antigen-generation theory would say that cells able to produce such antibody simply do not exist before antigen stimulation. (There will be some exceptions to this: occasional antigens will correspond well to antibodies coded by germ-line genes, and the B cell pool will be expanded by contact with environmental antigens in conventionally reared animals.) A fairly high proportion of B cells would have receptors of *low* affinity for any antigen, but stimulation might require multipoint binding to antigen held on the surface of a macrophage. Mutants would appear which could produce antibody with sufficient affinity to give a serological effect. Members of these clones would persist as memory cells which could be immediately activated in a secondary response.

The conventional theories see antigen interacting with an enormous spectrum of B cells ranging in affinity from very low to very high. On the simplest model, all above a certain level are activated immediately, and the lag phase is explained as the time required for small numbers of cells to proliferate to numbers able to give detectable antibody. Such an argument is possible to sustain when serum antibody levels are measured, but difficult when plaque-forming cells are counted. In effect, plaquing lowers the threshold for detection of new antibody synthesis to zero. The fact that the lag phase is real for some antigens even when plaque-forming cells are measured (Merchant and Hraba, 1966; Kishimoto *et al.,* 1968; Golub *et al.,* 1968) suggests that cells releasing antibody of detectable affinity must first be generated as variants within clones whose antibody is of affinity too low to cause plaque formation.

This objection can be countered by postulating that a critical number of antigen-induced handling cells (e.g., specific T cells) must be present before B cells can be stimulated. These cells, it could be said, may be available from the beginning of a secondary response. However, there is some evidence (Steiner and Eisen, 1967; Paul *et al.,* 1967; Rittenberg and Campbell, 1968; Claflin and Merchant, 1973) that a secondary response to a hapten can be induced more rapidly even when the hapten is attached to a carrier protein different from that used in priming. More data on this point, especially with plaque counts, would be interesting. The conventional theory must explain this accelerated secondary response as an increase in the number of B cells able to be activated directly by antigen, or by antigen plus nonimmune handling cells. If no entirely new cell types are produced by immunization, then a finite number of such cells must have been present initially. But none at all can be detected using the plaque technique, which has no sensitivity limitations.

This kind of argument should not be pressed too hard in dealing with cell interactions as complex as those of the immune system. It is no doubt possible to construct more elaborate models to answer the objections raised here to the conventional scheme. However, it does seem that the lag phase is more simply explained by the antigen-generated-diversity theory.

C. Specificity

The antibody produced during an immune response tends to become increasingly cross-reactive with time (Eisen *et al.,* 1969). This section will discuss two recent papers by Gershon and Kondo (1972a,b) which show how such changes support the idea that antigen generates new high-affinity B cells.

Inbred mice immunized with sheep red cells made antibody of high avidity which agglutinated both sheep and horse erythrocytes. These cross-reactive antibodies appeared late in a primary response or early in a secondary. These observations are consistent with the gradual selection of preexisting high-affinity cells, present initially in very low numbers. However, three additional facts are difficult to explain in this way. First, there was no antihorse activity at all in serum after two weeks, when antisheep titers were already very high. This poses the same problem discussed earlier: if B cells capable of producing cross-reactive antibody do exist from the start, why are they not stimulated? Second, the time of appearance of cross-reactive antibody, and the titers it reached, varied greatly from one animal to another. The data show that some individuals had equally high titers against both sheep and horse at times when other genetically identical individuals had no antihorse reactivity at all. This does not sound like a relatively orderly process of selection of cells of progressively higher affinity. Third, the production of high-affinity cross-reactive antibodies was much more dependent on T cell help than was the antisheep specific response. This is the reverse of conventional predictions: absence of help should favor high-affinity B cells. This makes sense if T cells are needed to stimulate B-cell proliferation and so generate more mutants. Selective tolerization of high-affinity cells in the relative absence of T cells was unlikely in these experiments, since doses of antigen above the optimum did not depress the levels of cross-reactive antibody.

IV. NUMBERS OF B CELLS

Different theories on the origin of antibody diversity make very different predictions about the number and variety of B cells in an animal. According to conventional ideas, there should be cells with a continuous spectrum of avidities for any one antigen. Even in antigen-free animals, cells bearing high-affinity receptors should be present, and the total number reactive against any one antigen must be large enough to allow maturation of affinity from low to high by simply altering the proportions of preexisting cells.

If antigen generates diversity, an animal could start with a relatively small number (perhaps one thousand) of different types of B cells. In conventionally reared animals, this repertoire would be expanded by contact with environmental antigens. High-affinity B cells should not be present unless the animal had been immunized. From a population of 10^6 B lymphocytes, possibly 0.1–1% might have receptors of sufficient affinity to bind a random antigen (provided each molecule of antigen could bind to several receptor molecules), but among these only a small number would, by chance, produce mutant progeny able to release antibody of measurable affinity. According to this view, an estimate of the "number of specific B cells" will reflect the probability that such a detectable clone will emerge.

At present there are two ways of counting specific B cells. The first is by looking at antigen-binding cells. It is not completely clear what such counts mean, since the number detected depends on the concentration of antigen, as discussed recently by Ada (1970). At high concentrations, up to about 1% of cells may bind to radiolabeled antigen, to antigen attached to a solid support (Rutishauser et al., 1972). These are several orders of magnitude more B cells than are detected by functional tests.

The alternative way of counting antibody-forming precursors is to culture

Table I. Some Estimates of the Number of Specific B Cells in
Mouse Spleen or Bone Marrow[a]

Antigen	Method	Cell population tested	Immun- ized or not	Approx. number of precursor cells per 10^8	Refer- ences[d]
Heterologous erythrocytes[b]	Limit dilution in tissue culture	Spleen	−	33	1
			−	163 (chicken)	1
	Cloning *in vitro*	Spleen	−	500	2
	Focus formation in spleen	Spleen	−	200	3
			−	100	4
			−	40	5
	Clone formation in spleen	Spleen	−	50	6
	Focus formation in spleen	Spleen	+	240	7
	Limit dilution transfer *in vivo*	Bone marrow	−	200 or more (wide scatter)	8
			−	1000 (wide scatter, non-Poissonian)	9
			+	300	9
			−	250 (chicken)	9
DNP	Clonal cultures, spleen fragments *in vitro*	Spleen	−	300	
			+	1000	10
	Limit dilution transfers *in vivo*	Spleen	+	100	11
Poly-D-alanine	Limit dilution transfers *in vivo*	Spleen	−	3	12
NIP	Limit dilution transfers *in vivo*	Spleen	+	100	13
BSA	Adoptive transfer	Spleen	−	0[c]	14
HSA	Adoptive transfer	Spleen	−	0[c]	15

[a]Numbers calculated from authors' data.
[b]Sheep erythrocytes except where otherwise stated.
[c]No response to soluble antigen by unprimed cells. Good response with primed cells.
[d]Reference key: 1, Osoba (1969); 2, Lefkovits (1972); 3, Playfair *et al.* (1965); 4, Kennedy *et al.* (1966); 5, Claman *et al.* (1966); 6, Cunningham (1969); 7, Luzzati *et al.* (1970); 8, Playfair and Purves (1971); 9, Miller and Cudkowicz (1970); 10, Klinman (1972); 11, Roelants and Askonas (1971); 12, Bosma and Weiler (1970); 13, Kreth and Williamson (1973); 14, Makela and Mitchison (1965); 15, Celada (1967).

lymphoid cell populations (*in vitro* or in irradiated recipients) at limiting dilutions, or under conditions where single clones of antibody-forming progeny can be measured. References to such methods are given in Table I which lists some of the results. There are a number of problems here: (a) Factors other than the B cell may be limiting. (b) The efficiency of detection of B cells is usually uncertain. (c) A point often overlooked is that the cell population transferred may contain B cells at different stages of development, so the result of an assay will depend very much on the duration of the culture and on the time for which antigen persists. This becomes particularly important with cells such as those from bone marrow which contain many primitive elements. Stem cells may produce new specific B cells which will then score in a protracted culture. (d) Most of the cellular work has been done only in mice, while most of the antibody affinity studies come from rabbits and guinea pigs.

Bearing in mind the problems involved in counting specific B cells, do the available estimates discriminate between the two theories? The high concentrations (1%) of antigen-binding cells detected by some methods may well reflect the ability of very low-affinity antibody to bind to antigen provided the binding occurs at several points. Probably any antibody binds to almost any antigen, but with varying (and often extremely low) affinities. The real question is whether these cells in nonimmune animals represent relatively few different kinds, or a large variety with receptor affinities covering the full range which the animal can produce. To decide between these alternatives one would need data showing the avidity distribution of such binding cells from animals with different experience of antigen. For example, it would be interesting to compare cells from embryos, young and adult animals, and immunized adults. Such studies are likely to encounter the same problems discussed earlier for plaque-forming cell avidity work: avidity is a continuous variable, and it would probably be difficult to prove whether high-avidity binding cells were entirely absent or present in small numbers.

Table I lists results from functional tests. Most data come from work with heterologous erythrocytes, large complex antigens presumably capable of binding to antibodies of many different primary structures. In spite of this, the numbers of specific B cells are not very large. Those estimates which are probably most free from objection are derived from *in vitro* limit dilution and cloning work (Osoba, 1968; Lefkovits, 1972): numbers varied from 30 to 500 per 10^8 mouse spleen cells.

For haptens, the clonal fragment cultures of Klinman (1972) provide some of the best data. He found about 300 anti-DNP precursor cells per 10^8 in spleens of mice primed with the carrier but not with the hapten, and about three times more after immunization. It is rather surprising that this value should be so high compared with the much more complex red cell antigens, and also that the increment produced by priming was so small.

For another simple antigen, poly-D-alanine, the figures were much lower. Even after applying a 10% correction factor for the efficiency of transfer of lymphoid cells, Bosma and Weiler (1970) estimated that there were only 150 B cells for this antigen in a whole mouse.

Still more extreme cases exist where unprimed spleen cells transferred to irradiated recipient mice would not respond at all to protein antigens without adjuvant (see Makela and Mitchison, 1965; Celada, 1967), while primed cells, under the same conditions, responded well. This could be due to a total absence, in unprimed mice, of B cells with sufficient avidity to respond and give measurable products. More data are needed on the responsiveness of B cells from various sources under different conditions, e.g., in the presence or absence of immune T cells or mitogens.

The antigen-generated-diversity theory would be seriously weakened if it were possible to use antigen to preselect, from a population of unimmunized cells, a very small fraction which contained all the cells able to respond to that antigen. The experiments of Wofsy and his colleagues are the best of this kind so far (Henry et $al.$, 1972). They were able to obtain from approximately 5×10^8 unimmunized spleen cells, 6000 which bound to the lac hapten on a solid support. These 6000 cells, on transfer to irradiated recipients, gave a response almost as good as that of 2×10^7 unfractionated cells. This could be interpreted to mean that the animals used had at least 3000 (i.e., $2 \times 10^7/6000$) different "types" of B cells, one of which was reactive against the lac hapten. An obvious complication is that the mice may have been cross-primed with environmental antigens. Another is that 25 times more cells were needed to provide the hapten-reactive population than were used to inject the recipients of unfractionated cells. Nevertheless, if the technique could be refined to the extent that 10 or even 100 antigen-binding cells from an antigen-free (newborn?) animal gave as good a response as quickly as 10^7 normal cells, this would virtually rule out antigen-generated diversity.

It may be misleading to think of immunocompetent cells as an array of discrete types, each reactive against "its own" antigen: a more accurate picture might be a spectrum of cells, many of which can be activated by any one antigen but with different probabilities. The probability would be increased by optimal presentation of large amounts of antigen. Some antigens (e.g., DNP–gramicidin; Montgomery et $al.$, 1972), which are essentially monomeric with hapten present on a constant background, may bind sufficiently strongly to activate only a very restricted range of germ-line gene-coded receptors or near mutant forms. Others, such as hapten coupled randomly and at high density to proteins, may be able to bind to a wide variety of different initial receptor antibodies and mutants, thus generating a range of antibodies with greatly varying affinities for the hapten on any background. If this view is correct, then the concept of an absolute number of B cells reactive to a particular antigen has little meaning, unless one also specifies the conditions under which these cells are activated and the threshold of affinity above which any product will be detected. The available data do not help much to distinguish between the rival hypotheses, except that some of the estimates of B cell numbers seem uncomfortably low for conventional theories.

V. STUDIES ON SINGLE CLONES

A. Isoelectric Focusing

If an antigen acts on B cells to generate many new variants, then a study of the pattern of individual clones produced during the course of an immune response should show this. A recent paper by Kreth and Williamson (1973) seems to provide a direct demonstration of such generation of diversity. Mice were immunized with NIP–BGG, and at intervals after priming cells were transferred to irradiated recipients in sufficiently low numbers to allow an average of only one clone to develop in each recipient. Spleen cells from each of 4 donors were transferred to about 100 recipients. Recipient sera were tested by isoelectric focusing, giving a series of monoclonal spectra. These patterns were then compared to see what similarities existed in clones produced by cells from each of the 4 donors.

The results were striking. Of 337 different anti-NIP clones only 5 cases were found where a clone derived from one donor was indistinguishable from a clone produced by cells from another. This was a maximum estimate, since the technique might fail to distinguish antibodies of closely similar amino acid sequences. It appears that each donor mouse gave rise to an almost unique array of antibody-forming cell clones. Such a result is exactly what would be expected with a random generation of diversity, although the authors interpret it differently, The small proportion of common clones may represent the products of germ-line genes. That the vast majority of clones from each of four inbred mice is different is difficult to reconcile with the germ-line theory, which predicts that a similar array of specificities would be produced by all individuals of an inbred strain. To rescue the germ-line hypothesis, it is necessary to postulate (as the authors do) that there is a very large pool of different kinds of B cells in each animal, but that only a small proportion of these is ever selected by chance. At the phenotypic level this would be indistinguishable from somatic generation of diversity.

These experiments also seem to show directly that antigen stimulated the development of B cells producing new antibodies over a period of several weeks. Clonal precursors were first looked for at 9 days after priming, when the proportion was around 1 in 10^7 cells. (It would be interesting to know how many were present earlier than this.) The frequency of precursors rose to about 1 in 10^6 over the next 20 days, at which time the donor mice had also developed the capacity to produce many new types of antibody not formed earlier. This increase cannot reasonably be ascribed to development of specific T cells from limiting to nonlimiting numbers, since T memory develops much more rapidly than B (Mitchison, 1971; Cunningham and Sercarz, 1971).

B. Lymph Node Fragment Cultures

Macario *et al.* (1972) have recently published some data which suggest that the antibody produced by a single clone may change with time. They cultured small fragments of lymph node from rabbits immunized with β-galactosidase. A secondary response was started *in vitro*, and the affinity of synthesized antibody followed for several weeks. Many of the fragments probably contained single clones since the size of pieces was adjusted so that some were negative and some positive. At suitable doses of antigen, the affinity of the antibody released by such fragments increased several orders of magnitude during the test period. The authors discuss one possible objection, which is that B cells may not have been randomly distributed, so that any positive fragment contained several precursor cells. Another possibility is that cells other than the precursors were limiting. Both problems could be overcome by using allotype-marked clones, as Macario *et al.* point out. This kind of evidence, once the objections are dealt with, could well provide the most direct and unequivocal support for the antigen-generated-diversity hypothesis.

VI. GENETIC CONTROL OF ANTIBODY PRODUCTION

There are two kinds of observations which seem at first sight to contradict the idea that antigen stimulation generates antibody diversity. The first is the fact that certain antibody specificities can be shown to be under the control of single germ-line genes (Benacerraf and McDevitt, 1972). The second is the demonstration of restricted or homogeneous antibody patterns, particularly cases where these are identical between different related individuals of a species (Krause, 1970).

Most examples of genetic low responsiveness in fact are not caused by the presence or absence of a structural V gene in B cells, but reflect the inheritance of genes expressed in T cells (Benacerraf and McDevitt, 1972). However, there are some cases where injection of a complex antigen yields consistently different specificity patterns in different inbred strains of animals, which could denote different inherited populations of B cells (Pinchuck and Maurer, 1968; Mozes *et al.*, 1969; Bluestein *et al.*, 1972). When antigen XY produces only anti-X and not anti-Y in some strains of animals, the simplest interpretation is that the gene for anti-Y is missing. That this interpretation is not necessarily correct is shown by the work of di Pauli (1972) who found (using bacterial lipopolysaccharides in mice) that strains unable to produce anti-Y on injection of XY could produce anti-Y when YZ was used as antigen. This seems to mean that different ways of presenting the same antigenic determinants to the B cell population results in synthesis of different antibodies, as suggested by Bluestein *et al.* (1972).

An example of low responsiveness caused by absence of a structural V gene in B cells has been described by Weigert and his colleagues (Blomberg *et al.*, 1972; Carson and Weigert, 1973). The ability to respond well to dextran containing a-1,3-glucosyl linkages in mice depends on a single autosomal dominant locus linked to the gene of the constant region of the heavy chain. The existence of some such genes is predictable on any theory. What is intriguing about the dextran work is that the normal antibody response of high-responder mice can be greatly depressed by the absence of this single V gene. Carson and Weigert (1973) have suggested that the normal antidextran response involves a heterogeneous population of antibodies, implying that many different Ig chains are derived from mutants of the original gene.

Homogeneous and restricted antibody patterns also imply a strict genetic control of antibody specificity. For example, Montgomery and Williamson (1972) have demonstrated antibodies with similar and restricted isoelectric focusing properties in the different members of occasional litters of young rabbits. Undeniably this shows that certain antibody genes are transmitted in the germ line. Such homogeneity was uncommon, however. The authors point out that most littermates had distinct antibody spectra after immunization and that initially restricted responses could rapidly become heterogeneous after further injections of antigen. The conditions which favor homogeneous antibody responses are not fully understood as yet, but would seem to include choice of suitable antigens, route of immunization, physical state of the antigen, and genetic background of the animals treated (Krause, 1970).

The recent study of Chen *et al.* (1973) is a good example of the general rule that antibody responses are normally diverse and variable between different animals, not restricted and similar. Rabbits immunized with pneumococcal polysaccharides showed marked fluctuations in their serum antibody electrophoretic patterns when these were followed for several months. Many varied from very heterogeneous to restricted and back to heterogeneous again.

Stable clones of cells producing antihapten antibody (Askonas *et al.*, 1970) also seem to argue against a significant role for antigen in generating new antibodies. These may in fact be throwing off variants which fail to compete with the main clone. It is also fair to ask why, if "E9" is a germ-line gene product, this particular clone has only been isolated once. Similarly, the stability of myeloma products is a weak argument against antigen-generated diversity, since these are probably not continually stimulated by antigen, and may have an abnormal resistance to normal control mechanisms in any case.

To summarize this section, it is obvious that the antibody produced depends *ultimately* on the structural V genes in the germ line. It is also clear that many other levels of control are superimposed on V gene expression, notably ways of handling and presenting antigen to B cells. This complicates the genetic interpretation of antibody phenotype. Some examples of restricted or low responsiveness may indeed reflect absence of antibody structural genes, but overall, the enormous diversity and heterogeneity of immune responses, and the notorious variability between individual animals, is more compatible with random generation of diversity than with complete germ-line control.

VII. SELF-TOLERANCE

If antigen stimulation generates new specificities at random, then many of these will have anti-self-activity. What happens to these cells? Burnet's original explanation of the generation of diversity avoided this problem by assuming that all specificities were produced in a burst of hypermutation early in the development of an individual (Burnet, 1959). Any self-reactive cell met its corresponding antigen at that time and died. Cohn (1972) has pointed out that such a "time" model, where antigen-sensitive cells are tolerized by antigen in the young animal but stimulated in the adult, is unlikely to be correct, since it is now known that tolerance to many antigens can be readily induced in adults.

There are a number of mechanisms known which might inactivate anti-self-reactive cells as they arise. Bretscher and Cohn (1970), Cohn (1972), and Bretscher (1972) have put forward a comprehensive scheme to explain how any cell, whether T or B, is either tolerized or induced: they suggest that antigen by itself tolerizes a cell, while antigen plus associative antibody induces it. According to this idea, a mutant anti-self-reactive B cell would be quickly tolerized by contact with the self-antigen in the absence of T cells producing associative antibody against the same antigen. Other possibilities are (and see discussion by Allison, 1971): suppressor T cells might quickly abort a response where high levels of self-antigen are present continuously (Gershon and Kondo, 1970); enhancing antibody might protect a tissue against attack by anti-self-reactive mutant cells (Hellstrom et al., 1971). The role of such mechanisms in self-tolerance is still uncertain, but they at least create a precedent which makes it plausible that new mutant immunocompetent cells can safely be generated throughout life, and particularly after contact with antigen. In passing it may be noted that an upper limit to the possible affinity of any antibody may be set by the increasing likelihood that it will react against (cross-react with) self-components.

VIII. EXPERIMENTAL APPROACHES

Inferences about generation of diversity have been mainly based on studies of amino acid sequences of myeloma proteins. This has given an impression of the extent of the diversity, and has shown clearly that there must be more than one germ-line V gene for each Ig family (because of V region subgroups; Hood and Prahl, 1971). The main deficiency of these kinds of data is that the dimension of *time* is not controlled, and the debate between germ-line and somatic theories revolves mainly around the time during which most antibody specificities are generated. What in essence we need to know first is whether B cells late in a response are producing antibodies not produced earlier.

Since sequence analysis of a heterogeneous population of antibodies is impracticable, we must find some other way of distinguishing different Ig V regions. Four markers may be considered.

(a) Affinity. The average affinity of serum antibody may increase dramatically during an immune response. Possible interpretations of this phenomenon have been discussed in Section III, where it was pointed out that even studies of affinity at the level of inhibition of single plaques can not determine unequivocally whether the full range of antibody sequences is present before antigen. Affinity is a continuous variable: we need a marker which will give an "all or none" answer.

(b) Idiotype. The unique antigenic characteristics of a particular pair of V regions constitute a marker which can be used to describe the antibodies produced early or late in a response (Kuettner, 1972). It suffers from much the same drawback as affinity: it is probably impossible to say that there are no B cells producing antibody of a particular idiotype at any one time.

(c) Isoelectric Focusing. This is a powerful technique which can easily distinguish many hundreds of different Ig sequences which have activity against the same antigen. It has already been used to show that different individuals in an inbred strain of mice produce an almost entirely distinct range of antibodies (Kreth and Williamson, 1973). The main limitation is sensitivity: very small amounts of antibody are not detectable.

(d) Specificity. A very simple way to distinguish different V regions is to look at that antibody property which they directly control—specificity. This is a V region marker which has been neglected in studies on the sequence of appearance of different antibodies during the course of an immune response.

A convenient way to distinguish two different antibodies with similar specificities is by their *cross-reactivity.* The antibodies produced by stimulation with antigen X can be subdivided into groups using a second antigen, Y. There will be molecules able to react with both X and Y, others reacting against X and not Y, and even some which react with Y and not X (heteroclitic antibody; Makela, 1965). Provided these all belong to the same class, it is fair to assume that anti-(X+Y) has a different V region structure from anti-(X not Y), just as it is assumed that an antibody with affinity $10^7 M^{-1}$ has a different primary structure from one with affinity $10^8 M^{-1}$ for the same antigen.

In our laboratory we have used panels of erythrocytes from different species to do this kind of analysis. Mice injected with sheep erythrocytes produce plaque-forming cells which, when tested on a mixed monolayer of sheep and goat red cells, can be resolved into clear and partial plaques (i.e., those able to lyse both or only one kind of red cell; Cunningham and Szenberg, 1968). By increasing the phylogenetic distance between the erythrocyte types, one can define rarer subgroups of the antibody-forming cells stimulated by sheep erythrocyte antigens. Clear plaques on sheep-plus-cow monolayers are much less common than those on sheep-plus-goat mixtures, and cells producing antibody which lyse both sheep and pig or both sheep and horse are usually less than 1% of the total in a primary response (any one subgroup will, of course, include antibodies with a variety of different primary structures). Presumably, similar subdivisions could be obtained using any battery of protein or polysaccharide antigens.

The antibody-forming cell response of mice to sheep erythrocytes may now be analyzed with time in terms of these specificities. One of the most interesting questions concerns the uncommon cross-reactive specificities (Table II). If plaque-forming cells able to lyse sheep and pig erythrocytes appear in the spleen at the peak of a response, then small numbers of such plaques should also be present at early times (according to conventional ideas). In fact, examination of the *entire* spleens of 9 mice immunized two days earlier revealed no plaques at all which could lyse sheep and pig in 8 cases and 1 plaque in the remaining spleen. On sheep-plus-horse mixtures, 3 spleens had no clear plaques and one had 8. In this last case, an early mutation (or past experience with environmental

Table II. Specificity of Early Plaque-Forming Cells
Induced by Sheep Erythrocyte Antigen[a]

	Plaque-forming cells per spleen on Day 2 of the response		
	Total plaques on sheep rbc alone[c]	Clear plaques on	
		Sheep + pig	Sheep + horse
Primary	1445 (612–2592)	0, 0, 0, 0, 0, 0, 0, 0, 1	0, 0, 0, 8
Secondary[b]	2630 (408–18,000)	4, 15, 30, 60, 75, 105, 112, 120, 150, 165, 315	3, 7, 50 107

[a]5×10^8 Srbc 1/V.
[b]Secondary responses were measured in mice which had had either single or multiple injections of 5×10^8 Srbc 2–8 months earlier.
[c]Geometric mean and range.

antigen) may have generated a B cell with this specificity. It is an interesting example since it seems to show that if anti-(sheep + horse) B cells were present they would be stimulated within two days. These results should be contrasted with the pattern seen in secondary responses, where at two days after challenge there were roughly the same total number of antisheep plaques, but now a fair proportion with anti-(sheep + pig) or anti-(sheep + horse) specificities.

This difference between primary and secondary responses is reminiscent of that seen when affinity is measured (Section III). In a secondary response, high-affinity antibody or highly cross-reactive plaque-forming cells are produced immediately. In a primary response, such antibody takes longer to appear. With affinity measurements it is possible to argue that high-affinity cells are present early in the primary response, but in numbers too small to be detected. By examining the specificity of antibody released by single cells, this objection can be overcome. It could still be said that high-affinity (or highly cross-reactive) antibody is synthesized more quickly in a secondary response not because of any change in the B cell population, but because of antigen-induced changes in other "handling" cells. This is an *ad hoc* assumption which cannot be completely discounted but which seems unlikely, because (as discussed in Section III) it is those B cells with receptors of highest affinity or highest cross-reactivity which should be most easily stimulated by antigen.

Thus the specificity of antibody, when measured at the single cell level, has two main advantages over other V region markers. First, it is possible to count a definite *number* of cells in a piece of lymphoid tissue which are able to lyse, say, sheep and pig erythrocytes. This is in contrast with affinity data, where the *proportion* of plaque-forming cells inhibited by certain concentrations of antigen is recorded. Second, there are no real sensitivity limitations: it is fairly simple to search the entire spleen of a mouse for one plaque-forming cell of a particular specificity. (It cannot be argued that the whole mouse must be examined since clear plaques on sheep-plus-pig or sheep-plus-horse erythrocyte mixtures can be found in irradiated recipients after transfer of small numbers of spleen cells (Pilarski and Cunningham, 1974); that is, the *ultimate* precursor for this specificity must reside in the spleen.)

Because it is perilous to extrapolate from antibody phenotype to genotype (Section VI), the kind of evidence cited above, although suggestive, cannot be taken as proving conclusively that new genetic variant B cells arise during the course of an immune response. We are attempting to strengthen this idea in various ways. One approach involves studies on single clones of antibody-forming cells (Pilarski and Cunningham, 1974). Such clones can be grown *in vitro* in polyacrylamide rafts bathed in medium, each raft containing a number of small individual wells (Marbrook and Haskill, 1971). There is a linear single-hit dose-response relationship between the number of cells cultured per well and the number of wells containing one or more plaque-forming cells (when the frequency of "positives" is corrected for overlap). We have found that mouse

Table III. Association of Plaque-Forming Cells of Two Different Specificities in Limit-Dilution Clonal Cultures[a]

Number of culture wells tested	504
Number containing only partial plaques	91
Number containing only clear plaques	34
Number with both clear and partial plaques	27

Test of association between clear and partial:

$$\chi^2 = 16.8$$
$$p << 0.001$$

[a] Cells from each individual culture well were assayed on a mixture of red cells from sheep 1 and sheep 2. Each well was scored as containing no plaques, only "partials," only "clears," or both clear and partial plaques.

spleen cells may be cultured for 3 days without added sheep erythrocytes, but in medium containing 10 µg/ml of lipopolysaccharide from *E. coli,* to yield large numbers of anti-red-cell plaques. When approximately 10^4 spleen cells are cultured in each well, about one quarter of the wells contain from 1 to 30 plaques, and the rest have none. The dose-response properties, and the probable antigen independence of these colonies, strongly suggest that they are single clones.

One can test whether the members of such clones are homogeneous in their specificity by assaying on a mixture of two red cell types. Most are homogeneous: not only are all plaques clear or all partial, but in addition the individual plaques are often conspicuously similar in their morphology, all being the same size and having borders with the same degree of sharpness. However, some appear to be mixed. Table III shows an experiment in which the proportion of wells containing both clear and partial plaques was significantly higher than expected by chance. This is strong evidence for production of variants within a fairly high proportion of single clones. We have carried out similar experiments with clones grown *in vivo,* in the spleens of irradiated mice (Cunningham, 1969; Klinman, 1972), and have obtained similar results (Pilarski and Cunningham, 1974).

IX. DISCUSSION

Three theories can be distinguished by comparing the *time* over which they claim different antibody specificities are generated. Germ-line theories say this happens during evolutionary time, or at least over many generations of individuals, while somatic theories say during the life-span of the individual. The present model suggests an even more rapid development of new antibodies, within days after antigen stimulation. This is by no means a new idea, but it does not seem to have been seriously advocated except for a theoretical discussion by Makela and Cross (1970). Here, a case has been made mainly on the basis of patterns of antibody produced at different times during immune responses.

An obvious question concerns possible genetic mechanisms for antigen-driven generation of diversity. In view of our general ignorance of possible events in the genome of eukaryotic cells, and because the immune system has so many unusual features, it would be unreasonable to discount the present theory on the grounds that it must postulate special and rapid variation in somatic cells. If antigen-driven diversity can be proven phenotypically, then it will be necessary to investigate the genetic basis for it. At the moment it seems simplest to assume that the Ig genes of immunologically competent cells have a high rate of mutation, that antigens (or mitogens) stimulate cell proliferation and so variation, and that variants are selected by antigen according to binding affinity. It is, however, conceivable that all V genes are initially present in the genome of a B cell, and that after stimulation with antigen some members of a clone may switch from expression of one V gene to another.

If an animal's repertoire of immunologically competent cells were dependent largely on its past antigenic history, "wastage" could be cut to a minimum. The germ-line gene complement would stabilize at a number of V genes giving a few hundred or a few thousand different antibody receptors. Competing evolutionary pressures here (Cohn, 1970) are the probable loss of rarely used genes and retention of enough to provide almost any useful V region in a few mutational steps. The young animal expands its repertoire by contact with environmental antigens while losing a substantial proportion by reaction with self-antigens (Bretscher and Cohn, 1970).

A distinct advantage of the present theory is that it is testable. We need to know the number and particularly the *range* of antibody specificities which can be immediately produced by animals which have had different antigenic experience. One kind of test, described in Section VIII, is to examine the specificities of the antibody produced by normal adult animals at different stages of an immune response. Other predictions are as follows:

(a) Antigen-free animals should have a small number and range of immunologically competent cells. They should, for example, have no high-affinity antigen-binding cells against randomly chosen antigens. Their cells should be difficult to stimulate rapidly with antigen (because of their low-affinity receptors), especially under restrictive conditions such as tissue culture.

(b) Predictions for neonatal animals are similar. Two phases of development are expected in embryos and young animals, a "physiological" production of cells bearing germ-line-coded receptors, and an "immunological" phase during which environmental antigens cause massive proliferation and diversification of lymphoid cells. The transition period need not coincide with time of birth (Solomon, 1970), and many species may respond to antigens administered before birth (Sterzl and Silverstein, 1967), but in general, large numbers of easily stimulated cells should appear only after birth.

(c) Genetic unresponsiveness due to lack of structural V genes expressed in B cells should be overcome by repeated immunization, since mutants arising from other B cells less easily stimulated by the antigen will gradually compensate. Similarly, recovery from "suicide" or B cell tolerance should occur with repeated immunization.

(d) A similar prediction to (c) is that a small number of lymphoid cells should be able to produce as many different antibodies as a much larger population, given time. This explains why the competence of an animal does not depend on its size: du Pasquier (1970) showed that tadpoles with as few as 10^4 lymphocytes could respond to human and sheep red cells by producing plaque-forming cells and rosettes. Very recently, Haimovich and du Pasquier (1973) have demonstrated that the diversity of antihapten antibody produced by tadpoles with 2×10^6 lymphocytes is similar to that made by much larger animals. This is strong support for the idea that antigen generates antibody diversity. A further example of an animal with a very restricted initial population of specific lymphoid cells is the bursectomized anti-Ig-treated chicken (Kincade et al., 1973). Such birds have very few B cells, but can still give normal antibody titers to antigen, provided they are repeatedly stimulated. It would be interesting to compare the diversity of antibody in these birds with that in normal, immunized animals.

(e) Individual clones, while being stable to the extent that most daughter cells produce the same antibody as their parents, must throw off some variants. This seems to be borne out by experiment (Macario et al., 1972; Pilarski and Cunningham, 1974), but it is a crucial point which must be established beyond doubt. It is quite possible that clones may eventually become stable (Askonas et al., 1970), or at least evolve to a stage where variants are very unlikely to have a survival advantage and so are not selected.

Do T cells diversify after antigen stimulation in the same way as B cells? It is probable that they do, since the same arguments of economy (carrying few initial genes, yet being able to develop high-affinity responses to many antigens), apply to both cell lines. The fact that helper activity can sometimes appear very cross-reactive (see Falkoff and Kettman, 1972) does not necessarily mean that the repertoire of T cell specificities is different from that of a B cell: for example, arrangement of receptors in different patterns on the surface could produce quite different avidity for antigen. However, until single cell tests for active T cells are devised it will be difficult to examine their diversity directly, and for this reason the present discussion has been confined mainly to B cells.

Finally, what practical benefits would come from the knowledge that antigen stimulates generation of diversity? Would this provide a basis for more rational immunization regimes, for example? It has always been difficult to predict exactly the outcome of exposing an animal to an antigen because of the many chance factors involved. A lot must depend on the way the antigen is broken down and presented to cells, and on the chance that a relatively small number of cells will be in the right place at the right time for stimulation. Somatic mutation theories also attribute a major role to chance in the actual generation of antigen-reactive cells. The degeneracy exhibited by the immune system is obviously a way of compensating for these uncertainties. If antigen stimulates diversity, then the use of generalized vaccines (mitogens?) might be helpful to expand the repertoire of young or immunodeficient animals. In any case, a more rational approach to immunization and other practical problems associated with immune function will certainly be possible when germ-line genes have been identified, and when the rules governing their variation after antigen stimulation become clear.

X. SUMMARY

This chapter argues that antigen stimulation is necessary for the generation of most antibody diversity. The evidence cited is mainly data on the changes which take place in the antibody produced during the course of immune responses. That is, the argument is at the level of cellular phenotype.

Two apparent obstacles to the theory have been discussed: the fact that some aspects of immune responses are under direct genetic control, and the need to cope with anti-self-reactive cells which could arise during the course of an immune response. The theory is readily testable, and experimental approaches have been suggested.

ACKNOWLEDGMENTS

Many of the ideas expressed in this chapter were stimulated by reading the papers of Melvin Cohn. I am also grateful to Gordon Ada, Linda Pilarski, and Bob Blanden for helpful discussions.

REFERENCES

Ada, G. L., 1970, *Transplant. Rev.* **5**: 105.
Allison, A. C., 1971, *Lancet* **II**: 1401.
Andersson, B., 1972, *J. Exp. Med.* **135**: 312.
Askonas, B. A., Williamson, A. R., and Wright, B. E. G., 1970, *Proc. Nat. Acad. Sci. US* **67**: 1398.
Benacerraf, B., and McDevitt, H. O., 1972, *Science* **175**: 273.

Blomberg, B., Geckeler, W. R., and Weigert, M., 1972, *Science* 177: 178.
Bluestein, H. G., Green, I., Maurer, P. H., and Benacerraf, B., 1972, *J. Exp. Med.* 135: 98.
Bosma, M., and Weiler, E., 1970, *J. Immunol.* 104: 203.
Bretscher, P., 1972, *Transplant. Rev.* 11: 217.
Bretscher, P. A., and Cohn, M., 1970, *Science* 169: 1042.
Burnet, F. M., 1959, *The Clonal Selection Theory of Acquired Immunity,* Cambridge Univ. Press. Lond. and New York.
Carson, D., and Weigert, M., 1973, *Proc. Nat. Acad. Sci. US* 70: 235.
Celada, F., 1967, *J. Exp. Med.* 125: 199.
Chen, F. W., Strosberg, A. D., and Haber, E., 1973, *J. Immunol.* 110: 98.
Claflin, L., and Merchant, B., 1973, *J. Immunol.* 110: 252.
Claflin, L., Merchant, B., and Inman, J., 1973, *J. Immunol.* 110: 241.
Claman, H. N., Chaperon, E. A., and Triplett, R. F., 1966, *Proc. Soc. Exp. Biol. Med.* 122: 1167.
Clem, L. W., and Small, P. A., 1970, *J. Exp. Med.* 132: 385.
Cohn, M., 1970, *Cell Immunol.* 1: 461.
Cohn, M., 1972, *Cell Immunol.* 5: 1.
Cunningham, A. J., 1969, *Australian J. Exp. Biol. Med. Sci.* 47: 485.
Cunningham, A. J., and Sercarz, E. E., 1971, *Eur. J. Immunol.* 1: 413.
Cunningham, A. J., and Szenberg, A., 1968, *Immunology* 14: 599.
Davie, J. M., and Paul, W. E., 1972, *J. Exp. Med.* 135: 660.
Davie, J. M., Paul, W. E., Katz, D. H., and Benacerraf, B., 1972, *J. Exp. Med.* 136: 426.
Di Pauli, R., 1972, *J. Immunol.* 109: 394.
Doria, G., Schiaffini, G., Garavini, M., and Mancini, C., 1972, *J. Immunol.* 109: 1245.
du Pasquier, L., 1970, *Immunology* 19: 353.
Eisen, H. N., 1966, *Cancer Res.* 26: 2005.
Eisen, H. N., and Siskind, G. W., 1964, *Biochem.* 3: 996.
Eisen, H. N., Little, J. R., Steiner, L. A., Simms, E. S., and Gray, W., 1969, *Israel J. Med. Sci.* 5: 338.
Falkoff, R., and Kettman, J., 1972, *J. Immunol.* 108: 54.
Gally, J. A., and Edelman, G. M., 1972, *Ann. Rev. Genetics* 6: 1.
Gershon, R. K., and Kondo, K., 1970, *Immunology* 18: 723.
Gershon, R. K., and Kondo, K., 1972a, *J. Immunol.* 23: 321.
Gershon, R. K., and Kondo, K., 1972b, *J. Immunol.* 23: 335.
Gershon, R. K., and Paul, W. E., 1971, *J. Immunol.* 106: 872.
Golub, E. S., Mishell, R. I., Weigle, W. O., and Dutton, R. W., 1968, *J. Immunol.* 100: 133.
Haimovich, J., and du Pasquier L., 1973, *Proc. Nat. Acad. Sci. US* 70: 1898.
Hellstrom, I., Hellstrom, K. E., and Allison, A. C., 1971, *Nature* 230: 49.
Henry, C., Kimura, J., and Wofsy, L., 1972, *Proc. Nat. Acad. Sci. US* 69: 34.
Hood, L., and Prahl, J., 1971, *Advan. Immunol.* 14: 291.
Huchet, R., and Feldmann, M., 1973, *Eur. J. Immunol.* 3: 49.
Jerne, N. K., 1971, *Eur. J. Immunol.* 1: 1.
Kennedy, J. C., Till, J. E., Siminovitch, L, and McCulloch, E. A., 1966, *J. Immunol.* 96: 973.
Kincade, P. W., Self, K. S., and Cooper, M. D., 1973, in press.
Kishimoto, S., Tsuyuguchi, I., and Yamamura, Y., 1968, *Intern. Arch. Allergy Appl. Immunol.* 34: 544.
Klinman, N. R., 1972, *J. Exp. Med.* 136: 241.
Krause, R. M., 1970, *Advan. Immunol.* 12: 1.
Kreth, H. W., and Williamson, A. R., 1973, *Eur. J. Immunol.* 3: 141.
Kuettner, M. G., Wang, A. L., and Nisonoff, A., 1972, *J. Exp. Med.* 135: 579.
Lefkovits, I., 1972, *Eur. J. Immunol.* 2: 360.
Luzzati, A. L., Tosi, R. M., and Carbonara, A. O., 1970, *J. Exp. Med.* 132: 199.
Macario, A. J. L., deMacario, E. C., Franceschi, C., and Celada, F., 1972, *J. Exp. Med.* 136: 353.

Makela, O., 1965, *J. Immunol.* **95**: 378.
Makela, O., and Cross, A. M., 1970, *Progr. Allergy* **14**: 145.
Makela, O., and Mitchison, N. A., 1965, *Immunol.* **8**: 539.
Marbrook, J., and Haskill J. S., 1971, in *Cellular Interactions in the Immune Response,* Karger, Basel, p. 66.
Merchant, B., and Hraba, T., 1966, *Science* **152**: 1378.
Miller, H. C., and Cudkowicz, G., 1970, *J. Exp. Med.* **132**: 1122.
Miller, G. W., and Segre, D., 1972, *J. Immunol.* **109**: 74.
Mitchison, N. A., 1971, *Eur. J. Immunol.* **1**: 18.
Montgomery, P. C., Rockey, J. H., and Williamson, A. R., 1972, *Proc. Nat. Acad. Sci. US* **69**: 228.
Montgomery, P. C., and Williamson, A. R., 1972, *J. Immunol.* **109**: 1036.
Mozes, E., McDevitt, H. O., Jaton, J. C., and Sela, M., 1969, *J. Exp. Med.* **130**: 1263.
Osoba, D., 1969, *J. Exp. Med.* **129**: 141.
Paul, W. E., Siskind, G. W., Benacerraf, B., and Ovary, Z., 1967, *J. Immunol.* **99**: 760.
Pilarski, L., and Cunningham, A. J., 1974, (*Eur. J. Immunol.,* submitted).
Pinchuck, P., and Maurer, P. H., 1968, *in* Cinader, B. (ed.), *Regulation of the Antibody Response,* Charles C. Thomas, Springfield, Illinois, p. 97.
Playfair, J. H. L., and Purves, E. C., 1971, *Nature New Biol.* **231**: 149.
Playfair, J. H. L., Papermaster, B. W., and Cole, L. J., 1965, *Science* **149**: 998.
Rittenberg, M. B., and Campbell, D. H., 1968, *J. Exp. Med.* **127**: 717.
Roelants, G. E., and Askonas, B. A., 1971, *Eur. J. Immunol.* **1**: 151.
Rutishauser, U., Millette, C. F., and Edelman, G. M., 1972, *Proc. Nat. Acad. Sci. US* **69**: 1590.
Siskind, G. W., and Benacerraf, B., 1969, *Advan. Immunol.* **10**: 1.
Siskind, G. W., Dunn, P., and Walker, J. G., 1968, *J. Exp. Med.* **127**: 55.
Solomon, J. B., 1970, *Nature* **227**: 895.
Steiner, L. A., and Eisen, H. N., 1967, *J. Exp. Med.* **126**: 1185.
Sterzl, J. and Silverstein, A. M., 1967, *Advan. Immunol* **6**: 337.
Theis, G. A. and Siskind, G. W., 1968, *J. Immunol.* **100**: 138.
Urbain, J., van Acker, A., de Vos Cloetens, C. H., and Urbain-Vansanten, G., 1972, *Immunochemistry* **9**: 121.
Urbain-Vansanten, G., 1970, *Immunology* **19**: 783.
Weigle, W. O., and Dixon, F. J., 1957, *J. Immunol.* **79**: 24.
Weksler, M. E., Merritts, L. L., Werblin, T. P., and Siskind, G. W., 1973, *J. Immunol.* **110**: 897.
Yamada, H., Yamada, A., and Hollander, V. P., 1970, *J. Immunol.* **104**: 251.

Preparation and Properties
of Lymphocyte Plasma Membrane

Michael J. Crumpton and David Snary

National Institute for Medical Research
Mill Hill
London, England

I. INTRODUCTION

The cell surface (plasma) membrane plays a crucial role in many diverse aspects of the cell's behavior. Thus, the membrane acts not only as a barrier regulating the influx and efflux of ions, nutrients, and metabolites, but also provides the location for a multiplicity of molecules ("receptors") which monitor the external environment for "messengers" such as hormones, antigens, and the surface components of other cells. The surfaces of different cell types vary with respect to the nature of their receptors and their antigenic specificities. A well-documented example of these distinctions is provided by the lymphocyte. Lymphocytes comprise essentially two populations [thymus-derived (T) and bone-marrow-derived (B) cells; Roitt *et al.,* 1969] which can be distinguished functionally, antigenically, and in terms of their receptor activities. Thus, the surface of T lymphocytes plays major roles in cellular immunity, in immunosuppression by antilymphocytic serum, and in providing "help" in a humoral immune response, whereas the B-lymphocyte surface is primarily responsible for mediating humoral immunity (Greaves *et al.,* 1973). Also, T cells (mouse) possess an antigenic specificity (θ) which is not shared by B cells (Raff, 1971), whereas receptors for Fc (Basten *et al.,* 1972a,b) and the activated C3 component of complement (Nussenzweig and Pincus, 1972) are unique for B cells. Apart from these differences, the surfaces of T and B cells share histocompatibility antigens, mediate antigen recognition although not necessarily via an identical receptor, and possess receptors for plant lectins (Greaves and Janossy, 1972), polypeptide hormones [insulin (Hadden *et al.,* 1972; Gavin *et al.,* 1973) and

27

growth hormone (Lesniak *et al.*, 1973)], and small pharmacologically active molecules such as histamine (Melmon *et al.*, 1972; Shearer *et al.*, 1972).

In order to understand how the surface membrane controls cell behavior it is essential to be able to relate the surface-mediated biological activities to the molecular structure of the membrane. A variety of molecular models have been proposed for the structure of cell membranes (Hendler, 1971). The most attractive is that due to Singer and Nicolson (1972), who view the membrane as a two-dimensional solution of oriented globular proteins in a lipid matrix. The main features of this model are illustrated in Fig. 1. The basic structural framework and barrier function of the membrane are attributed to an interrupted lipid bilayer. On the other hand, the mediators of the membrane's biological functions are equated with the proteins and glycoproteins, which are represented as a heterogeneous collection of molecular species. Although the number of species varies for different cell types, it is invariably large; for

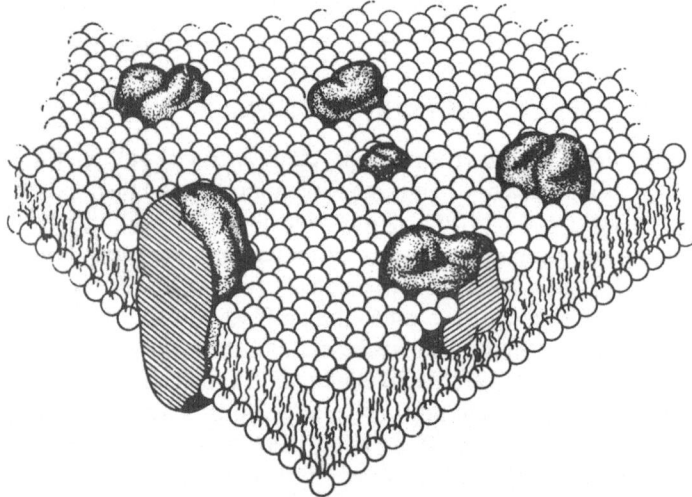

Figure 1. Schematic three-dimensional and cross-sectional views of the lipid-globular protein mosaic model of membrane structure proposed by Singer and Nicolson (1972). The lipids are arranged as a discontinuous bilayer; the circles represent the ionic and polar head groups that make contact with the aqueous environment, whereas the lines represent nonpolar fatty acid chains that are sequestered within the bilayer and are out of contact with water. The integral membrane proteins are depicted as globular molecules partially embedded in and partially protruding from the lipid bilayer and are distributed randomly in the plane of the membrane. The degree to which they penetrate the lipid layer and whether they actually span the membrane depends on their hydrophobicity and size. Peripheral membrane proteins which are superficial to the lipid layer and which may be bound electrostatically to the polar head groups are not shown.

instance, the surface membrane of chicken peripheral blood lymphocytes contains approximately thirty different proteins (Ragland *et al.,* 1973). The membrane proteins are frequently differentiated into two groups depending on whether they are peripheral (extrinsic) to the lipid bilayer or form an integral (intrinsic) part of the membrane continuum (e.g., Capaldi and Vanderkooi, 1972). If this distinction has reality, then the peripheral proteins are most probably attached by electrostatic interactions and should be relatively soluble in neutral aqueous buffers; in view, however, of their superficial location it is questionable whether such proteins play any dominant role in membrane function. In contrast, the integral proteins penetrate and, in some cases, span the lipid bilayer (Bretscher, 1971; Marchesi *et al.,* 1972), are bound primarily by hydrophobic interactions, are readily solubilized by detergents, and form aggregates in neutral aqueous buffers. The extent to which these protein molecules dip into the lipid layer, and whether they span the entire membrane, depends on the proportion of their surface that is nonpolar and their molecular size. Although integral proteins are essentially anchored in the membrane, it appears that they are bound relatively loosely to the lipids and that, apart from some structurally integrated complexes, the majority interact only weakly with each other. Furthermore, various results suggest that the lipid layer is fluid under physiological conditions and that the integral proteins are free to diffuse laterally in the plane of the membrane. Some of the most convincing evidence in support of this suggestion is provided by the intermixing of cell surface antigens after the formation of mouse–human heterokaryons (Frye and Edidin, 1970) and the redistribution of lymphocyte surface antigens ("capping") on addition of antisera to surface components (Taylor *et al.,* 1971; de Petris and Raff, 1973).

One approach to the problem of elucidating the relationship between the structure of the cell surface and cell behavior is initially to separate the plasma membrane and subsequently to isolate the individual membrane components in a biologically active form. The isolation of the native plasma membrane, however, poses a number of problems. For instance, the above model of membrane structure predicts that some membrane proteins will be loosely bound and will have a finite solubility in the aqueous phase. In this case the exact protein composition of the native membrane will be difficult to define, especially since the presence or absence of the peripheral proteins will depend upon the washing procedures used during the preparation of the membrane. This explanation may account for the reported variations in the lipid-to-protein ratio (1:1 compared with 3:7) of erythrocyte ghosts (Van Deenan, 1972) and in the protein compositions of erythrocyte membranes (Kobylka *et al.,* 1972) isolated using different procedures.

The purpose of this article is to review the methods which have been used to prepare the plasma membrane of lymphocytes, to compare the nature of the products, and to emphasize the advantages and disadvantages of the different methods. Although microsomal fractions separated from disrupted lymphoid cells have been frequently used as a source of histocompatibility antigens (e.g., Manson, 1972) and for the production of antilymphocytic serum, such preparations have rarely been either extensively purified or well characterized and will not be included in this review. The isolation of lymphocyte plasma membranes is based on the same principles that have been exploited for the separation of the surface membrane from various cell types. These principles and the methods used have been critically discussed in a number of recent reviews (Steck and Wallach, 1970; de Duve, 1971; Warren and Glick, 1971; DePierre and Karnovsky, 1973; Wallach and Lin, 1973).

II. ISOLATION OF PLASMA MEMBRANE

The isolation in good yield of highly purified preparations of undamaged plasma membrane depends on three events: firstly, the availability of a fresh, homogeneous cell population; secondly, the disruption of the maximum number of cells concurrent with minimal damage to the membrane; and thirdly, the separation of the plasma membrane from subcellular components and especially other membranes. In general, well-established, efficient methods based on differential centrifugation and/or density-gradient centrifugation are available for the separation of the plasma membrane from the cell homogenate. Unfortunately, the other two requirements are less readily satisfied. Thus, lymphocyte populations comprising only one cell type are difficult to obtain and few methods exist for efficiently disrupting cells in a reproducible and controlled manner.

A. Source of Lymphocytes

Sources of lymphocyte plasma membrane have varied from solid tissues, such as pig lymph node and pig and human thymus (Allan and Crumpton, 1970, 1972), to free cells, obtained either in the form of a mouse ascites lymphoma (Wolf and Avis, 1970), a mouse leukemia cell line (Dods et al., 1972), and a human lymphoblastoid cell line (Kennel and Lerner, 1973) or by mincing/macerating human tonsil (Demus, 1973; Lopes et al., 1973), pig lymph node (Ferber et al., 1972), mouse thymus (Lance et al., 1968), and calf thymus (Van Blitterswijk et al., 1973). Although these sources vary in their suitability, none is ideal. There seems to be little doubt that solid tissue represents the least suitable source because of fairly extensive contamination with cells other than small lymphocytes (e.g., large lymphocytes, plasma cells, and, particularly, connective tissue) whose surface membranes undoubtedly possess different protein components (Ragland et al., 1973), enzymic activities (Lauter et al., 1972), and antigenic specificities. Purified cell suspensions obtained by filtering through Perlon wool (Ferber et al., 1972) or silk (Demus, 1973), or by centrifuging on a Ficoll-

Hypaque gradient (Lopes *et al.*, 1973), represent an improvement but are often still contaminated with other cell types; for example, Demus (1973) and Lopes *et al.* (1973) reported that only 90% of their purified cells were lymphocytes. Purer lymphocyte suspensions can be obtained by using various procedures based on differences in density, size, charge, and adherence to an inert, insoluble material (e.g., cotton wool), or by cannulation of lymphatic vessels (for references see Zettergren *et al.*, 1973, and review by Denman, 1973). However, such procedures are often tedious, not readily adaptable to processing large numbers of cells, and frequently give a functionally and antigenically heterogeneous product. The problem of functional and antigenic heterogeneity can be circumvented in a number of ways. Thus, murine B cells free from T cells can be obtained from congenitally athymic ("nude") mice (Raff and Wortis, 1970), whereas avian B and T lymphocytes can be separated from the bursa of Fabricus and thymic tissues respectively (Ragland *et al.*, 1973). Alternatively, cultured lymphoblastoid cell lines (mouse and human) provide very convenient sources of large numbers of similar cells. These cells suffer, however, from at least two disadvantages: firstly, it is evident from the variation in the expression of surface-located immunoglobulin (Buell and Fahey, 1969) and histocompatibility antigens (Cikes and Friberg, 1971; Pasternak *et al.*, 1971; Pellegrino *et al.*, 1972) with the cell cycle that synchronous cultures must be employed if the cells are to possess identical surface structures; and secondly, since the surface antigenic patterns of cultured and normal cells differ (Moore and Woods, 1972; Rogentine and Gerber, 1970), the plasma membrane of lymphoblastoid cells will not be characteristic of normal lymphocytes. Indeed, the most promising current source of functionally and antigenically homogeneous lymphocyte populations appears to be provided by those methods which exploit particular surface receptors (e.g., C3 and Fc receptors and membrane-bound IgM) or antigenic specificities for cell fractionation (Paris and Hayward, 1974).

Another way of circumventing heterogeneity is afforded at the level of the disrupted cell by the selection of only those membrane fragments bearing a particular receptor/antigen. This approach has been promoted particularly by Wallach *et al.* (1972), who have termed their technique "affinity-density-perturbation." In this technique membrane vesicles bearing a given receptor are bound by the specific ligand covalently attached to a high-density particle and are separated from non-receptor-containing fragments in a centrifugal field according to their different densities. The applicability of the technique has been illustrated by using pig lymphocyte plasma membrane and Concanavalin A attached to coliphage K29 as the ligand. Although the results were somewhat disappointing in that essentially all the membrane fragments were bound and little fractionation was achieved, this result is not unexpected in view of the report that Concanavalin A binds all of the lymphocyte plasma membrane glycoproteins (Allan *et al.*, 1972). However, given more specific ligands, this approach holds considerable potential.

B. Disruption of Lymphocytes

The method employed for cell breakage influences not only the subsequent procedure used for separating the plasma membrane but also the yield and properties of the purified membrane, particularly its physical state (i.e., whether "ghosts," sheets, or vesicles; the size of fragments; the orientation of vesicles) and its biological activities (see Table I). Thus, the different distributions of rat liver plasma membrane on centrifugation reported by different workers most probably reflect the variation in the disruption conditions used, in that the more vigorous the homogenization the higher the gravitational field required to sediment the membrane (Coleman *et al.*, 1967). An example of the dependence of the membrane's biological activities upon the disruption procedure is provided by the work of Oye and Sutherland (1966), who showed that gross fragmentation of the avian erythrocyte membrane by nitrogen cavitation was associated with a loss of the adenyl cyclase response to epinephrine, whereas large membrane fragments obtained by hypotonic lysis or with a Dounce homogenizer retained the epinephrine-stimulated adenyl cyclase activity characteristic of the whole cell. Similarly, the retention of adenyl cyclase activity by isolated leukocyte membranes relies upon careful disruption (Polgar *et al.*, 1973).

Methods currently employed for cell disruption depend upon mechanical (shear) forces (Potter–Elvehjem and Dounce homogenizers, and various types of presses), osmotic forces (hypotonic shock), pressure (nitrogen cavitation), or a combination of the above, especially osmotic and mechanical forces. The choice of method depends upon the source of lymphocytes in that certain methods are not applicable to both solid tissue and free cells; for instance, disruption by pressing lymph node or thymus tissue through a perforated plate (Allan and Crumpton, 1970, 1972) is not suitable for free lymphocytes, whereas nitrogen cavitation is applicable only to cell suspensions. Another important factor is that the applicability of a particular method may be considerably influenced in various ways by the nature of the solvent. A dramatic example of the effect of the solvent is provided by the importance of the Ca^{2+} ion concentration in maintaining membrane integrity (Ray, 1970). Another is provided by the work of Steck *et al.* (1970) and Kant and Steck (1972), who observed that the inside-out orientation of erythrocyte membrane vesicles promoted by disruption in 0.5 mM sodium phosphate buffer, pH 8.0–8.5, was prevented by the presence of divalent cations (0.1 mM Mg^{2+}). Similarly, the presence of Mg^{2+} in concentrations higher than 0.25 mM during the disruption of pig lymphocytes gave indiscriminate aggregation of subcellular components (cf. the effect of Ca^{2+} in rat liver homogenates; Nigam *et al.*, 1971), whereas sucrose caused irreversible aggregation of the nuclei (Allan and Crumpton, 1970; Ferber *et al.*, 1972).

The magnitude of the problem of cell disruption is evident from Fig. 2, which shows an electron micrograph of a cultured, human lymphoblastoid cell

Table I. Relationship between Cell-Disruption Method Used, Extent of Nuclear Breakage, and Size, Yield, and Degree of Purification of Isolated Plasma Membrane Vesicles

Cells	Disruption	Solvent	Nuclear breakage (%)[a]	Yield (% total protein)	Plasma membrane			Reference[c]
					Yield (% total 5'-nucleotidase)	Vesicle size (nm diameter)	Purification[b]	
Pig lymphocytes	Mince/press[d]	10 mM tris 0.15 mM NaCl	4	1.3	15	100–800	12	1
	N$_2$ cavitation (50 atm, 15 min)	2 mM hepes 0.13 M NaCl 0.5 mM MgCl$_2$ 0.25 M sucrose	30	1.7	45	50–300	25	2
Human tonsils	Dounce	10 mM tris 0.2 mM DTT	–	0.7	8	300–600	13	3
	Potter–Elvehjem	10 mM tris 0.15 M NaCl	30	0.9	12	–	13	4
Calf thymus	N$_2$ cavitation (36 atm, 15 min)	Hanks	4	0.7	5.4	100–200	8	5
Human lymphoblastoid cell line	Shear by a mechanical pump[e]	Eagle's	9	0.6	41	100–300	49	6

[a] Assessed in terms of the fraction of total DNA that did not sediment with the nuclei.

[b] Assessed in terms of specific activity of 5'-nucleotidase.

[c] Reference key: 1, Allan and Crumpton (1970); 2, Ferber et al. (1972); 3, Lopes et al., (1973); 4, Demus (1973); 5, Van Blitterswijk et al. (1973); 6, Snary and Crumpton (unpublished observations).

[d] Solid tissue (mesenteric lymph node) was used; similar results were obtained using another solid tissue (human thymus; Allan and Crumpton, 1972). In all other cases suspensions of free cells were employed.

[e] Disruption of 8 × 10⁹ BRI 8 cells suspended in 100 ml at 0°C by pumping at a rate of about 400 ml/hr through a small orifice under a pressure of about 750 lb/in² against a spring-loaded ball [developed from a design by Dr. B. M. Wright (Wright et al., 1974; M. J. Crumpton, unpublished observations)].

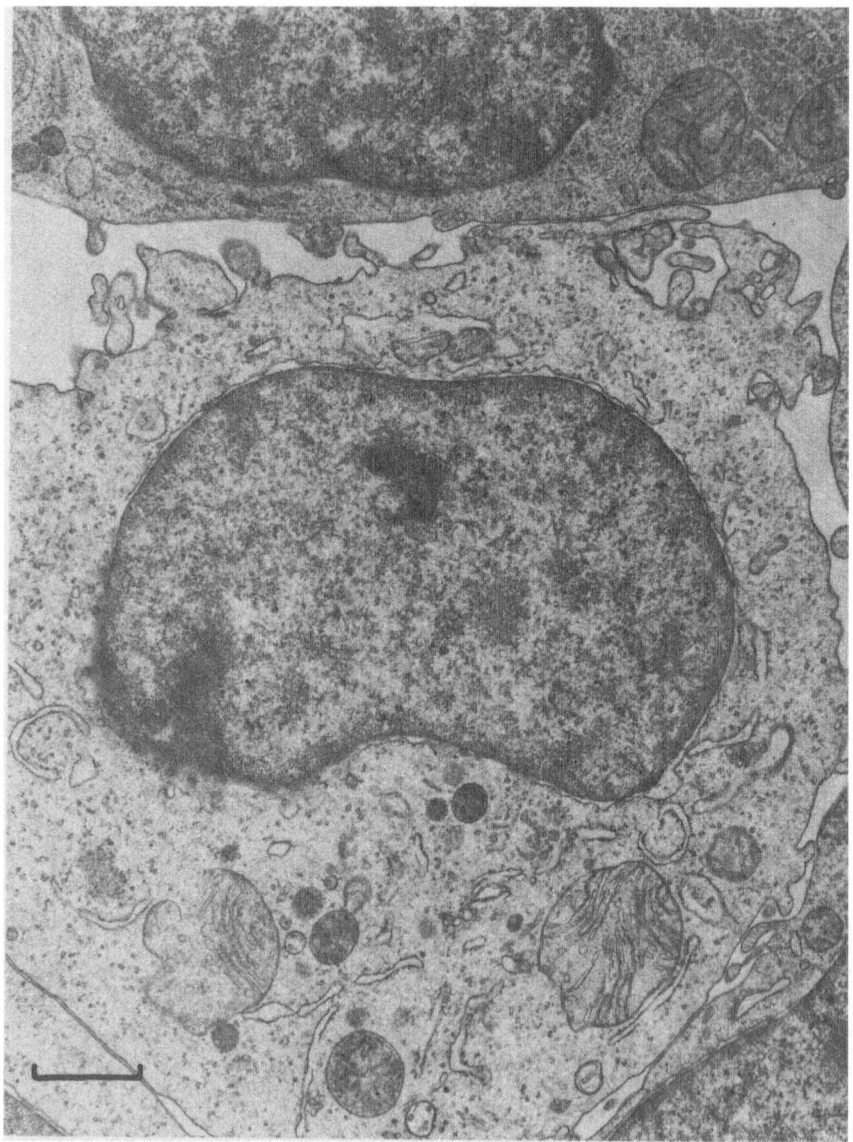

Figure 2. Electron micrograph of cultured, diploid, lymphoblastoid BRI 8 cells derived from normal human peripheral blood (Searle Diagnostics, High Wycombe, U.K.). Magnification: bar represents 1 μm. Individual cells showed some variation in size, degree of surface crenulation, and presence of electron-dense cytoplasmic bodies.

(normal lymphocytes possess a similar morphology; e.g., see Allan and Crumpton, 1970, Plate 1). Apart from the plasma membrane each intracellular organelle (nucleus, mitochondrion, lysosome, Golgi apparatus, and endoplasmic reticulum) possesses a membrane with a characteristic composition and biological function. Ideally, homogenization should rupture the surface membrane but should not disrupt the cell organelles, especially the nucleus, since this not only provides for ease of fractionation and increased resolution of fractions but also reduces the risk of degradation of the membrane by, for instance, lysosomal enzymes. It may also be desirable to avoid the vesiculation of membrane fragments that accompanies the more vigorous disruption procedures, since extraneous material may thereby be occluded within the vesicles. The monitoring of disruption is unfortunately difficult in that no one technique provides an exact measure of the ideal breakage, although a combination of the following methods gives a reasonable assessment: extent of fragmentation as judged by phase contrast microscopy, decrease in cell viability and number, distribution of subcellular markers on subsequent fractionation, and the yield of purified plasma membrane.

The relationships between the various methods which have been used to disrupt lymphocytes and the extents of nuclear breakage, the sizes of the membrane fragments, and the yield and degree of purification of the plasma membrane are summarized in Table I. Plasma membranes have also been isolated from suspensions of mouse thymocytes disrupted by nitrogen cavitation (Lance et al., 1968), and in the form of "ghosts" from mouse ascites lymphoma and leukemia cells by gentle homogenization (Dounce or a syringe) in hypotonic medium (Wolf and Avis, 1970, and Dods et al., 1972, respectively). The latter methods are not included in Table I due to the lack of detailed information.

Solid lymph node and thymus were disrupted by pressing coarsely chopped tissue through a perforated plate (Allan and Crumpton, 1970, 1972). During disruption the connective tissue present formed a pad on the perforated plate, and it was suggested that as the cells were squeezed through the pad they were stressed sufficiently for fragmentation of the surface membrane to occur. This procedure apparently ruptured the majority of the cells in that only 4% of a marker for surface membrane (5'-nucleotidase) sedimented at $300g_{av}$ on subsequent fractionation, but did not cause gross disruption of the nuclei (96% of the DNA sedimented at $300g_{av}$). On the other hand, the number of intact nuclei recovered was only 26% of the initial cell number, which suggests that the homogenate probably contained significant amounts of nuclear membranes. This method has the advantages that large amounts of tissue (about 500 g wet weight containing roughly 10^{12} lymphocytes) can be readily processed within a short period and that the isolated plasma membrane is of good quality. It suffers from the disadvantages that the membrane vesicles varied greatly in size and that the yield of purified membranes was lower than is desirable.

Of the methods available for homogenizing suspensions of free cells, nitrogen cavitation (Hunter and Commerford, 1961; Wallach and Kamat, 1966; Gahmberg and Simons, 1970) appears to be one of the least deleterious. In this procedure cells are subjected within a pressure vessel to a positive nitrogen pressure for about 15 min and are then driven by the internal pressure through a small orifice. Although it has been proposed that as the cells return to atmospheric pressure nitrogen dissolved in the cytoplasm forms bubbles causing rupture of the surface membrane, it seems equally plausible that the cells are subject to shear as they pass through the orifice. This method has been used to disrupt pig lymphocytes (Ferber et al., 1972) and calf thymocytes (Van Blitterswijk et al., 1973), although the actual procedures employed differed in two respects. Firstly, the pig lymphocytes were carefully suspended in 0.25 M sucrose prior to cavitation, whereas the calf thymocytes were ruptured in the absence of sucrose since sucrose had been shown to cause leakage of DNA due to an increase in the cell's fragility (Van Blitterswijk et al., 1973). Secondly, the nitrogen pressure used varied from 50 atm (Ferber et al., 1972) to 36 atm (Van Blitterswijk et al., 1973). These variations are undoubtedly responsible for the observed differences in the degrees of disruption, the amounts of DNA released, and the yields of plasma membrane. Thus, the use of sucrose by Ferber et al. (1972) was probably responsible for the incomplete sedimentation of DNA (only 70%) in the nuclear fraction, whereas the less vigorous disruption conditions employed by Van Blitterswijk et al. (1973) were probably not sufficient to break all the cells (about 40% of the surface marker enzyme sedimented at $13,500g_{av}$) and most probably accounted for the poor yield of plasma membrane. On the other hand, Ferber et al. (1972) obtained a very good yield of highly purified membrane.

Suspensions of lymphocytes in hypotonic and isotonic media have also been disrupted by using glass homogenizers (Lopes et al., 1973, Dounce homogenizer, hypotonic medium; Demus, 1973, Potter–Elvejem homogenizer, isotonic medium). As assessed by various criteria, these procedures were harsher than nitrogen cavitation. Thus, Demus (1973) reported that the nuclear fraction contained only 70% of the DNA, that DNA was present in all the subcellular fractions, and that a large fraction (22%) of the surface membrane marker enzyme was not sedimented even after centrifuging at $250,000g_{av}$ for 2 hr. These methods would also appear to be relatively inefficient in that the plasma membrane was recovered in low yield (8% and 12% respectively).

Recently, a general method was described in which cells were disrupted by pumping a suspension at a controlled pressure through a small orifice occupied by a spring-loaded ball bearing (Wright et al., 1974; M. J. Crumpton, unpublished observations). The pressure was adjusted by means of the tension on the spring so that the viability of the cell suspension, as judged by Trypan Blue exclusion, and the cell number were reduced by about 95% and about 50% respectively. A somewhat higher pressure was required to disrupt (as defined above) lymph node and thymus cells (approximately 1000 lb/in^2) than to disrupt cultured lymphoblastoid BRI 8 cells (approximately 750 lb/in^2); this difference probably reflects the difference between the cell diameters (< 8 μm compared with about 10 μm). Under the above conditions, nuclear breakage was apparently reduced to a minimum ($< 9\%$ of the DNA was not sedimented with the nuclear fraction; Table II). Furthermore, electron micrographs of the homogenate suggested that the surface membrane had been preferentially stripped from the cells, because many nuclei were still surrounded by cytoplasm containing mitochondria and other organelles (Fig. 3). If this interpretation of the disruption process is correct, then the lack of dissociation of the cell contents should promote the isolation of plasma membrane free from cellular contaminants. This method has the advantages that it is easily controlled, is continuous, and gives highly purified plasma membrane vesicles (49-fold purification) with a fairly uniform size. It has also proven applicable to small (10^7) and large (10^{11}) numbers of lymphocytes, although for cell numbers within the range $10^{10} - 10^{11}$ the yield of membrane was apparently inversely related to the number of cells disrupted (41% and 24% respectively).

A comparison of the various disruption methods which are applicable to free cells suggests that the pump method and nitrogen cavitation are generally superior. It would, however, appear that the pump is more easily controlled than nitrogen cavitation, gives less extensive disruption of the cells, and, being a continuous flow process, is more suitable for handling the very large numbers of cells (probably about 10^{12}) which would be required for the isolation of particular membrane receptors or antigens in amounts sufficient for structural studies.

Each of the above methods converts the plasma membrane into a polydisperse population of small vesicles. A general alternative approach, which has the advantage of yielding large membrane fragments or whole cell ghosts, is to strengthen or stabilize the surface membrane prior to cell disruption by using various fixatives (Warren et al., 1966). This method has been utilized by Kennel and Lerner (1973) who fixed cultured lymphocytes in 1mM zinc chloride before homogenization. Alternatively, Dods et al. (1972) added glutaraldehyde to the homogenate of mouse leukemic cells before separating the plasma membrane fragments. This approach is, however, fraught with a number of problems. For instance, glutaraldehyde fixation apparently destroyed 60–90% of the enzymic activity (Dodds et al., 1972) and may have attached extraneous protein to the membrane; furthermore, fixed membranes are unlikely to prove as amenable to the isolation of the individual membrane components as the membranes from untreated cells.

C. Subcellular Fractionation

Although the above homogenates are suitable for fractionation by zonal centrifugation, this technique has not been exploited apart from mouse thymocytes (Lance et al., 1968) and lymphoma ascites cells (Wolf and Avis, 1970).

Table II. Chemical Composition and Histocompatibility Antigenic Activity (HL-A2) of Subcellular Fractions[a]

	Protein	DNA		RNA		Cholesterol		HL-A2 activity	
	(mg total)	(mg total)	(μg/mg protein)	(mg total)	(μg/mg protein)	(mg total)	(μg/mg protein)	total (Id$_{50}$)	specific (Id$_{50}$/mg protein)
Homogenate	5520	645	117	595	108	100	18	3.5×10^7	6.3×10^3
Nuclear	2610	410	157	162	62	40	15	1.4×10^7	4.2×10^3
Mitochondrial	800	59	74	48	60	21	26		
Supernatant	2190	0	0	186	85	15	7	3.5×10^6	1.6×10^3
Endoplasmic reticulum	54	0	0	1.8	35	14	250	n.d.	n.d.
Plasma membrane	34	0	0	0	0	9	260	5.1×10^6	1.5×10^5

[a] Chemical assays were carried out as described by Allan and Crumpton (1970); DNA was used as a marker for nuclei and RNA as a marker for nuclei, ribosomes, and rough endoplasmic reticulum. HL-A2 activity was assessed by inhibition of fluorochromasia cytotoxicity as described previously (Snary et al., 1974); Id$_{50}$ represents the amount of antigen giving 50% inhibition. The results represent the average of two fractionations using batches of 4×10^{10} cells. n.d. means not determined. A value of 0 indicates that no material or activity was detected under the assay conditions used.

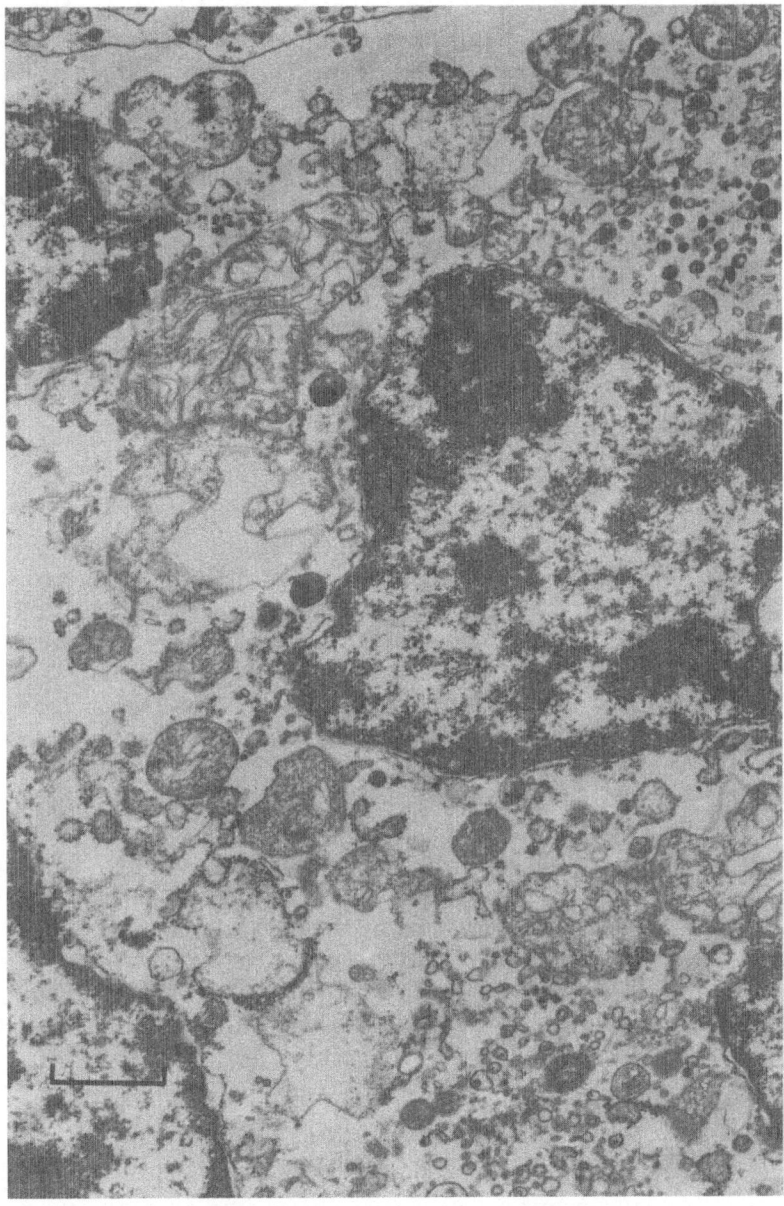

Figure 3. Electron micrograph of human, cultured, lymphoblastoid BRI 8 cells disrupted by extrusion under pressure through a small orifice occupied by a spring-loaded ball. Magnification: bar represents 1 μm.

Alternatively, the plasma membrane has been isolated by a combination of differential and density-gradient centrifugation. The fractionation schemes adopted by different workers differ primarily with respect to the centrifugal forces used to sediment the microsomal fraction and in the nature of the density gradients. Thus, after disruption by nitrogen cavitation the microsomes were sedimented at $100,000g_{av}$ for up to 90 min (Ferber et $al.$, 1972; Van Blitterswijk et $al.$, 1973), whereas 20,000 to $30,000g_{av}$ for up to 60 min was sufficient after other methods of disruption. These variations reflect the different sizes of the plasma membrane fragments (Table I) and the presence or absence of other cellular components and, in this sense, depend on the methods employed for cell disruption. In all cases, the fractionation is monitored by the distribution of chemical, enzymic, and/or antigenic markers for the various cellular components, although different markers have been employed in different studies. For example, markers for lymphocyte plasma membrane include 5'-nucleotidase, the adsorption of lymphoagglutinating antibodies from antilymphocytic sera (Allan and Crumpton, 1970), and the adsorption of the mitogenic and lymphoagglutinating activities of $Phaseolus$ $vulgaris$ phytohemagglutinin (Allan et $al.$, 1971), whereas more recent results suggest that histocompatibility antigens and (Na^+, K^+) ATPase are uniquely located in the surface membrane. The use of markers is not, however, without its pitfalls. Thus, although glucose 6-phosphatase, NADH-oxidoreductase, and lysolecithin acyltransferase have been considered to be markers for the endoplasmic reticulum of liver homogenates, in lymphocytes and thymocytes glucose 6-phosphatase activity was low and generally failed to show a consistent or reproducible distribution pattern, whereas the specific activities of NADH-oxidoreductase and lysolecithin acyltransferase were highest in the plasma membrane fraction (Ferber et $al.$, 1972; Van Blitterswijk et $al.$, 1973). Similarly, 5'-nucleotidase is not necessarily located exclusively in the surface membrane but has been detected in the rough endoplasmic reticulum of liver cells (Widnell, 1972); also, established markers for some components, especially Golgi and nuclear membranes, are lacking, although it appears that nuclear membranes may share glucose 6-phosphatase with the endoplasmic reticulum (Kay et $al.$, 1972) and that UDP-galactose N-acetylglucosamine galactosyl transferase is a reliable marker for Golgi membranes (Fleischer et $al.$, 1969).

1. Differential Centrifugation

A typical fractionation scheme adopted for the purification of the surface membrane of cultured BRI 8 cells is summarized in Fig. 4, and the distributions of the chemical, antigenic, and enzymic markers are given in Tables II and III. One notable feature of these distributions relative to those of other studies is the large proportion of the markers for mitochondria, lysosomes, and endoplasmic

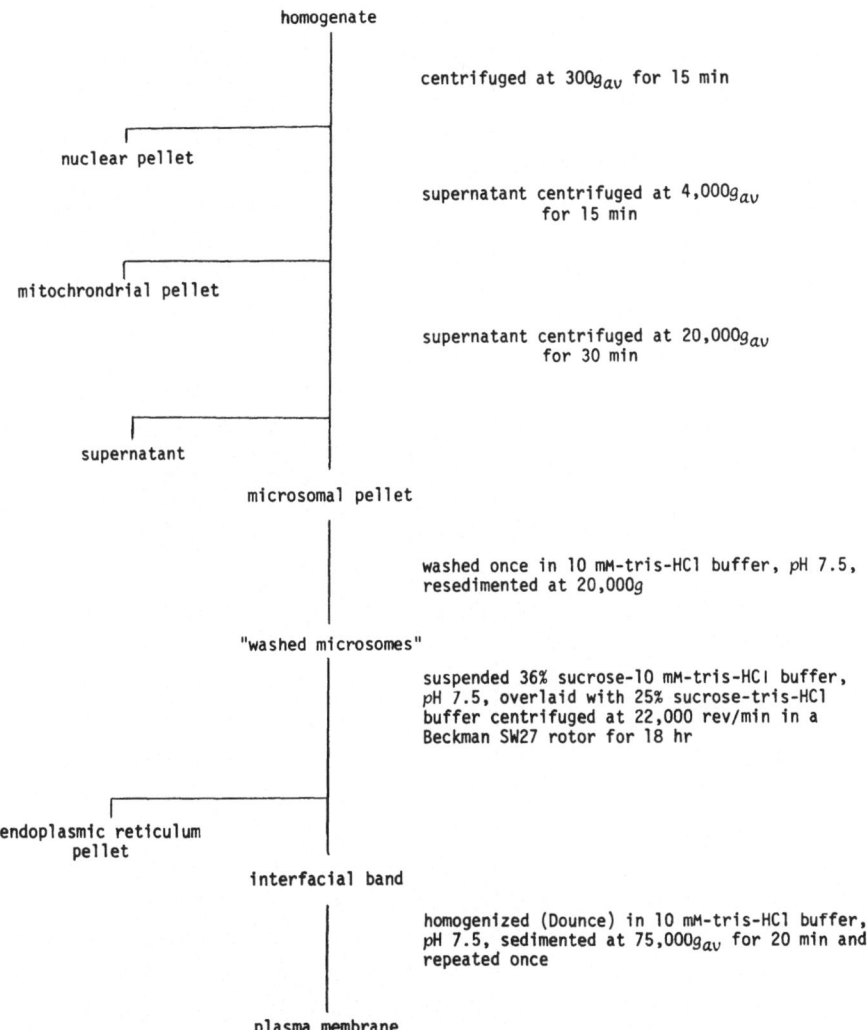

homogenate

centrifuged at 300g_{av} for 15 min

nuclear pellet

supernatant centrifuged at 4,000g_{av}
for 15 min

mitochrondrial pellet

supernatant centrifuged at 20,000g_{av}
for 30 min

supernatant

microsomal pellet

washed once in 10 mM-tris-HCl buffer, pH 7.5,
resedimented at 20,000g

"washed microsomes"

suspended 36% sucrose-10 mM-tris-HCl buffer,
pH 7.5, overlaid with 25% sucrose-tris-HCl
buffer centrifuged at 22,000 rev/min in a
Beckman SW27 rotor for 18 hr

endoplasmic reticulum
pellet

interfacial band

homogenized (Dounce) in 10 mM-tris-HCl buffer,
pH 7.5, sedimented at 75,000g_{av} for 20 min and
repeated once

plasma membrane

Figure 4. Fractionation scheme for isolation of plasma membrane from a homogenate of lymphoblastoid BRI 8 cells produced by extrusion of a cell suspension (10^8 cells/ml of Eagle's medium) through a small orifice at a pressure of about 750 lb/in².

reticulum which are associated with the nuclear fraction; in particular, this fraction contained the major portion (about 50%) of the glucose 6-phosphatase whereas in other studies this enzyme was primarily confined (about 40%) to the supernatant fraction (Allan and Crumpton, 1970; Demus, 1973; Van Blitterswijk *et al.*, 1973). While the relevance of this dramatic difference is not clear, the overall results are consistent with the previous suggestion that the pump-disrup-

Table III. Enzyme Activities of Subcellular Fractions[a]

	5'-Nucleotidase		(Na+, K+) ATPase		Glucose 6-phosphatase		Acid phosphatase		Succinic dehydrogenase		Lactic dehydrogenase	
	Total	Specific	Total	Specific	Total	Specific	Total	Specific	Total	Specific	Total	Specific
Homogenate	608	0.11	990	0.18	1480	0.25	3540	0.64	1730	0.33	26200	4.76
Nuclear	157	0.06	340	0.13	756	0.29	1180	0.45	625	0.24	2760	1.06
Mitochondrial	56	0.07	144	0.18	345	0.43	1310	1.64	408	0.51	608	0.76
Supernatant	44	0.02	88	0.04	131	0.06	830	0.38	373	0.17	23000	10.5
Endoplasmic reticulum	49	0.91	59	1.1	17	0.32	14	0.21	10	0.19	38	0.7
Plasma membrane	184	5.4	296	8.7	6	0.18	0	0	0	0	0	0

[a] Assays were carried out as described by Allan and Crumpton (1970) except that (Na+, K+) ATPase and lactic dehydrogenase were determined in the presence of 0.2% (w/v) sodium deoxycholate in 10 mM tris–HCl, pH 8.9. 5'-Nucleotidase was used as a marker for surface membrane, glucose 6-phosphatase for endoplasmic reticulum, succinic dehydrogenase for mitochondria, acid phosphatase for lysosomes, and lactic dehydrogenase for cytosol. Total enzymic activities are expressed as μmole of product liberated/hr and specific activities as μmole of product liberated/hr mg of protein. Activities were assayed at 37°C except for glucose 6-phosphatase which was measured at 30°C. The results represent the average of two fractionations using batches of 4×10^{10} cells. A value of 0 indicates that no activity was detected under the assay conditions used.

tion method stripped the plasma membrane from the cell but caused little dispersion of the intracellular contents. On the other hand, the proportions of the surface membrane markers that sedimented with the nuclear fraction (about 25%) were higher than desirable, and it would appear that slightly more vigorous disruptive conditions should have been employed.

2. Density-Gradient Centrifugation

Separation of the plasma membrane from the contaminating membranes of the microsomal fraction is based upon their different buoyant densities. Thus, Golgi membranes have a lower density than plasma membrane (Fleischer and Fleischer, 1970), whereas results obtained with hen erythrocytes suggest that the nuclear membranes possess a higher density (Zentgraf et al., 1971); the densities of smooth and rough endoplasmic reticulum are also higher than that of the plasma membrane. An example of the application of this approach to the purification of the BRI 8 cell plasma membrane is illustrated in Fig. 5, which shows the complete separation of the surface membrane marker, 5'-nucleotidase, from a protein band of higher sucrose density that possesses the marker, glucose 6-phosphatase, and the morphology (Fig. 6a) of rough endoplasmic reticulum. The significance of the association of 5'-nucleotidase with only the leading edge of the asymmetric protein peak with a sucrose density of 1.14 g/ml is difficult to assess, but it may represent an impurity or express a heterogeneity in structure of the plasma membrane.

Similar procedures to that described in Fig. 5 have been exploited by all workers. Thus, Van Blitterswijk et al. (1973) layered the "washed microsomes" onto a Ficoll cushion of density 1.05 g/ml, whereas Ferber et al. (1972) used a shallow dextran gradient (density 1.088–1.092 g/ml) containing 1 mM Mg^{2+}. Although Mg^{2+} ions have been reported (Kamat and Wallach, 1965) to improve the separation of plasma membrane by binding preferentially to the endoplasmic reticulum, it appears that, under some circumstances, Mg^{2+} and also Ca^{2+} promote microsomal aggregation resulting in increased contamination of the plasma membrane with RNA (Allan and Crumpton, 1970; Demus, 1973). In both of the above procedures the plasma membrane collected at the buffer–gradient (cushion) interface while the endoplasmic reticulum was pelleted. Gradients of sucrose have been employed in all other instances. In general, the results of continuous gradients have been subsequently used to construct step gradients which are much better suited to the isolation of large amounts of membrane. Thus, a step gradient (36% sucrose overlaid by 25%) based on the data shown in Fig. 5 has been employed routinely to purify the BRI 8 plasma membrane. Lopes et al. (1973) have also used a step gradient (30% to 40% sucrose) whereas Demus (1973) employed a multistep gradient such that the plasma membrane was distributed in a ratio of about 4:1 at the interfaces between 24 to 33% and

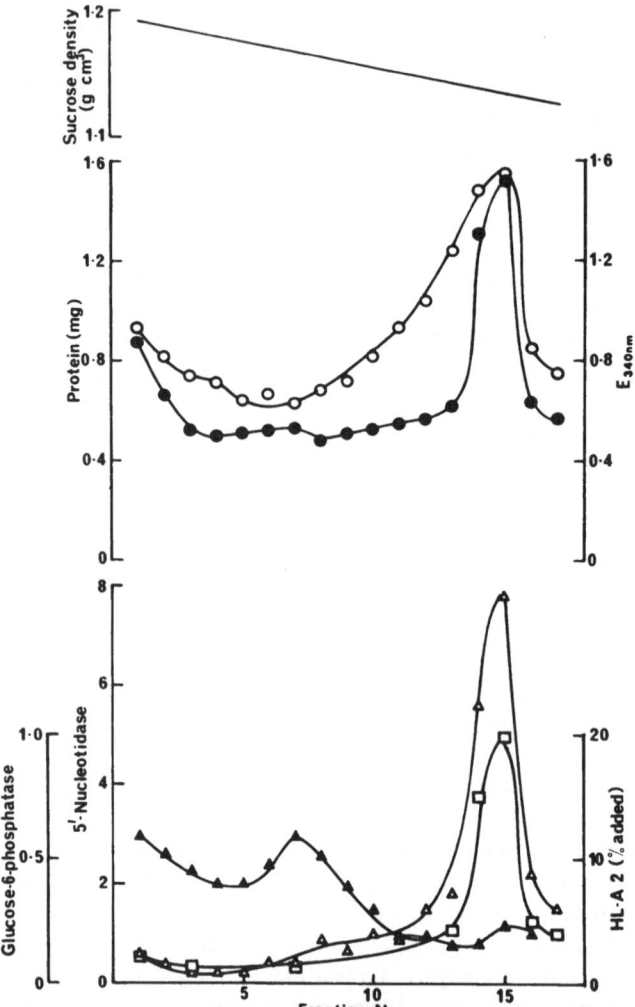

Figure 5. Fractionation of "washed microsomes" from disrupted BRI 8 cells by sucrose density-gradient centrifugation. The microsomes were resuspended in 10 mM tris–HCl buffer, pH 7.4, by using a tight-fitting homogenizer, and 1.0 ml samples were layered onto continuous sucrose gradients (8 ml of 25% (w/v) against 8 ml of 42%). After centrifuging at 22,000 rev/min for 18 hr in a Beckman SW27 rotor, 1.0 ml fractions were removed from just above the small pellet by using a "Perpex" pump. Samples were analyzed for sucrose density, turbidity (●, E_{340} nm), protein (○), 5'-nucleotidase (△, μmole product/mg protein/hr), glucose 6-phosphatase (▲, μmole product/mg protein/hr) and HL-A2 activity (□).

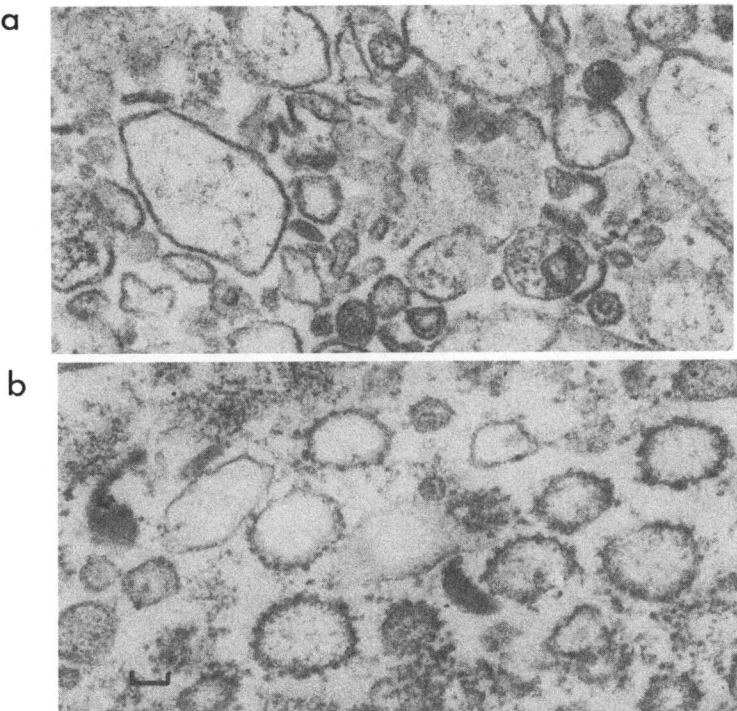

Figure 6. Electron micrographs of membrane fractions recovered from "washed microsomes" of BRI 8 cells after centrifuging on a continuous sucrose density gradient. (a) fractions 12–16 of Fig. 5 and (b) fractions 5–10 of Fig. 5. Pooled fractions were recovered by addition of 5 volumes of 10 mM tris–HCl buffer, pH 7.4, and sedimenting at 75,000g for 20 min. Magnification: bar represents 0.1 μm.

16 to 24% sucrose. It seems likely that this distribution is not indicative of distinct entities but is an expression of the polydisperse nature of the membrane fragments. This interpretation is supported by the observation that the yield of the lighter material was reduced by more vigorous disruption conditions. Apart from the light fraction of Demus (1973), the positions occupied by plasma membrane on sucrose gradients corresponded to densities within the range 1.10–1.15 g/ml. This value is significantly higher than that found with dextran and Ficoll gradients. Although membrane density is influenced by the physical state (whether sheets or vesicles, size of vesicles, and whether vesicles are inside-out or right-side-out; see Kant and Steck, 1972), it seems likely that the above variation is a function of the different media rather than an intrinsic property of the different membrane preparations.

The plasma membrane fraction is normally recovered by addition of slightly alkaline, low-ionic-strength buffer and sedimentation at high speed. In our experience the membrane (pig lymph node, human thymus, and BRI 8 cells) recovered under these conditions appears, morphologically, to be associated with a relatively large amount of amorphous material (Fig. 6a). It seems likely that this appearance is related to the report that microsomal vesicles contain up to 60% cytoplasmic protein (Wallach and Kamat, 1966). This suggestion is in agreement with the change in appearance of the BRI 8 plasma membrane on hypotonic shock (compare Fig. 7b with Fig. 6a), which was carried out by resuspending the membrane twice in 10 mM tris–HCl buffer, pH 7.4, in a tight-fitting glass homogenizer and sedimenting at $75,000g_{av}$ for 20 min. It is also supported by the observation that similar treatment of BRI 8 plasma membrane which had been biosynthetically labeled with [^{35}S] methionine released about 40% of the radioactivity (D. Snary, unpublished observations). The almost complete removal of cytoplasmic protein under these conditions is shown by the absence of lactic dehydrogenase activity in the washed membranes. The efficacy of this treatment is, however, questionable since it probably solubilizes at least some of the extrinsic membrane proteins. On the other hand, the wash fluids from the BRI 8 membrane contained no detectable 5′-nucleotidase, (Na^+, K^+) ATPase, or histocompatibility antigen (HL-A) activities.

One notable feature of the results summarized in Tables II and III and Fig. 5 is the close parallel between the distribution of the histocompatibility antigen activity and those of the well-recognized markers of the surface membrane, 5′-nucleotidase and (Na^+, K^+) ATPase; a similar association of histocompatibility antigens with the cell surface has been reported recently (Wilson and Amos, 1972; Molnar et al., 1973). These results suggest strongly that histocompatibility antigens are located primarily, if not exclusively, in the plasma membrane. This suggestion is in agreement with the observations that lymphocyte disruption was not associated with any significant changes in the H-2 and HL-A activities (Haughton, 1966; Snary et al., 1974), but is contrary to previous reports that histocompatibility antigens are also expressed on intracellular membranes [summarized by Edidin (1972) and Manson and Palm (1972)].

3. Yield and Degree of Purification

The yield is usually expressed in terms of the fraction of the total 5′-nucleotidase activity recovered in the plasma membrane. This value varies within fairly wide limits (5.4% to 45%) for the different preparations (Table I) and appears to be related principally to the conditions used for cell disruption. If it is assumed that these values are realistic estimates of the yields, then given the fraction of the homogenate protein recovered in the plasma membrane fraction, it is possible to calculate the percentage of the total cellular protein contained in the surface membrane. The results showed considerable variation (from 1.5% for

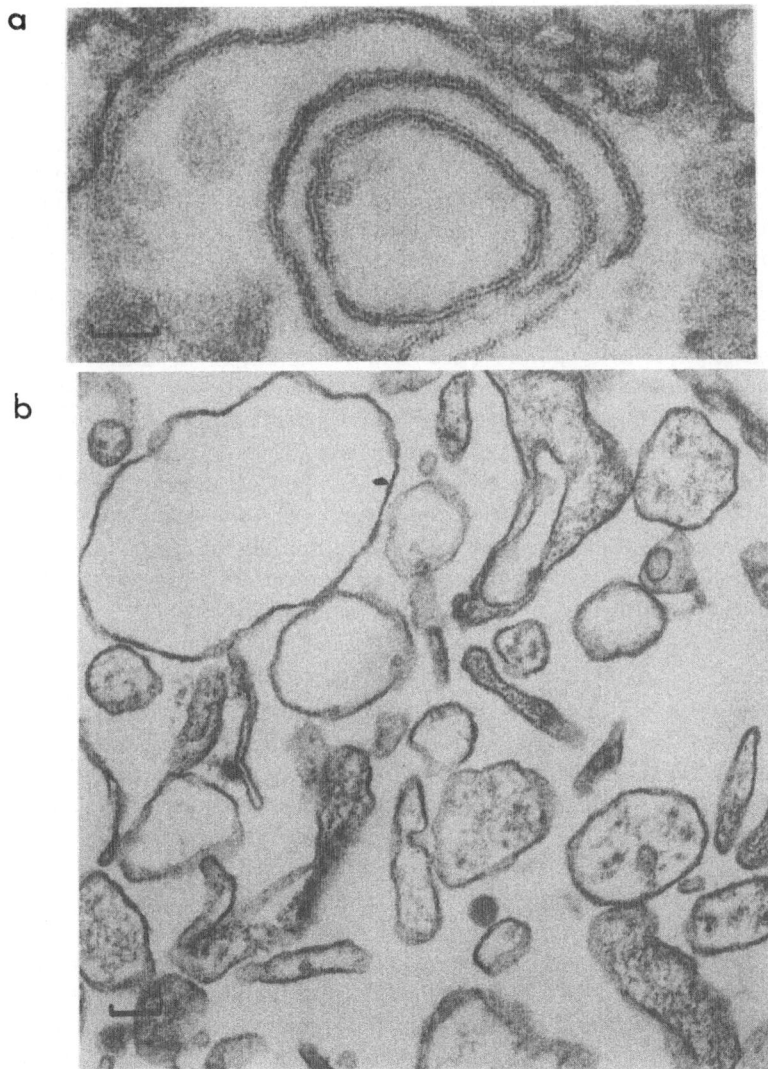

Figure 7. Electron micrographs of washed plasma membrane (fractions 12–16 of Fig. 5). The membrane was washed twice by homogenizing in a tight-fitting glass homogenizer with 10 mM tris–HCl buffer, pH 7.4, and sedimenting at 75,000g for 20 min. Magnification: (a) bar represents 50 nm and (b) bar represents 0.1 μm.

BRI 8 cells to 13.8% for calf thymocytes), which implies considerable differences in the purities of the various preparations.

The degree of purification is generally assessed in terms of the increase in specific activity of a surface marker, especially 5'-nucleotidase, relative to the cell homogenate (Table I). The lower degree of purification obtained by Allan and Crumpton (1970) for the pig lymphocyte membrane compared with that reported by Ferber et al. (1972) (12-fold versus 25-fold) may be related to the suggestion that tris buffer depresses the activities of membrane-associated enzymes (Ferber et al., 1972). Although this explanation is at variance with the lower specific activity of 5′-nucleotidase reported by Ferber et al. (1972) (7.5 μmole versus 10.1 μmole of product liberated/hr per mg of protein; Table IV), it is consistent with the much higher purification (about 28-fold) calculated from the capacities of the pig membrane to adsorb the lymphoagglutinating activity of antilymphocytic serum and the lymphoagglutinating and mitogenic activities of P. vulgaris phytohemagglutinin (Allan and Crumpton, 1970; Allan et al., 1971). If this explanation is correct then the degree of purification and possibly the yield achieved by Allan and Crumpton (1970) compare favorably with those reported by Ferber et al. (1972). The exceptionally high degree of purification of the BRI 8 membrane determined using 5′-nucleotidase (49-fold) is most probably related to the larger diameter of BRI 8 cells, compared with small lymphocytes and thymocytes, and the consequent decrease in the ratio of cell surface area to cell mass; similar degrees of purification were calculated for (Na^+, K^+) ATPase (48-fold) and histocompatibility antigenic activity (25-fold).

4. Storage

Most workers agree that the purified plasma membrane can be stored at −70°C for fairly prolonged periods without significant alteration. In contrast, storage of the BRI 8 membrane at 0°C or successive freezing and thawing were associated with marked reductions in histocompatibility antigenic activity and solubility in sodium deoxycholate. These changes are most probably partly due to proteolysis since, as shown in Fig. 8, the aged membrane gave on polyacrylamide gel electrophoresis in sodium dodecylsulfate fewer high-molecular-weight protein bands and more intensely staining low-molecular-weight bands than the fresh membrane. Similar changes in the nature of the membrane have been detected when BRI 8 cells from a terminal culture were used to prepare membrane and when the time required for membrane preparation was prolonged. Attempts to minimize proteolysis during preparation by adding diisopropylfluorophosphonate dissolved in isopropanol to the microsomal fraction (1 μl of 1 M soln/ml) were discontinued when it was noticed to cause aggregation of membrane vesicles, and it has generally proven more satisfactory to carry out all operations as quickly as possible at 0°C.

III. PROPERTIES OF PLASMA MEMBRANE

A. Purity

The establishment of the purity of the membrane preparation is an essential prerequisite to the characterization of the plasma membrane and the correlation

Table IV. Compositions and Properties of Lymphocyte Plasma Membrane Preparations[a]

	Pig lymph node		Human tonsil	Human	Human thymus	Calf thymus	Mouse leukemia cell
	Allan and Crumpton (1970)	Ferber et al. (1972)	Demus (1973)	BRI 8 cells[b]	Allan and Crumpton (1972)	Van Blitterswijk et al. (1973)	Dobs et al. (1972)
Protein (% dry wt.)	57	n.d.	n.d.	42	n.d.	n.d.	n.d.
Lipid (% dry wt.)	42	n.d.	n.d.	51	n.d.	n.d.	n.d.
Cholesterol	217	285	210	260	197	390	147
Phospholipid	438	563	608	510	540	1287	316
Cholesterol/phospholipid molar ratio	1.01	1.03	0.69	1.02	0.75	0.61	0.77
Neutral sugar	59	n.d.	n.d.	117	n.d.	n.d.	778
Sialic acid	11	n.d.	n.d.	14	n.d.	18	10
RNA	28	25	15	17	25	30	1.5
DNA	0	10	10	0	0	0–0.2	n.d.
5'-Nucleotidase	10.1	7.5	13.5	5.6	3.9	2.6	1.6
(Na+, K+) ATPase	n.d.	n.d.	n.d.	8.7[c]	n.d.	0–4	12.7
Succinic dehydrogenase	0	0[f]	0.01	0	n.d.	0[d]	0.27
Acid phosphatase	0.51	0	1.51	0	0.22	10.4[e]	0.61
Lactic dehydrogenase	n.d.	n.d.	0.1	0[c]	n.d.	n.d.	n.d.
Glucose 6-phosphatase	0.30	n.d.	0.98	0.18	0.02	0.56	0.81
NADH-oxidoreductase	n.d.	41.2	n.d.	n.d.	n.d.	29.8	n.d.

[a] Chemical compositions are expressed, except where otherwise stated, as μg/mg protein and enzymic activities as μmole of product liberated/hr per mg protein. A value of 0 indicates that no material or activity was detected under the assay conditions used; n.d. means not determined.

[b] D. Snary and M. J. Crumpton, unpublished observations.

[c] Measured in the presence of 0.2% sodium deoxycholate in order to expose the (Na+, K+) ATPase located on the inner membrane surface (see Rostgaard and Moller, 1971) and to ensure there was no latent lactic dehydrogenase occluded within the membrane vesicles.

[d] Determined as succinate: cytochrome c oxidoreductase.

[e] Estimated using disodium p-nitrophenyl phosphate as substrate whereas in all other cases β-glycerophosphate was used.

[f] Lysosomal contamination was evaluated using β-glucuronidase.

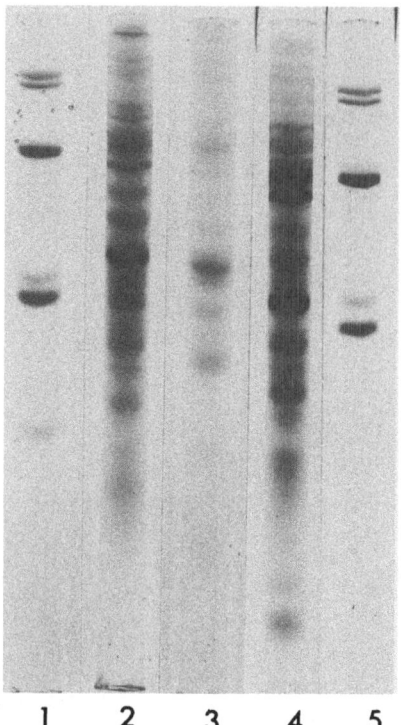

1   2   3   4   5

Figure 8. Protein patterns given by lymphocyte plasma membrane on electrophoresis in 7.5% polyacrylamide gel containing 0.1% sodium dodecylsulfate and 2-mercaptoethanol; the experimental details were as described previously (Allan and Crumpton, 1971). Gels 1 to 3 were run at the same time as were gels 4 and 5. Gels 1 and 5 are reovirus marker proteins; molecular weights in order of increasing mobility were 15.5, 14.0, 7.2, 3.8, and 3.4 × 10^4. Gel 2 is fresh plasma membrane from BRI 8 cells. Gel 3 is a glycoprotein fraction from BRI 8 plasma membrane prepared as described by Hayman and Crumpton (1972); about 10 bands can be distinguished, each of which also stains for carbohydrate and which, collectively, account for all of the carbohydrate-staining bands of the membrane (cf. Allan *et al.*, 1972). Gel 4 is BRI 8 plasma membrane after storage at 2°C for 7 days. A comparison of gels 2 and 4 reveals some marked differences, especially with respect to the relative mobilities and staining intensities of the low-molecular-weight bands.

of molecular structure with biological function. The assessment of the purity presents a number of problems, however. For example, the exact level of contamination with other subcellular components is very difficult to estimate using enzymic markers since the specific enzymic activity of the corresponding highly purified organelle is usually not available. In spite of these difficulties a reasonable evaluation of purity can generally be made from a consideration of various criteria, namely, morphology, enzymic and antigenic markers, and chemical composition, whereas the buoyant density, sialic acid content, and ratio of cholesterol to phospholipid can provide additional useful parameters (see Wallach, 1967, and Emmelot and Bos, 1972). Thus, morphologically the plasma membrane should appear free from subcellular components such as lysosomes, and electron-dense particles such as ribosomes, and the membrane vesicles should not contain amorphous material although microfilaments attached to the interior of the membrane are commonly visible (Fig. 7b); also, at higher magnification the distinct trilamellar appearance characteristic of cell membranes should be revealed (Fig. 7a).

The compositions and properties of the various preparations of lymphocyte plasma membranes are compared in Table IV. This comparison reveals a number of notable features. Firstly, the purities of the human tonsil, calf thymus, and mouse leukemia membranes, as assessed by marker enzyme activities for mitochondria, lysosomes, and endoplasmic reticulum, compare unfavorably with those of the other membranes. Secondly, the mouse leukemia membrane showed an exceptionally high carbohydrate content. The significance of this is uncertain, but it may be related to the glutaraldehyde fixation step during the preparation of the membrane. Thirdly, the human tonsil and calf thymus membranes possessed unusually low cholesterol-to-phospholipid molar ratios, whereas the calf thymus membrane had an abnormally high phospholipid content. The reason for these differences is not known but they could have arisen in various ways, such as contamination with extraneous phospholipid or loss of protein due to degradation or to overvigorous cell disruption conditions. It may, however, be significant that neither the human tonsil nor the calf thymus membrane vesicles had been subjected to hypotonic shock. As a result, both of these membrane preparations would be expected to be contaminated with soluble components (Wallach and Kamat, 1966). This association is supported in the case of the human tonsil membrane by the presence of some soluble protein (serum albumin and lactic dehydrogenase; Demus, 1973).

On the other hand, the variation in specific activity of 5'-nucleotidase for the different preparations is most probably of little, if any, significance since this has been shown to vary greatly for the same tissue from different species and for different tissues (Lauter et al., 1972). Finally, the pig lymphocyte membranes prepared by Allan and Crumpton (1970) and Ferber et al. (1972) and the BRI 8 cell membrane appear to possess similar purities and to share many of the features, such as a buoyant sucrose density close to 1.14 g/ml and a cholesterol-to-phospholipid ratio close to 1.0, that have come to be associated with highly purified preparations of plasma membranes.

B. Composition

Lymphocyte plasma membrane is composed of approximately equal amounts (by weight) of protein and lipid and a much smaller amount of carbohydrate (about 6% by weight). The protein fraction is seen by polyacrylamide gel electrophoresis in sodium dodecylsulfate (Fig. 8; Ragland et al., 1973) to comprise a large variety of polypeptide chains (> 30) with various molecular weights within the range 2×10^5 to 1.5×10^4. A comparison of the protein electrophoretic patterns given by the plasma membranes from chicken bursa and thymus tissues (Ragland et al., 1973) suggests that only a very small number of these polypeptide chains (4 and 3 respectively) are unique for B and T lymphocytes. An indication of the actual number of protein molecules present in the surface membrane of one lymphocyte can be derived in the following way: the relative capacities of whole pig lymphocytes and of the plasma membrane to reduce the mitogenic activity of *P. vulgaris* phytohemagglutinin by 50% indicate that 10^9 cells are equivalent to 1 mg of membrane protein (Allan *et al.*, 1971). If it is assumed that the membrane proteins have an average molecular weight of 5×10^4, as suggested by sucrose density-gradient centrifugation of deoxycholate-solubilized membrane (Allan and Crumpton, 1971), then the plasma membrane of a lymphocyte with a diameter of 8 µm and a smooth surface contains about 10^7 protein molecules.

Although a detailed analysis of the carbohydrate composition of the lymphocyte membrane is lacking, the results of a preliminary survey of the pig lymphocyte plasma membrane (M.J. Crumpton, unpublished observation) suggest that the carbohydrate (neutral sugars, amino sugars, and sialic acid) is distributed approximately equally between the lipid and protein fractions. The distributions of the individual sugars, however, showed some interesting differences. Thus, all of the glucose and the majority of the *N*-acetylgalactosamine were present in the lipid fraction, all of the mannose and fucose and most of the *N*-acetylglucosamine were associated with the protein, whereas the lipid and protein contained similar amounts of galactose and sialic acid. The separation of the glycoproteins from the nonglycosylated proteins, by affinity chromatography of deoxycholate-solubilized plasma membrane (pig lymphocyte and BRI 8 cells) on a column of *Lens culinaris* phytohemagglutinin covalently attached to Sepharose, revealed that 10–15% of the membrane protein is glycosylated (Hayman and Crumpton, 1972). This amount corresponds to about 1.2×10^6 molecules/cell, assuming the above calculation of the number of protein molecules is correct. The glycoprotein fraction of the BRI 8 cell membrane included all of the histocompatibility (HL-A) antigenic activity and the 5'-nucleotidase (Snary *et al.*, 1974), whereas polyacrylamide gel electrophoresis revealed at least ten protein-staining bands (Fig. 8; Hayman and Crumpton, 1972). It has recently been suggested on the basis of ruthenium red staining, which is claimed to be specific for glycoproteins and acid mucopolysaccharides, that T lymphocytes possess a thicker surface glycoprotein "coat" than B lymphocytes (28.7 nm *versus* 16.5 nm) (Santer *et al.*, 1973). This distinction is interesting, but it is desirable that it should be confirmed by using alternative approaches, such as a comparison of the carbohydrate compositions of highly purified preparations of the T and B cell plasma membrane.

Little definitive information is at present available on the distribution of the proteins and glycoproteins between the membrane's inner and outer surfaces, and on which molecules correspond to the peripheral and the integral membrane proteins. However, by analogy with the distributions of glycoproteins in the plasma membranes of other cell types, especially erythrocytes, it seems likely that the carbohydrate moieties are preferentially located on the outside surface, where they may play major roles in cell adhesion, cell recognition, lympho-cyte–lymphocyte (macrophage) interaction, and in the migratory behavior of lymphocytes (Winzler, 1970; Nicolson and Singer, 1971; Hirano *et al.*, 1972). Freeze-fracture studies (Mandel, 1972; Loor, 1973) have revealed the presence of relatively few intramembranous particles in the lymphocyte surface mem-brane. The results further suggest that the distribution of particles differs for T and B lymphocytes in that larger clusters were detected in T than in B cells (Mandel, 1972). The particle density was 350 and $150/\mu m^2$ respectively for the inner and outer fracture faces of the surface membrane of mouse lymphocytes (Loor, 1973). These densities correspond to no more than 7×10^4 molecules for a lymphocyte with a diameter of 8 μm and a smooth surface. Presumably the intramembranous particles extend across the central hydrophobic plane of the lipid bilayer and, in some cases, may span the membrane; also, they are most probably glycoproteins since their distribution was dramatically altered by a mitogenic dose of *P. vulgaris* phytohemagglutinin (Loor, 1973). Molecules which traverse the lipid bilayer represent strong potential candidates for the transfer of information across the membrane. As a result, identification and characteriza-tion of the lymphocyte intramembranous particles are of considerable interest.

Nucleic acid analyses of the various membrane preparations have revealed the presence of variable amounts of RNA (15–30 $\mu g/mg$ of protein), whereas amounts of DNA varied from 10 $\mu g/mg$ of protein to being undetectable. The significance of the presence of RNA is not possible to assess at present. Undoubtedly, the most likely explanation is that it represents, at least partly, ribosomal contamination. However, several investigators (Shapot and Davidova, 1971; Juliano *et al.*, 1972) have proposed that the cell surface membrane contains a unique, nonribosomal RNA which may be associated with the synthesis of membrane protein. In view of the recent results of Stevens and Williamson (1974) it seems possible that in the case of the lymphocyte plasma membrane this RNA may include the immunoglobulin H-chain messenger. The significance of the DNA values is also difficult to assess, especially in relation to the reports that a unique species of DNA, corresponding to 0.5% of the total cell DNA, is associated with the plasma membrane of cultured, human, lympho-blastoid cells (Lerner, 1972); this DNA has been ascribed an important role in the linkage between gene expression and the membrane immunoglobulin. If these reports are correct, then 0.5% of the total DNA of disrupted human lymphoblastoid BRI 8 cells (645 mg; Table II) should be present in the plasma membrane fraction. This would correspond to 20 μg of DNA/mg of membrane protein, assuming a 25% recovery of the purified membrane. In contrast, the isolated plasma membrane contained no detectable DNA (Table II). It seems very unlikely that this discrepancy can be ascribed to the sensitivity of the assay procedure, although it is conceivable that the surface membrane DNA is only loosely associated with the membrane and has been lost during purification. Further work is essential to resolve this notable difference.

IV. SUMMARY

The various methods which have been employed to isolate the surface membrane of lymphocytes have been compared, as have the characteristics of the purified membrane preparations. The role of cell disruption in determining the procedure subsequently used to fractionate the homogenate and the yield and purity of the purified plasma membrane have been emphasized. Disruption of free lymphocytes by nitrogen cavitation or by extrusion under pressure through a small orifice was superior to the use of glass homogenizers or pressing solid tissue through a perforated plate. The use of markers to identify the surface membrane and to assess the degree of contamination by subcellular components has been discussed. The results suggest that $5'$-nucleotidase, (Na^+, K^+) ATPase, and histocompatibility (HL-A) antigen are located primarily, if not exclusively, in the plasma membrane. The most notable features of the purified plasma membrane preparations are as follows: firstly, DNA is undetectable in the membrane from a cultured human lymphoblastoid cell line; secondly, $10-15\%$ of the membrane protein is glycosylated; thirdly, the membrane apparently contains more than 30 different types of polypeptide chains of which about 10 are glycosylated; fourthly, only a very small fraction of the total protein (less than 1%) apparently traverses the center plane of the lipid bilayer.

ACKNOWLEDGMENT

The authors are grateful to Dr. J. A. Armstrong for the electron micrographs.

REFERENCES

Allan, D., and Crumpton, M.J., 1970, *Biochem. J.* **120**: 133.
Allan, D., and Crumpton, M.J., 1971, *Biochem. J.* **123**: 967.
Allan, D., and Crumpton, M.J., 1972, *Biochim. Biophys. Acta* **274**: 22.
Allan, D., Auger, J., and Crumpton, M.J., 1971, *Exp. Cell Res.* **66**: 362.
Allan, D., Auger, J., and Crumpton, M.J., 1972, *Nature New Biol.* **236**: 23.
Basten, A., Miller, J.F.A.P., Sprent, J., and Pye, J., 1972a, *J. Exp. Med.* **135**: 610.
Basten, A., Warner, N.L., and Mandel, T., 1972b, *J. Exp. Med.* **135**: 627.
Bretscher, M.S., 1971, *Nature New Biol.* **231**: 229.
Buell, D.N., and Fahey, J.L., 1969, *Science* **164**: 1524.
Capaldi, R.A., and Vanderkooi, G., 1972, *Proc. Nat. Acad. Sci. U.S.* **69**: 930.
Cikes, M., and Friberg, S., 1971, *Proc. Nat. Acad. Sci. U.S.* **68**: 566.
Coleman, R., Michell, R.H., Finean, J.B., and Hawthorne, J.N., 1967, *Biochim. Biophys. Acta* **135**: 573.
Demus, H., 1973, *Biochim. Biophys. Acta* **291**: 93.
Denman, A. M., 1973, *J. Immunol. Meth.* **2**: 331.
DePierre, J.W., and Karnovsky, M.L., 1973, *J. Cell Biol.* **56**: 275.

Dods, R.F., Essner, E., and Barclay, M., 1972, *Biochem. Biophys. Res. Commun.* **46**: 1074.

de Duve, C., 1971, *J. Cell Biol.* **50**: 20D.

Edidin, M., 1972, in Kahan, B.D., and Reisfeld, R.A. (eds.), *Transplantation Antigens,* Academic Press, New York-London, p. 125.

Emmelot, P., and Bos, C.J., 1972, *J. Membrane Biol.* **9**: 83.

Ferber, E., Resch, K., Wallach, D.F.H., and Imm, W., 1972, *Biochim. Biophys. Acta* **266**: 494.

Fleischer, B., and Fleischer, S., 1970, *Biochim. Biophys. Acta* **219**: 301.

Fleischer, B., Fleischer, S., and Ozawa, H., 1969, *J. Cell Biol.* **43**: 59.

Frye, L.D., and Edidin, M., 1970, *J. Cell Sci.* **7**: 319.

Gahmberg, C.G., and Simons. K., 1970, *Acta Path. Microbiol. Scand.* Sec. B **78**: 176.

Gavin, J.R., Gorden, P., Roth, J., Archer, J.A., and Buell, D.N., 1973, *J. Biol. Chem.* **248**: 2202.

Greaves, M.F., and Janossy, G., 1972, *Transplant. Rev.* **11**: 87.

Greaves, M.F., Owen, J.J. T., and Raff, M.C., 1973, *T and B Lymphocytes: Origins, Properties, and Roles in Immune Responses,* Excerpta Medica, Amsterdam.

Hadden, J.W., Hadden, E.M., Wilson, E.E., Good, R.A., and Coffey, R.G., 1972, *Nature New Biol.* **235**: 174.

Haughton, G., 1966, *Transplantation* **4**: 238.

Hayman, M.J., and Crumpton, M.J., 1972, *Biochem. Biophys. Res. Commun.* **47**: 923.

Hendler, R.W., 1971, *Physiol. Rev.* **51**: 66.

Hirano, H., Parkhouse, B., Nicolson, G.L., Lennox, E.S., and Singer, S.J., 1972. *Proc. Nat. Acad. Sci. U.S.* **69**: 2945.

Hunter, M.J., and Commerford, S.L., 1961, *Biochim. Biophys. Acta* **47**: 580.

Juliano, R., Ciszkowski, J., Waite, D., and Mayhew, E., 1972, *FEBS Lett.* **22**: 27.

Kamat, V.B., and Wallach, D.F.H., 1965, *Science* **148**: 1343.

Kant, J.A., and Steck, T.L., 1972, *Nature New Biol.* **240**: 26.

Kay, R.R., Fraser, D., and Johnston, I.R., 1972, *Eur. J. Biochem.* **30**: 145.

Kennel, S.J., and Lerner, R.A., 1973, *J. Mol. Biol.* **76**: 485.

Kobylka, D., Khettry, A., Shin, B.C., and Carraway, K.L., 1972, *Arch. Biochem. Biophys.* **148**: 475.

Lance, E.M., Ford, P.J., and Ruszkiewicz, M., 1968, *Immunology* **15**: 571.

Lauter, C.J., Solyom, A., and Trams, E.G., 1972, *Biochim. Biophys. Acta* **266**: 511.

Lerner, R.A., 1972. in Inman, F.P. (ed.), *Contemporary Topics in Immunochemistry,* Vol. 1, Plenum Press, New York-London, p. 111.

Lesniak, M.A., Roth J., Gorden, P., and Gavin, J.R., 1973, *Nature New Biol.* **241**: 20.

Loor, F., 1973, *Eur. J. Immunol.* **3**: 112.

Lopes, J., Nachbar, M., Zucker-Franklin, D., and Silber, R., 1973, *Blood* **41**: 131.

Mandel, T.E., 1972, *Nature New Biol.* **239**: 112.

Manson, L.A., 1972, in Kahan, B.D., and Reisfeld, R.A. (eds.), *Transplantation Antigens,* p. 227, Academic Press, New York-London, p. 227.

Manson, L.A., and Palm, J., 1972, in Kahan, B.D., and Reisfeld, R.A. (eds.), *Transplantation Antigens,* Academic Press, New York-London, p. 141.

Marchesi, V.T., Tillack, T.W., Jackson, R.L., Segrest, J.P., and Scott, R.E., 1972, *Proc. Nat. Acad. Sci. U.S.* **69**: 1445.

Melmon, K.L., Bourne, H.R., Weinstein, J., and Sela, M., 1972, *Science* **177**: 707.

Moore, G.E., and Woods, L., 1972, *Transplantation* **13**: 155.

Molnar, J., Klein, G., and Friberg, S., 1973, *Transplantation* **16**: 93.

Nicolson, G.L., and Singer, S.J., 1971, *Proc. Nat. Acad. Sci. U.S.* **68**: 942.

Nigam, V.N., Morais, R., and Karasaki, S., 1971, *Biochim. Biophys. Acta* **249**: 34.

Nussenzweig, V., and Pincus, C.S., 1972, in Hanna, M.G. (ed.), *Contemporary Topics in Immunobiology,* Vol. 1, Plenum Press, New York-London, p. 69.

Oye, I., and Sutherland, E.W., 1966, *Biochim. Biophys. Acta* **127**: 347.

Parish, C.R., and Hayward, J.A., 1974, *Proc Roy. Soc.(London), Ser.B* in press.

Pasternak, C.A., Warmsley, A.M.H., and Thomas, D.B., 1971, *J. Cell Biol.* **50**: 562.

Pellegrino, M.A., Ferrone, S., Natali, P.G., Pellegrino, A., and Reisfeld, R.A., 1972, *J. Immunol.* **108**: 573.

de Petris, S., and Raff, M.C., 1973, *Nature New Biol.* **241:** 257.
Polgar, P., Vera, J.C., Kelley, P.R., and Rutenburg, A.M., 1973, *Biochim. Biophys. Acta* **297:** 378.
Raff, M.C., 1971, *Transplant. Rev.* **6:** 52.
Raff, M.C., and Wortis, H.H., 1970, *Immunology* **18:** 931.
Ragland, W.L., Pace, J.L., and Doak, R.L., 1973, *Biochem. Biophys. Res. Commun.* **50:** 118.
Ray, T.K., 1970, *Biochim. Biophys. Acta* **196:** 1.
Rogentine, G.N., and Gerber, P., 1970, in Terasaki, P.I. (ed.), *Histocompatibility Testing 1970,* Munksgaard, Copenhagen, p. 333.
Roitt, I.M., Greaves, M.F., Torrigiani, G., Brostoff, J., and Playfair, J.H.L., 1969, *Lancet* **2:** 367.
Rostgaard, J., and Moller, O.J., 1971, *Exp. Cell Res.* **68:** 356.
Santer, V., Cone, R.E., and Marchalonis, J.J., 1973, *Exp. Cell Res.* **79:** 404.
Shapot, V.S., and Davidova, S.Y., 1971, in Davidson, J.N., and Cohn, W.E. (eds.), *Progress in Nucleic Acid Research and Molecular Biology,* Vol. XI, Academic Press, New York-London, p. 81.
Shearer, G.M., Melmon, K.L., Weinstein, Y., and Sela, M., 1972, *J. Exp. Med.* **136:** 1302.
Singer, S.J., and Nicolson, G.L., 1972, *Science* **175:** 720.
Snary, D., Goodfellow, P., Hayman, M.J., Bodmer, W.F., and Crumpton, M.J., 1974, *Nature* **247:** 457.
Steck, T.L., and Wallach, D.F.H., 1970, *Meth. Cancer Res.* **5:** 93.
Steck, T.L., Weinstein, R.S., Straus, J.H., and Wallach, D.F.H., 1970, *Science* **168:** 255.
Stevens, R.H., and Williamson, A.R., 1974, mRNA for H and L Chains of Immunoglobulin: Specific Control of H-Chain Production, in Ada, G.L. (ed.), *Contemporary Topics in Molecular Immunology,* Vol. 3, Plenum Press, New York-London, p. 85–110.
Taylor, R.B., Duffus, P.H., Raff, M.C., and de Petris, S., 1971, *Nature New Biol.* **233:** 225.
Van Blitterswijk, W.J., Emmelot, P., and Feltkamp, C.A., 1973, *Biochim. Biophys. Acta* **298:** 577.
Van Deenan, L.L.M., 1972, *Chem. Phys. Lipids* **8:** 372.
Wallach, D.F.H., 1967, in Davis, B.D., and Warren, L. (eds.), *The Specificity of Cell Surfaces,* Prentice-Hall, Englewood Cliffs, N.J., p. 129.
Wallach, D.F.H., and Kamat, V.B., 1966, *Methods Enzymol.* **8:** 164.
Wallach, D.F.H., and Lin, P.S., 1973, *Biochim. Biophys. Acta* **300:** 211.
Wallach, D.F.H., Kranz, B., Ferber, E., and Fischer, H., 1972, *FEBS Lett.* **21:** 29.
Warren, L., and Glick, M.C., 1971, in Manson, L. (ed.), *Biomembranes,* Vol. 1, Plenum Press, New York-London. p. 257.
Warren, L., Glick, M.C., and Nass, M.K., 1966, *J. Cell Physiol.* **68:** 269.
Widnell, C.C., 1972, *J. Cell Biol.* **52:** 542.
Wilson, L.A., and Amos, D.B., 1972, *Tissue Antigens* **2:** 105.
Winzler, R.J., 1970, *Intern. Rev. Cytol* **29:** 77.
Wolf, A., and Avis, P.J.G., 1970, *Transplantation* **9:** 18.
Wright, B.M., Edwards A.J., and Jones, V.E., 1974, *J. Immunol. Meth.* **4:** in press.
Zentgraf, H., Deumling, B., Jarasch, E.D., and Franke, W.W., 1971, *J. Biol. Chem.* **246:** 2986.
Zettergren, J.G., Luberoff, D.E., and Pretlow, T.G., 1973, *J. Immunol.* **111:** 836.

Immunogenicity In Vitro: *Structural Correlation*

Marc Feldmann[1]

Imperial Cancer Research Fund Tumour Immunology Unit
Department of Zoology, University College
London, England

I. INTRODUCTION

Immunologists strive to understand the mechanism by which lymphoid cells are stimulated by antigen to produce antibody. One approach to this problem is the identification of particularly immunogenic molecules. By comparing the structures of immunogenic and nonimmunogenic molecules possessing the same antigenic determinants, some of the details of the "key" which turns lymphocytes on should be revealed.

Since the development of successful tissue culture techniques for the induction of antibody responses *in vitro* by Mishell and Dutton (1967), Marbrook (1967), and Diener and Armstrong (1967), it has become possible to directly study the manner in which antigen interacts with lymphoid cell surface receptors in an immunogenic way. The uniform concentration of antigen *in vitro*, the capacity to vary antigen concentrations precisely over very wide ranges, the ability to alter these at will, as well as the ability to use defined (and purified) cell populations, has made *in vitro* studies of lymphocyte stimulation much easier to interpret than previous work *in vivo*. For this reason, and since a whole book on immunogenicity *in vivo* has recently been published (Immunogenicity, edited by F. Borek, 1972), as well as a thought-provoking conceptual review by Mitchison (1971a), only aspects of immunogenicity *in vitro* will be reviewed here. Only two aspects of the molecular biology of immunogenicity will be considered: firstly, the importance of "polymeric" antigenic determinants for effecient stimulation of B cells,[2] be it with antigens or mitogens; secondly, the

---

[1] C.J. Martin Fellow of the National Health and Medical Research Council (Australia).
[2] A list of abbreviations used in this article is included for convenient reference. The list is located at the end of this article.

role of the density of antigenic determinants on a polymeric antigen in influencing the discrimination between immunity and tolerance in B cells. Since recent
studies on the chemical basis of immunogenicity have been elegantly reviewed
(Gill, 1972; Borek, 1972; Leskowitz, 1972; Sela, 1969, 1973), they will not be
considered in detail.

II. DIRECT STIMULATION OF B CELLS

A. Thymus Independence

While the role of T helper cells in the induction of antibody responses is
widely acknowledged (reviewed by Claman and Chaperon, 1969; Miller, 1972;
Katz and Benacerraf, 1972), such cells are not invariably needed. Responses
which are not impaired in the absence of T cells have been termed "thymus-independent." Antigens which elicit these responses include pneumococcal polysaccharide type III (SIII) (Davies *et al.,* 1970), *Escherichia coli* endotoxin (LPS)
(Andersson and Blomgren, 1971), polyvinyl pyrrolidone (PVP) (Andersson and
Blomgren, 1971), polymeric flagellin (POL) (Feldmann and Basten, 1971), levan
(LE) (Miranda, 1972), and their haptenic conjugates (see Feldmann and Basten,
1971; del Guercio and Leuchars, 1972).

For some antigens, stringent criteria for the absence of T cells have been
met. For example, spleen cells from "nude" mice (with thymic aplasia) respond
normally to DNP POL (Feldmann *et al.,* 1972) *in vitro,* as do spleen cells from

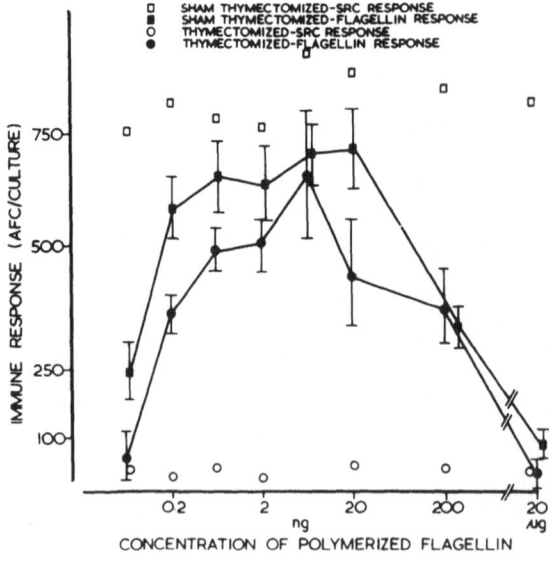

Figure 1. The immune response
of ATXBM and XBM cultures to
POL. Each point represents the
arithmetic mean of 10–20 cultures ± the standard error of the
mean. The mean of the response
of these cultures to SRC is indicated by the open symbols. (Reproduced from Feldmann and
Basten, 1971, *J. Exp. Med.* **134:**
103)

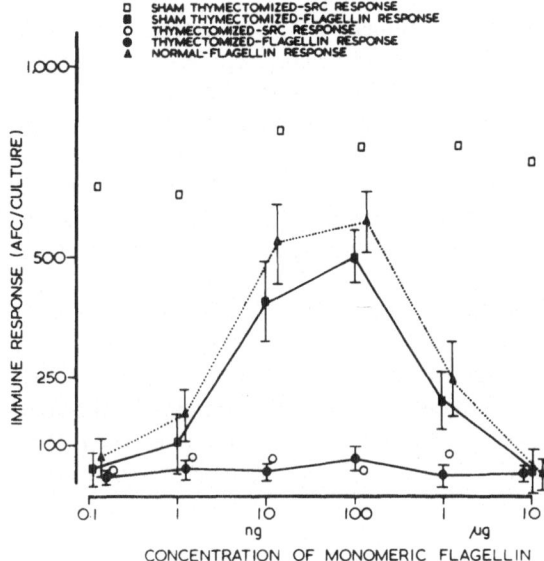

Figure 2. The immune response of ATXBM, XBM, and normal spleen cultures to MON. Each point represents the arithmetic mean ± the standard error of the mean of 8–16 cultures. The mean of the response to SRC is indicated by the open symbols. (Reproduced from Feldmann and Bastens, 1971, *J. Exp. Med.* **134**: 103)

adult thymectomized, irradiated, and bone-marrow-injected mice (ATXBM), which have been further depleted of T cells by drainage from the thoracic duct for several days and by treatment with anti-θ serum and complement (Feldman and Basten, 1971).

The molecular structure of all these thymus-independent antigens is remarkably similar, since they are all polymers with repeating antigenic determinants. The critical importance of the repeating determinants for thymus independence is illustrated by comparing two physical forms of the protein flagellin from *Salmonella adelaide:* the monomeric form (MON) and the polymeric (POL) as shown in Figs. 1 and 2. However there are other factors involved in thymus independence, especially *in vivo*. Antigen persistence has been emphasized (Mitchell *et al.*, 1973; Sela, 1973). Langman (personal communication) has found that in some strains of mice *in vivo* both MON and POL are thymus *dependent* while in others they are thymus independent. These experiments are difficult to interpret because flagellin is a nonpersisting antigen (Shellam, 1970), and difference in responses may be related to antigen handling.

B. Macrophage Independence

Diener *et al.* (1970) first reported that the antibody response to POL *in vitro* was normal despite deletion of cells which adhered to glass bead columns, while the response to particulate sheep red cells (SRC) was not. Subsequently these results were extended by Shortman and Palmer (1971), who demonstrated by reconstitution experiments and by the use of antimacrophage serum (AMS) that the macrophage was the essential adherent cell needed for the response to SRC, and by Feldmann and Palmer (1971), who demonstrated that the requirements for macrophages were qualitatively the same in the secondary response as in the primary response to these antigens. Dinitrophenylated conjugates of POL and levan were also found to immunize in the absence of macrophages (Feldmann, 1972a, Desaymard, 1974, unpublished). Palmer (personal communication) found that sonication of SRC membranes could produce a soluble SRC antigen which was immunogenic in the absence of macrophages, as illustrated in Tables I and II.

Thus certain antigens may immunize lymphoid cell suspensions markedly depleted of macrophages. Whether these antigens can immunize in the *total* absence of macrophages cannot be proven, but since the combined use of two techniques, each effective by itself, does not diminish the response, it seems likely that they do.

C. Correlation of Macrophage and Thymus Independence

Since POL is both thymus and macrophage independent *in vitro*, the only cells necessary for a response to this antigen are the B lymphocytes, the

Table I.   Immune Response to Soluble SRC Antigen

		Immune response (AFC[a]/culture ± SE)		
Cells	Antigen	SRC	DNP	POL
ATXBM	Intact SRC	240 ± 110	< 20[c]	0[d]
	Sonicated SRC	1265 ± 260	< 20[c]	0[d]
	DNP POL	110 ± 20[b]	820 ± 160[e]	640 ± 105
XBM	Intact SRC	2845 ± 620	< 20[c]	0[d]
	Sonicated SRC	1645 ± 310	< 20[c]	0[d]
	DNP POL	310 ± 105[b]	1060 ± 240[e]	580 ± 95

[a] Each value represents the arithmetic mean of four cultures ± the standard error of the mean. Similar results were obtained in four other experiments. Period of culture was four days.

[b] Background anti-SRC response of cultures was not challenged with SRC.

[c] Background anti-DNP response was always < 20 AFC/culture.

[d] Background response to POL was zero.

[e] Immune response to DNP (after subtracting SRC background response). (From Byrd, Feldmann, and Palmer, 1974.

Table II.　Macrophage Independence of the Response to
Sonicated SRC

Cells	Immune response (AFC/10^6 cultured cells ± SE)		
	Intact SRC	Sonicated SRC	POL
Spleen with NRS[a]	132 ± 16	86 ± 22	42 ± 8
Filtrate[b] with NRS[a]	3 ± 1	79 ± 11	52 ± 12
Filtrate with AMS[a]	0	67 ± 20	39 ± 21

[a] 10% serum present throughout. AMS (antimacrophage serum)
prepared as described by Feldmann and Palmer (1971). NRS is
normal rabbit serum.
[b] Filtrate compound of macrophage-depleted cells by technique of
Shortman et al. (1971).
(Data from Feldmann and Palmer, unpublished)

precursor of AFC. In an analogous way, solubilized SRC antigen, a macrophage-independent antigen, was also found to be thymus independent in vitro (Byrd et al., 1974). Nonpolymeric antigens of low molecular weight, such as MON, DNP FγG, and DNP KLH, were found to be macrophage dependent (Feldmann, 1972a) as well as T-cell dependent (see above).

The correlation of T-cell and macrophage dependence (or independence) with antigen structure suggested that macrophages participate in the process of cell cooperation, as discussed previously, and that the capacity to stimulate B cells directly was related to the physical structure of antigens and did not depend on the nature of their individual antigenic determinants.

Immunization of populations of B lymphocytes depleted of other cells need not imply that cell cooperation does not occur. Cooperation between two sets of B lymphocytes remains possible. Certain results of del Guercio suggest that this may occur in mice. It was found that the induction of tolerance in mice to LE prevented their subsequent response to DNP LE (del Guercio and Leuchars, 1972). However, Klaus and Humphrey (1974) have not been able to reproduce these results with DNP LE in vitro, nor could Desaymard and Feldmann (1974) either in vivo or in vitro, using a variety of tests for B–B cooperation. In contrast, using POL in vitro, it was not possible to demonstrate that the induction of tolerance to POL, or even the presence of POL in great molar excess (10^4-fold), had any influence on the response to DNP POL in primed or unprimed spleen cell suspensions (Feldmann, 1972b), whereas both these procedures completely abolished the response to DNP MON (which is carrier dependent and T-cell and macrophage dependent). In an analogous way, priming to

POL did not influence the response to DNP POL, whereas priming to DNP (on any carrier) markedly augmented the response. The reasons for these conflicting results are not known.

Other evidence against B–B collaboration in the response to T-independent antigens, even DNP levan, is the failure to demonstrate carrier dependence as witnessed by the lack of memory after carrier priming in that system, or with other polysaccharides, such as SIII (del Guercio, 1972; Howard, 1972). Furthermore, B–B cooperation is difficult to envisage as a general principle with T-independent antigens, since some of these, such as native LE or PVP, are monodeterminant antigens (Basten and Howard, 1973).

III. STRUCTURE–ACTIVITY RELATIONSHIPS

A. Antigens

Results with several series of immunogens bearing the same antigenic determinants have been alluded to previously. They are summarized in Table III. Two classes of T-cell- and macrophage-independent (T- and M-independent) antigens have been found—polymers, as detailed above, and surfaces, such as those of beads (Sepharose or acrylamide) or plastic dishes.

Particulate antigens of cell size, such as red cells, are T and M dependent (Mosier, 1967; Claman and Chaperon, 1969); Salmonella are M dependent (Shortman and Palmer, 1971). To my knowledge, it has not been tested whether these bacteria are also T dependent. However, this has been investigated with other bacteria, e.g. the streptococcal polysaccharide A response to the whole bacteria is T dependent (Braun et al., 1972). Polymers of protein (e.g., POL) or polysaccharide (SIII dextran or LE) also act as carriers which can make other determinants act in a T-independent manner, establishing that there is nothing special about the determinants on these polymers which confers T and M independence. Taken together, these studies emphasize that the physical structure of the antigen is of marked importance in determining the cellular pathway of immune induction.

Proteins, such as serum globulins and albumins and keyhole limpet hemocyanin (KLH), have been identified by many investigators as being T dependent in vivo (Miller and Warner, 1971; Taylor, 1969; Kruger and Gershon, 1971; Unanue, 1970) as well as in vitro (Cheers et al., 1971; Bullock and Rittenberg, 1971). Several of these have been demonstrated to be M dependent—DNP MON, MON, DNP FγG, dissociated DNP KLH (Feldmann, 1972a) as well as associated TNP KLH (Feldmann et al., 1974).

Table III. Summary of M- and T-Independence–Size Relationships

Determinant	Large M- and T-dependent	M- and T-independent	Small M- and T-dependent
		Polymers	
SRC	Whole SRC	Sonicated SRC (Byrd et al., 1973)	SRC antigen in serum (Sjöberg and Britton, 1972)
Flagellin	Bacteria[a] (Shortman and Palmer, 1971) MON red cells	POL, flagella (Feldmann and Basten, 1971)	MON (Feldmann and Basten, 1971)
FγG	FγG red cells	FγG–POL[b] (Schrader and Feldmann, 1973a)	FγG (Schrader and Feldmann, 1973a)
DNP	DNP red cells (Feldmann and Basten, 1971)	DNP POL (Feldmann and Basten, 1971)	DNP MON (Feldmann and Basten, 1971)
		DNP SIII[c] (Mitchell et al., 1973)	DNP FγG (Feldmann, 1972a)
		DNP LE[c] (del Guercio and Leuchars, 1972)	DNP KLH (Feldmann and Basten, 1972)
		DNP Dextran (Desaymard and Feldmann, 1974)	
		Surfaces	
TNP		TNP KLH-Sepharose and TNP-acrylamide (Feldmann et al., 1974)	TNP KLH (Rittenberg and Bullock, 1972)

[a] T dependence not known.
[b] M dependence not clear.
[c] Levan is a branched polysaccharide of mol.wt. $\simeq 2 \times 10^7$; SIII is a linear polysaccharide of mol.wt. $2 \times 10^5 - 2 \times 10^6$.

T- and M-dependent antigens, such as TNP KLH, have been converted to T-and M-independent antigens by conjugation to the surface of Sepharose beads, in analogy with previous work with mitogens (Greaves and Bauminger, 1972). Since this work has not yet been published, an experiment illustrating the T and M independence of the TNP KLH–sepharose 4B beads compared with the same antigen not coupled to Sepharose beads is described in Table IV. These Sepharose-bound antigens are capable of stimulating normal B cells, as well as primed B cells.

There are several other examples of the influence of antigen structure on the cellular requirements for immunogenicity. Shortman and Palmer (1971) described sonicated SRC membranes that were M independent. Subsequent work has demonstrated that these same sonicated SRC preparations ("soluble SRC antigen") were also T independent *in vitro* (Table I taken from Byrd *et al.*, 1974). Electron microscopy revealed that these were membrane fragments ranging in size from 0.05 to 0.3 μm in diameter, a sufficient size for these to contain repeating determinants.

Schrader and Feldmann (1973a) have found that FγG–POL complexes are

Table IV. Immune Response to TNP KLH Coupled to Sepharose

Cells	Antigen	Antibody response (AFC/culture)	
		DNP	SRC
Normal spleen	Nil	8	
	DNP POL	415	
	TNP KLH	10	
	TNP KLH + Sepharose[a]	15	
	TNP KLH – Sepharose[b]	275	
	SRC		1645
Anti-θ-treated spleen	Nil	12	
	DNP POL	509	
	TNP KLH	10	
	TNP KLH – Sepharose	315	
	SRC		125
Macrophage-depleted	Nil	0	
	DNP POL	358	
	TNP KLH	0	
	TNP KLH – Sepharose	215	
	SRC		42

[a] TNP KLH (0.1 μg/ml), Sepharose equivalent number of unconjugated beads corresponding to b.
[b] Optimal number of TNP KLH-conjugated beads.

T independent, inducing antibody responses in thymectomized and nude mice. These complexes are large aggregates, and it has not been possible to convincingly show M independence in the primary response, although this is possible in the secondary response. The reasons for this difference are not yet clear. In contrast, FγG and FγG–SRC are T- and M-dependent antigens in cultures of spleen cells from primed or unprimed mice (Schrader and Feldmann, 1973a).

B. Mitogens

Isolated populations of T cells, but not B cells, are triggered by PHA and Con A (reviewed by Greaves and Janossy, 1972; Andersson et al., 1972). By altering the physical form of these mitogens, Greaves and Bauminger (1972) and Andersson et al. (1972) demonstrated that these mitogens, if surface-bound to either Sepharose beads or to plastic dishes, were capable of triggering B cells as efficiently as intrinsic B cell mitogens, such as LPS. These observations form a remarkable parallel with those found with antigens, as detailed above. The similarities even extend to the requirement for the correct degree of conjugation for optimal triggering (Greaves, personal communication).

The marked analogies between the structural requirements for B cell triggering by two different "T cell mitogens," and also by antigens, emphasize the fundamental importance of repeating determinants in the process of B-cell induction.

A further example of the importance of polymerization for the triggering of B-cell transformation was provided by comparing the effectiveness of univalent (Fab') anti-rabbit Fab preparations with divalent $F(ab')_2$ preparations. Univalent anti-Fab did not stimulate until it was polymerized (Fanger, 1972). These results are in close agreement with those discussed above for other mitogens or antigens.

IV. A SPECIAL EXAMPLE OF THYMUS-INDEPENDENT ANTIGENS–ANTIGEN BOUND TO MACROPHAGES VIA IgT

In some ways this proposition is logically inconsistent. However, it does serve to provide an example of the penultimate stage of immunization of B cells, after the involvement of T cells. Antigen bound by IgT is capable of immunizing isolated B-cell suspensions, e.g., macrophage-depleted spleen cells of nude mice (Feldmann, 1972c). Thus analysis of the localization of the antigen on the macrophage should provide clues to the mechanism of triggering of B cells responding to T-dependent antigens.

Radiochemical and autoradiographic studies by Cone et al. (1974) have indicated that ^{125}I-labeled IgT, obtained from virgin thymocytes or ATC, binds efficiently to the surface of macrophages. The criteria for this conclusion were (a) trypsin sensitivity of binding of ^{125}I-IgT (which was performed at $4°C$)

confirming prior functional studies which indicated that the immunogenic antigen was surface bound (Feldmann, 1972c), (b) recovery of ^{125}I-IgT from the macrophage membrane, (c) autoradiographs indicating that most, but not all, macrophages which bound the ^{125}I-IgT were labeled at only one or a few surface patches.

These studies do not prove whether IgT—antigen binds to the macrophage membrane to form local matrices or binds uniformly across the whole surface. However, recent studies on the mechanism of antigenic competition in mice (or in cultures sequentially immunized with two IgT—antigen complexes) have suggested that local matrices of antigen are formed. The initial model studied was an antigenic competition induced by the injection of red cells in mice which had been immunized a few months earlier with a carrier protein (FγG or KLH). Several days later, antigenic competition was expressed *in vitro* or *in vivo*, as witnessed by the diminished response to the haptenated protein, e.g., DNP FγG. The cellular basis of the diminished response was studied. It was found that very small numbers of anti-θ and complement-treated peritoneal exudate cells circumvented the antigenic competition, as did trypsinization of the spleen cells prior to culture (Schrader and Feldmann, 1973b). These observations indicate that there was no irreversible cellular deficit in this form of antigenic competition and that the locus of inhibition was at the macrophage level. These experiments have one important corollary: they stress the importance of the macrophage surface in cooperative responses (to the competing red cell antigen) induced *in vivo* and support the concepts derived from *in vitro* experiments. Further analysis of this work indicated that supernatants from activated T cells may also induce antigenic competition (Table V). Furthermore, the active principle in the competition was Ig-like in nature and cytophillic for macrophages, thus resem-

Table V. Antigenic Competition with Helper Cell Products

Macrophages incubated with:	Antibody response	
	DNP	FγG
I. ATC$_{KLH}$ + DNP KLH	720	0
II. ATC$_{FγG}$ + FγG	0	470
III. I & II Separately	495	310
Together	55	75
Together and I	395	50

10^6 Macrophages incubated for 2 hr at 4°C with supernatants I or II, obtained from 2×10^6 ATC. The macrophages were washed and 10^5 or 3×10^5 were cultured with 1.5×10^7 DNP-POL-primed spleen cells for four days. (Data from Feldmann and Schrader, 1974)

Table VI. Ig Nature of Helper and Competitive Material from
ATC

Macrophages incubated with supernatants from:	Antibody response	
	DNP	FγG
I. ATC$_{FγG}$ & FγG	0	445
II. ATC$_{KLH}$ & DNP KLH	720	0
III. I and subsequently II	80	400
IV. I and II simultaneously	65	55
V. I incubated anti-Ig beads	0	0
VI. V and then II	375	0

10^6 Macrophages incubated for 2 hr at $4°C$ with supernatants I or II, obtained from 2×10^6 ATC. The macrophages were washed and 10^5 or 3×10^5 were cultured with 1.5×10^7 DNP-POL-primed spleen cells for four days. (Data from Feldmann and Schrader, 1974)

bling the specific helper material (Feldmann and Schrader, 1974). Table VI summarizes some of these results and indicates that ATC products which are allowed to bind to the macrophage surface first, while initiating the events which lead to a response to that antigen, concurrently block the response to another ATC supernatant reactive to another antigen. These results, together with others which demonstrate that the ATC supernatant, administered second is adsorbed by macrophages, but *not* in an immunogenic manner, *suggest* that lattices of antigenic determinants must be formed on the macrophage surface prior to immune induction (Feldmann and Schrader, 1974).

The antigenic competition experiments are of interest with respect to the mechanism of B-cell triggering in T-dependent antibody responses, both primary and secondary (IgM and IgG). They indicate that lattices *are* of importance in the generation of these responses. They do not, however, exclude a more active participation of macrophages in these responses, as suggested by Waldmann and Munro (1973) and Schrader (1973a). These workers have suggested that macrophages produce factors which may facilitate the triggering of at least some B cells. Clearly, since macrophages do not seem to be required for the IgM responses to POL, DNP POL, DNP LE, DNP SIII, TNP KLH–Sepharose, and soluble SRC antigen, macrophage products are *not essential* for triggering of all B cells reactive to these antigens. The effect of IgT purified from the θ positive cultured lymphoma cell lines, El4 and WEHI 22 in augmenting IgG response *in vitro* (Feldmann, Boylston, and Hogg, 1974) is consistent with the concept of macrophage-released factors influencing B-cell immunization.

V. CAN NONPOLYMERIC ANTIGENS INDUCE B-CELL RESPONSES?

Many laboratories have reported failures in inducing primary *in vitro* responses to nonpolymeric antigens, such as FγG, BSA, and DNP HGG. In contrast, polymers containing the same antigenic determinants are immunogenic *in vitro* (e.g., DNP POL, DNP LE, DNP red cells, FγG POL). This is one of the observations which prompted the postulate that polymerization of antigenic determinants (or lattice formation) was an essential step in B-cell induction (prior observations discussed by Mitchison, 1971a). However, the induction of responses with nonpolymeric antigens, if demonstrated under some experimental circumstances, merely suggest that the requirement for polymerization may be bypassed or mimicked in these circumstances. Several investigators have obtained results which they have interpreted as triggering with nonpolymeric antigens.

(a) *Ultracentrifuged FγG.* It has been reported that high concentrations of ultracentrifuged FγG may, in the presence of high concentrations of POL, induce a response to FγG in spleen cells from nude mice (Schrader, 1972b). While this antigen is not a polymer, it is certainly *not monovalent.* Chicken globulin also has a tendency to aggregate, and may bind to lymphocytes or macrophages via Fc receptors. Hence, it will be difficult to ever conclusively prove that it interacts with FγG-reactive B cells in a nonpolymeric form. Furthermore, spleen cells from nude mice do *not* behave *in vitro* in the same way as B cells from other mice (Wagner, 1972).

Even if FγG *does* react with B cells in a nonpolymeric manner, other considerations cast some doubt upon the relevance of the conclusion based on this form of triggering to other antibody responses. The doses of FγG and POL required are very high, of the order of 10 μg POL/ml and 100 μg FγG/ml. Since the concentrations of POL used (10 or 100 μg/ml) induce POL *tolerance* in flagellin-reactive B cells, the mechanism by which POL facilitates a response of FγG cannot be the same as that by which POL immunizes flagellin-reactive B cells. Furthermore, macrophages seem to be essential for this POL-mediated FγG response (Schrader, personal communication) whereas they are not essential for a response to POL itself (Diener *et al.,* 1970; Shortman *et al.,* 1971). Thus, it could be argued that in these experiments the step at which polymeric antigens were required is being replaced or *bypassed* by a factor produced by a cell, presumably a macrophage, in response to POL.

(b) *DNP amino acids in the presence of mixed lymphocyte reaction (MLR) supernatants or cyclic GMP.* It has been reported that DNP lysine may induce anti-DNP responses in the presence of MLR supernatants (see Dennert and Lennox, 1973; Watson, unpublished) or the appropriate concentrations of cyclic GMP (Watson and Cohn, personal communication). These experiments have been interpreted to suggest that triggering of B cells may occur with antigens which interact with B cells in a monomeric way. However, these interpretations are open to doubt due to the same arguments advanced with FγG (above). DNP lysine aggregates at high concentrations or may bind to various molecules, e.g., albumin or cell surfaces. It is not possible to categorically argue that these components react with the cell surface in a monovalent manner. Furthermore, it is obviously not possible to extrapolate from these findings that this sort of factor acts under other experimental conditions.

Nevertheless, these observations are of interest, and perhaps the value of studying such "bypass factors" is that they may shed some insight into the mechanism by which membrane-receptor—antigen interactions are translated by an antigen-reactive B cell to initiate the biochemical events of antigen-induced differentiation. It is perhaps *not* a coincidence, that in the presence of POL, FγG remains on the B-cell surface for long periods (Schrader, 1974a) just as DNP Fla does (Wilson and Feldmann, 1972).

(c) *Highly conjugated hapten conjugates.* Aird (1971) reported that heavily conjugated NIP conjugates of BSA in mice were relatively T independent. On this basis, she concluded that intrinsically high conjugates may bind well enough to B cells to stimulate them. These experiments, performed *in vivo*, do not, however, establish that nonpolymeric antigens are involved in T-independent triggering. Heavily coupled NIP proteins are almost universally aggregated and tend to persist in mice for long periods of time (Mitchell, Klaus, and Kontiainen, personal communication). Thus, the exact manner of binding to B cells (polymeric or nonpolymeric) cannot be ascertained. Furthermore, heavily conjugated NIP or DNP conjugates are by no means universally T independent, as the reverse has usually been found *in vivo* (Kontiainen and G. Möller, personal communication) and *in vitro* (Feldmann, unpublished). In view of accruing evidence for the heterogeneity of B cells (see below) it is possible that the population of B cells triggered by the nonpolymeric reagents is different to the one triggered by polymers. Regardless of whether nonpolymers trigger B cells, the conclusion cannot be avoided that some B cells are triggered in a highly preferential way by the large polymers described above.

The above discussion on whether nonpolymeric antigens may directly trigger B-cell responses raises the question of what is a polymeric antigen? How long (or large) does it have to be? This question is not trivial, since it may elucidate the extent of crosslinking of receptors necessary for triggering to occur. Furthermore, these studies (currently in progress) may elucidate some differences between the requirements for B-cell triggering and tolerance induction.

VI. RELATIONSHIP OF B-CELL DIFFERENTIATION TO INDUCTION

It has been proposed that there are B-cell subpopulations which may differ in their mechanism of triggering. For example, Playfair and Purves (1972) postulated on the basis of their *in vivo* results that bone marrow contains a cell, termed B_1 which responds to SRC in the absence of thymus cells, whereas the spleen contains B_2 cells which require cooperation. These results remain to be confirmed. In contrast, Gorczynski (1973) has found that B cells purified from marrow responded to SRC only if *both* T-cell-dependent nonspecific factors and *specific T cells* were present. However, the concept of "T-independent B cells"

(B_1) and "T-dependent B cells" (B_2) has been experimentally clarified by Gorczynski and Feldmann (1974), who found that these two populations of cells from the spleen were separable by physical means (velocity sedimentation). Shortman *et al.* (1971) and Schrader (1974b) have suggested that there may be two subpopulations of B cells in spleen differing in adherence properties with "primed" B cells being less adherent to glass than virgin cells. Thus, the possibility remains that B cells at different stages in their differentiation, since they possess different receptors (discussed in Greaves *et al.*, 1973), may have somewhat different metabolic and/or antigenic requirements for induction into antibody-forming cells or tolerance and that conclusions reached with any one antigen and a single type of B cell may not be universally applicable.

VII. RELATIONSHIP OF EPITOPE DENSITY TO THE INDUCTION OF IMMUNITY AND TOLERANCE

During studies with DNP POL as an immunogen *in vitro*, it was noted that the immunogenicity of different batches varied and that immunogenicity correlated with the degree of DNP conjugation. It was found that high conjugates (> 3/40,000 daltons) were poorly immunogenic or nonimmunogenic, regardless of antigen dose over a wide dose range, whereas low conjugates (< 0.3/40,000 daltons) were suboptimally immunogenic. These results are summarized in Fig.

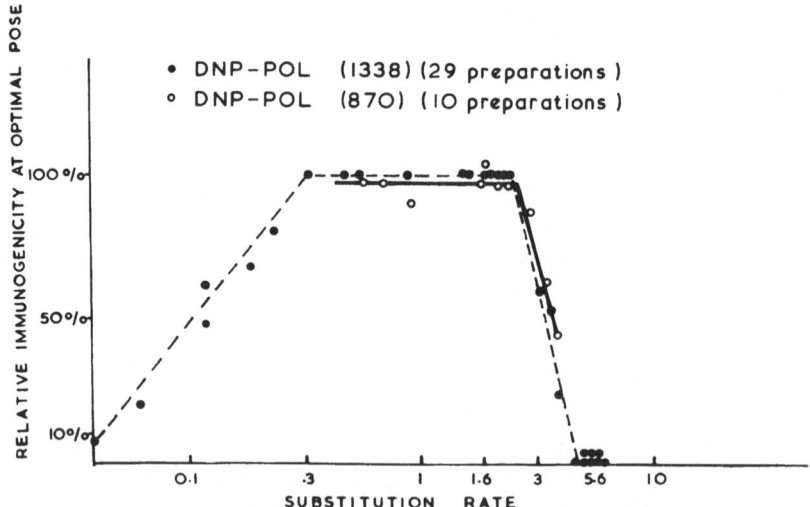

Figure 3. The effect of DNP substitution on the anti-DNP response elicited by DNP POL *in vitro*. Summary of data with all the batches of DNP POL prepared. DNP flagella (14 batches) behave in a similar fashion. The data is only plotted until 6 groups/mole because of depolymerization. (Reproduced from Feldmann, 1972d, *J. Exp. Med.* **135**: 735)

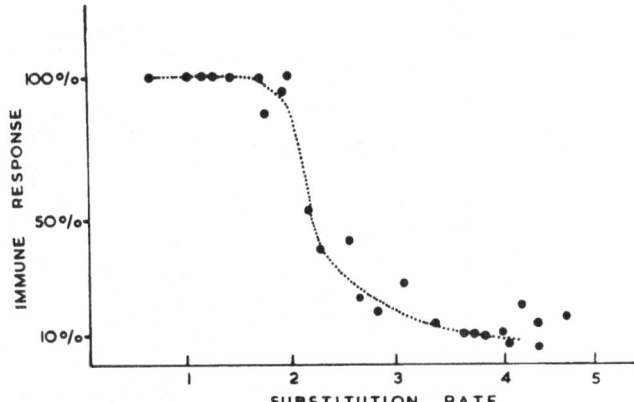

Figure 4. The pooled results of the effect of DNP conjugation rate on the capacity to induce immunological tolerance *in vitro*. Each point represents the average residual anti-DNP response obtained in various experiments in which normal spleen cells were treated with 100 μg/ml of $DNP_{3.8}$ POL *in vitro*. (Reproduced from Feldmann, 1972d, *J. Exp. Med.* **135**: 735)

3. An inverse correlation was found with the capacity to induce B-cell tolerance *in vitro*. High conjugates were tolerogenic (> 3), whereas low conjugates were not (< 2), as summarized in Fig. 4.

Many possible explanations for the nonimmunogenicity of high DNP POL conjugates may be proposed. For example, high conjugates may have become depolymerized into the monomeric form which is a T-dependent antigen (Feldmann and Basten, 1971). Evidence against this explanation was obtained both by electron microscopy and by centrifugation analysis (Feldmann, 1972d). Alternatively it may be suggested that the conjugation may so alter its properties, i.e., charge, that it no longer binds effectively to B cells. However, since DNP_3 dansyl$_1$ POL induces responses to dansyl, but not to DNP (Feldmann, 1972d), its structure cannot be too grossly altered. This experiment also emphasizes the *specificity* of the epitope density phenomenon. In a similar way, DNP_3 POL at low doses induces responses (admittedly not normal) to the flagellin determinants but not to the DNP (unpublished data).

Since none of the above possible reasons for nonimmunogenicity of high conjugates appears to be valid, nonimmunogenicity is almost certainly based on the tolerance-inducing properties of these compounds. Attempts to reproduce the phenomenon with other T-independent antigens are in progress. For example, the immunogenicity of TNP KLH—sepharose depends on the degree of conjugation (Feldmann *et al.*, 1974), as does DNP LE, DNP SIII, DNP dextran,

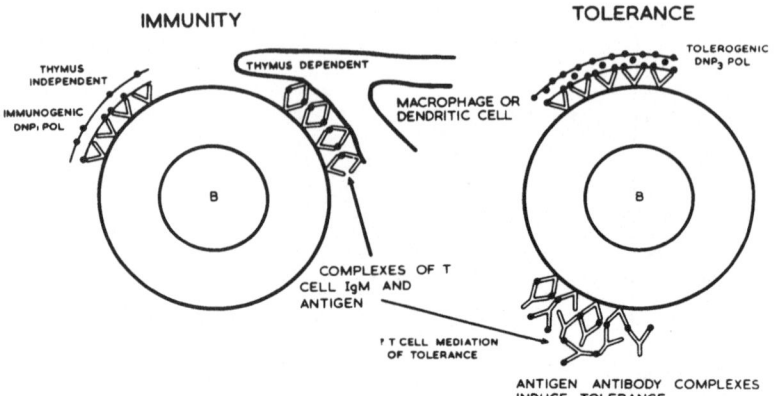

Figure 5. Representation of the mechanism of B-cell signal discrimination, based
on the epitope density and competitive inhibition data obtained using DNP POL.
Note that the lattice of DNP determinants on immunogenic DNP POL may
resemble the lattice of T-cell IgM—antigen bound on the macrophage surface, as
occurs in T-dependent responses. Similarly, the surface of antigenic determinants
on tolerogenic DNP_3 POL resembles that which may be formed by complexes of
antibody and antigen. T cells also mediate tolerance by the release of complexes
of T-cell monomeric IgM and antigen. (Reproduced from Feldmann, 1972e, *J.
Exp. Med.* **136**: 532).

and DNP D-GL (Desaymard and Feldmann, 1974), confirming the results obtained with DNP POL.

    With mitogens, Greaves and Bauminger (personal communication) have also
found that the degree of PHA conjugation of sepharose was of signal importance
in establishing its mitogenic properties for B cells.

    The effect of epitope density on the induction of B-cell tolerance has also
been noted in a variety of systems. Highly conjugated DNP D-GL, i.e., 37
DNP/110,000 mol. wt., produces B-cell tolerance (Katz *et al.,* 1972) in close
analogy to DNP POL. Borel (1971) has found that DNP mouse IgG induces
B-cell tolerance. Subsequent studies have revealed some interesting aspects of
this form of tolerance. Firstly, the degree of DNP conjugation was critical; with
insufficient DNP, tolerance did not occur. Furthermore, the class of the IgG
injected was of importance. IgG_1 and IgG_{2a} myelomas were especially tolerogenic, while IgG_{2b} was not. Since IgG_1 and IgG_{2a} are cytophilic in the mouse
(Herzenberg *et al.,* 1968; Basten *et al.,* 1972; Greaves *et al.,* 1973), these results
suggest that matrix formation on a cell surface of a sufficient epitope density
may also be of importance in the induction of tolerance in this system. It should
be pointed out that the *in vivo* half lives of the DNP myelomas have been
studied, and differences in this respect cannot explain these results.

    The induction of tolerance in B cells with antigen—antibody complexes
(Diener and Feldmann, 1972a) may also be interpreted in terms of epitope
density. Complexes of antigen and antibody may enable determinants to be

more closely clustered than with free antigen. Some evidence that this explanation may be partly true comes from the fact that preliminary experiments indicated that it is *not* possible to induce antibody-mediated tolerance with very lightly conjugated hapten protein conjugates (Feldmann, unpublished data). A contributory factor to the tolerance induced with antigen—antibody complexes would also be the greater total binding and the increased stability of binding to the B-cell surface, as suggested by Diener and Feldmann (1970), on the basis that antibody converted monomeric antigens (which by themselves were incapable of inducing B-cell tolerance) into polymer-like complexes which were tolerogenic. The relative contribution of these influences cannot be ascertained until the stability (e.g., reversibility by trypsinization or other means) of antibody-mediated tolerance is compared with that of other tolerance-inducing regimes.

An analogous situation to tolerance induction by antigen—antibody complexes has recently been described with complexes of antigen and IgT under a number of conditions (Feldmann, 1973, 1974). Tolerance occurred in the absence of adherent cells (including macrophages), in the presence of antimouse macrophage serum, or with supraimmunogenic doses of activated T-cell supernatants. Since these supernatants contain complexes of antigen with a presumably divalent antibody (IgT), the mechanism may be similar to antibody-mediated tolerance with humoral antibody. Some of these essential features of specific T-cell suppression are summarized in Table VII.

Table VII. Summary of Specific T-Cell Suppression

Source of suppressor material

Thymocytes	(Tada and Okamura, 1973)
ATC	(Feldman, 1973)
Primed T cells	(Waldmann and Munro, 1974)

Nature of suppressor

Thymocyte extract	(Tada and Okamura, 1973)
IgT—antigen complex	(Feldmann, 1974)

Target

T or B cells	(Feldmann, 1974)

Mechanism
? Antibody-mediated tolerance
Specific suppressive factor

Significance
Unknown (A) Likely role in regulation of immune response,
        preventing overrecruitment of cells
    (B) Possible role in induction of tolerance
        (Gershon and Kondo, 1971)

The degree of conjugation needed for the induction of tolerance with DNP POL was 3/MON unit. This contrasts with the fact that each unit of MON, which is a single polypeptide chain, could have only one determinant of any given specificity. Two reasons may contribute to this difference. Firstly, many DNP groups chemically coupled may not be accessible to DNP-specific receptors, e.g., if they lie in the same plane as the protein. Secondly, if there must be at least one DNP group/MON for a given length of POL, the average conjugation ratio must be greater than one.

Thus, the phenomenon of epitope density in the induction of immunity and tolerance seems to be of importance in a variety of circumstances, although current data do not permit generalizations for all B cells or exact conclusions about the *spacing* of determinants for the induction of immunity or tolerance. For these answers, more chemically defined, possibly synthetic, polymers may be necessary.

VIII. DISCUSSION

From the above data two major points emerge for discussion. One is the mechanism by which polymers stimulate B cells. The second is how the density of antigenic determinants on a polymer dictates the mechanism of "signal discrimination" between immunity and tolerance in B cells.

A. How do Polymers with Repeating Determinants Stimulate B Cells?

The first point to establish is whether the experiments with T cell and macrophage depletion permit the conclusion that *direct* B-cell triggering can occur. A consideration of the total evidence permits this conclusion, although each of the points taken individually is not sufficient to establish this as fact.

(a) *T depletion,* even by two or three *concurrent* means does not diminish the IgM response to T-independent antigens, such as DNP POL (see above). The depletion techniques used were adult thymectomy, lethal irradiation and bone marrow replacement (ATXBM), chronic thoracic duct drainage, and treatment with anti-θ serum and complement (Feldmann and Basten, 1971), or the use of spleen cells from genetically "athymic" nude mice, treated with anti-θ and complement (Feldmann et al., 1972).

(b) *Carrier independence.* Large doses of unconjugated POL, e.g., 100 μg/ml, do not inhibit the *primary or secondary* responses *in vitro* to DNP POL in either T-containing or T-depleted spleen cell populations (Feldmann, 1972b). In contrast, the response to DNP MON, which is T dependent, and is also carrier dependent, was abolished. It should be stressed that POL *readily* induces tolerance in flagellin-reactive T cells (Feldmann and Nossal, 1972) within a few hours at doses of 1 μg/ml or greater, and thus even if sufficient T cells, after T depletion, remain to "help" a response to DNP POL (but not to DNP MON), they will be rendered tolerant by high concentrations of POL. The same general argument applies to the polymeric T-cell mitogens—activation of B cells with PHA—Sepharose is unlikely to involve T cells, because spleen cells from ATXBM mice respond so much better to bound PHA than to soluble PHA. In contrast, T cells respond much less to the surface-bound PHA (Greaves and Bauminger, 1972).

(c) *Macrophage independence.* Macrophages are not only essential for the stimulation of B cells with IgT—antigen (Feldmann, 1972c; Feldmann and Nossal, 1972), but if they are *diminished* in number, B-cell tolerance occurs (Feldmann, 1973). Because of this, it is difficult to envisage how T cells could cooperate in a response to, say, DNP POL in the absence of macrophages, such as occurs with macrophage-depleted, T-depleted lymphocytes ·from nude mice (Feldmann and Basten, 1972; Schrader, personal communication).

Cohn (1972) has pointed out that point (a) above does not permit a *definite* conclusion of "T independence." However, he has not assessed the remainder of the evidence for direct triggering of B cells; namely, the carrier independence, M independence, the capacity of IgT—antigen to induce T-cell tolerance in the absence of macrophages, and the capacity of these polymers to readily induce T-cell tolerance. It is thus simply not possible to be certain, as Cohn is in "Genetic Control of Immune Responsiveness," p. 424, 1972, that polymeric T-independent antigens as such merely require *less* "associative antibody" (Cohn's terminology for IgT) than do other antigens. In view of the fact that excess carrier (see Feldmann, 1972a) should preferentially bind (and functionally inactivate the associative antibody), that excess carrier can be shown to induce T-cell tolerance (Feldmann and Nossal, 1972), and that IgT—antigen complexes in the presence of reduced numbers of macrophages actually induce *B-cell tolerance* (Feldmann, 1973), it seems possible to conclude that direct triggering of the B-cell populations studied by polymeric antigens can occur. Furthermore, since B cells may be triggered by polymeric mitogens such as PHA or Con A (Greaves and Bauminger, 1972; Andersson et·al., 1972a), which in their monomeric form do not trigger B cells, and by divalent anti-Fab antisera (Fanger, 1972), it seems reasonable to conclude that direct triggering of B cells by polymeric reagents seems to be a *general property of B cells.* *

However, the mechanism by which these polymers trigger B cells is not yet known in detail. The consequences of binding of a polymeric reagent with B cells are predictable. Binding occurs via several Ig receptors which become agglutinated into patches and then migrate to form a "cap" (Wilson and Feldmann, 1972; Taylor *et al.,* 1971; Raff *et al.,* 1973). In contrast "monomeric" reagents bind only via a single receptor, only remain on the cell surface for short periods of time (Wilson and Feldmann, 1972), and do not agglutinate receptors or form caps (Taylor *et al.,* 1971). Diener and Paetkau (1972) reported that after a cycle of capping and the subsequent loss of receptors and antigen

---

* This conclusion seems valid for most B cells, but may not be true for all B cell subpopulations or differentiation stages.

from the cell surface (they considered shedding as a more likely mechanism of loss of receptor–antigen complexes than endocytosis), receptors were regenerated within 6 hours and within 24 hours were present in increased numbers. With tolerogenic concentrations of POL, capping did *not* reoccur, but with immunogenic concentrations, there were further cycles of capping. Whether the details of this sequence is applicable to all polymeric antigens, is not known, although capping occurs with cells bound to surfaces (Kiefer, 1973). Other consequences of the binding of polymers to surfaces may be of importance in the mechanism of triggering. For example, the increased stability and duration of binding to the cell surface (Wilson and Feldmann, 1972) and the increased avidity of the cell for the antigen, resulting in greater total binding at $37°C$, may be of importance for triggering. The increased binding energy of combined receptors for the antigen may be of importance. Cross-linking of receptors by these polymers has been previously postulated by Diener and Feldmann (1970), Mitchison (1971a), and Feldmann and Nossal (1972) to be of importance in B-cell triggering. At present it is only possible to speculate how cross-linking of receptors (Ig or lectin receptors) by polymeric reagents activates B cells. It does *not* seem likely that any mere form of cross-linking of receptors is sufficient, since in the mouse, anti-Ig, which cross-links receptors, does *not* usually activate B cells, but in contrast often suppresses responsiveness (Lesley and Dutton, 1970; Feldmann and Diener, 1971b; Katz and Unanue, 1973), and there is no correlation between capping and triggering (discussed in Greaves *et al.*, 1973). It seems likely that combination with the Fab fragment of an Ig receptor is also required for antigen-induced triggering, which with polymeric antigens would obviously happen. This *suggests* that an allosteric signal may be transmitted via the Fe segment of the receptor Ig as proposed on theoretical grounds by Bretscher and Cohn (1968). By analogy with the work on complement fixation (Hyslop *et al.*, 1971), and as suggested by hapten-inhibition studies (Feldmann, 1972e), combination with *both* Fab segments of the receptor Ig may be necessary for the generation of an allosteric conformational change which participates in the initiation of triggering. The findings that only bivalent anti-Fab stimulates rabbit B cells (Fanger, 1972) and that anti-Fab, but not anti-hinge region or anti-Fc, stimulates increased receptor density (Diener and Pernis, 1973) are also consistent with the notion of a conformationally induced allosteric signal as a consequence of binding in the Fab region, probably involving both Fab's of a receptor Ig.

Klinman (1972) and Wilson and Feldmann (1972) have suggested that another consequence of the binding of polymeric reagents to the B-cell surface may also be of importance, namely, the stabilization of antigen binding. The rapid turnover of membrane Ig by shedding (Wilson *et al.*, 1972; Cone *et al.*, 1971, and by endocytosis (Taylor *et al.*, 1971), would not permit antigen–receptor interactions by a nonmultivalent antigen at a single receptor from triggering cells. Thus, a *surface* of determinants, which "anchor" receptors in the membrane and which prevent the above two forms of clearance of antigen from the cell membrane, may facilitate triggering. In keeping with this notion, Schrader (1973a) has found suggestive evidence that some macrophage-derived factors which augment responses appear to increase the persistence of antigen on the cell membrane.

Other theories have been proposed to explain some aspects of the direct triggering of B cells. Sela (1973), noting that polymeric synthetic polypeptides made up of D amino acids were T independent, whereas those made up of L amino acids were T dependent, suggested that T independence was linked to the incapacity to degrade these antigens. This idea is not at variance with the above concepts, because lack of degradation would lead to antigen persistence, and hence to the capacity to bind in a polymeric manner with the B-cell surface. However, antigen persistence is not the only factor in T independence, as *in vitro* essentially all antigens persist but many are T dependent. Polymeric flagellin is rapidly degraded *in vivo* (Shellam, 1970) and some D amino acids are not T independent (Roelants and Goodman, 1970). Mitchell *et al.* (1973) have also proposed a version of this antigen-persistence concept of T independence.

Dukor and Hartmann and their colleagues (1973) have suggested that T-independent antigens may be such, because, since they activate the complement bypass pathway, C3b will be generated and may bind to the C3 receptors on B cells. Binding to the C3 receptor was envisaged as a "signal" which activates B cells. Although some evidence in keeping with this concept is being generated, in that Sepharose-bound cobra-venom factor augments SRC responses *in vitro* (Dukor *et al.*, 1974), evidence against the *general validity* of this mechanism for the triggering of B cells in response to all T-independent antigens is also accruing. For example, Pepys has shown in mice that C3 depletion by purified cobra-venom factor or anti-C3 antibody does *not* diminish responses to two T-independent antigens (SIII and PVP), one of which, PVP, does not activate the complement bypass system (Pepys, 1972; Pepys, personal communication). *In vitro*, purified anti-C3 antibody suppresses T-dependent anti-DNP responses (DNP KLH) but not T-independent responses to DNP POL (Feldmann and Pepys, 1974). At this moment, it is too early to critically evaluate the role of C3 in lymphocyte triggering.

Coutinho and Möller (1973) have suggested that T-independent antigens may behave as such *because* they are also B-cell mitogens. They found that, in serum-free medium, at high concentrations ($200-1000 \mu g/ml$), essentially all the various polymeric T-independent antigens reported in the literature (e.g., SIII, POL, LE, Dextran, PVP) were B-cell mitogens. Coutinho and Möller also found that NNP-conjugated LPS was thymus-independent at low doses. While the latter studies were interpreted as demonstrating the role of "mitogens" in T-independent B-cell triggering, their relevance to the mechanism of B-cell triggering is not entirely clear. An interpretation in terms of binding of repeating determinants seems just as plausible. Coutinho and Möller (1973, personal communication) found that NNP–LPS reacted with B cells via NNP-specific receptors, since NNP-caproic acid blocked the response. Hence, there is no evidence that at low doses (approximately 10^{-2}–10^{-3} μg/ml) NNP–LPS reacted with B cells in the manner that induces mitogenicity, i.e., via mitogenic receptors.

This argument is supported by two lines of experimental evidence. First, Möller et al. (1972) have estimated the number of mitogen receptors on T and B cells and the number of mitogen molecules which need to be bound in order to activate lymphocytes. For surface-bound Con A, this was 10^5–10^6 molecules per cell, corresponding to 3–10% of the available receptors. For LPS, the number of molecules bound was less (not calculated by the authors), but at the optimally stimulating doses ($\sim 10^2$ μg/ml) about 2–10% of the available receptors ($\sim 10^6$/cell) were bound. Since all T and B cells have equal numbers of receptors for LPS, and a large proportion have to be bound for stimulation, it is very unlikely that NNP–LPS which was immunogenic at low concentrations ($\sim 10^{-3}$ μg/ml) would be present at high enough concentration, even on NNP-specific cells, and in a form free to react with enough mitogenic receptors, to activate the cell in that manner. It should be remembered, also, that most of the NNP–LPS would bind to other cells, all of which have receptors for LPS and, since LPS is polymeric, it would bind avidly to these cells, since multiple bonds would form.

Secondly, with POL, even at 26–30 μg/ml, Diener and Paetkau (1972) and Raff et al. (1973) have demonstrated that antigen is only detectable on a small proportion of cells and that on these cells the antigen forms caps concurrent with surface immunoglobulin. Thus there is as yet no evidence that T-independent antigens at immunologically relevant doses react significantly with "mitogenic" receptors of B cells. Furthermore, the doses of these antigens which were mitogenic were concentrations at which these compounds induce *tolerance*, and not immunity, in the corresponding specific B cells (Britton, 1969; Diener and Armstrong, 1969; Howard, personal communication). Alternatively, it could be argued that the mitogenic responses, observed by Coutinho and Möller, to very large doses of T-independent antigen may have been due to products of macrophages; Gery et al. (1972) and Gery and Waksman (1972) showed that macrophages incubated with LPS produce a "lymphocyte-activating factor" which augmented, and also stimulated, responses in thymocytes. Since macrophages are not essential for triggering with POL, DNP POL, soluble SRC antigen, or TNP KLH sepharose, an indirect mechanism of this kind must be ruled out before it can be assumed that mitogenicity may be of relevance to T independence. In my opinion, the interesting conclusion from this line of work, rather than implying a critical role for mitogenicity in T-independent triggering, is that it provides further evidence for the concept that cross-linking of *any* surface structure on B cells is a stimulus for triggering. In this case, cross-linking caused by high concentrations of polymeric T-independent antigens resulted in DNA synthesis, in the manner previously described for PHA Sepharose and Con A–plastic (see above). This conclusion is also supported by some of the newer data on the "artificial" production of T-independent antigens–by sonication from SRC into smaller membrane fragments (Table I), and also by conjugation of TNP KLH onto Sepharose (Table IV) or NIP directly onto Sepharose (M. Virolainen, personal communication). The concept of "mitogenicity" fails to explain the epitope density effects described above. Furthermore, no evidence of mitogenicity has been found with some T-independent antigens, such as DNP-Ficoll (Mosier, personal communication) or TNP-acrylamide (Parker, personal communication). Clearly, further work is needed to establish or refute this hypothesis.

B. Discrimination Between Immunization and Tolerance Induction of B Cells

A striking feature of the above data review is that the compounds which readily induce B-cell tolerance are the same or closely resemble those which also directly immunize B cells.

Some polymeric natural antigens can both induce or tolerize, e.g., POL, SIII, LE. Synthetic or conjugated antigens may only do one, e.g., DNP POL, DNP SIII, DNP LE, or TNP KLH-Sepharose, depending on the degree of hapten conjugation.

In order to evaluate the mechanisms which distinguish between immunity and tolerance, it is necessary to briefly recapitulate our knowledge of the factors which influence B-cell signal discrimination in mature B cells.

(a) *Antigen dose*. POL, for example, immunizes *in vitro* at less than 1 μg/ml and tolerizes at greater concentrations (rapidly at greater than 30 μg/ml) (Diener and Armstrong, 1969). Similar considerations also apply to other antigens.

(b) Presence of *antibody* in low doses. This is the phenomenon of "antibody-mediated tolerance" (reviewed by Diener and Feldmann, 1972a), in which low concentrations of antibody facilitate the induction of B-cell tolerance, with immunogenic (or subimmunogenic) doses of antigen.

(c) Chemical characteristics. A high degree of hapten conjugation causes DNP POL to act as a tolerogen, never as an antigen. This phenomenon is *hapten-specific*, since $DNP_3 POL$ induces tolerance to DNP, but not to POL, and $DNP_3 dansyl_1 POL$ causes tolerance to DNP but immunizes for dansyl. Analogous results have been found with DNP SIII by Mitchell *et al.* (1973). Conversely, a low degree of conjugation results in compounds unable to induce tolerance, even in very high doses (Feldmann, 1972d). This "epitope density" phenomenon has recently been confirmed using TNP-coated Sepharose or acrylamide beads (Feldmann, *et al.*, 1974) and also with DNP LE, DNP SIII, DNP dextran, and DNP-D-GL (Desaymard and Feldmann, 1974).

(d) Certain agents, e.g., LPS mitogens, may prevent tolerance induction *in vivo* (Golub and Weigle, 1966; Chiller and Weigle, 1973). These experiments are of importance, as they suggest that factors apart from antigen may influence the decision between immunity and tolerance.

(e) Cells at an early stage of differentiation may be paralyzable but not inducible, as proposed by Lederberg (1959). Nossal and his colleagues (personal communication) have some results which support this concept of "clonal abortion." This phenomenon has obvious relevance to tolerance with self antigens. However, these experiments do not clarify the events which discriminate between these two states in mature B cells, which may be *both* induced and paralyzed.

These considerations led to the concept that the *amount* of antigen bound to the surface was of importance, as was the *density* of antigen–receptor interactions in a certain region (Feldmann, 1972d; Diener and Feldmann, 1972a; Feldmann and Nossal, 1972, discussed also by Cooper, 1973). This concept, which basically only summarizes the results, does not imply that we understand the detailed mechanism by which tolerance, rather than immunity, is mediated. Several possibilities may be suggested. For example, a high density of bonds/unit may deform the membrane, leading to permeability changes. Second messengers, such as cyclic AMP, may be involved (Watson *et al.*, 1973). Alternatively, as suggested by Howard (Basten and Howard, 1973), cells coated with a lot of antigen may be phagocytosed. However, it is difficult to understand how macrophages distinguish between B cells coated with tolerogenic doses and those coated with immunogenic doses of antigen in the absence of an active B-cell contribution. Muller-Eberhard and his colleagues (personal communication) have found that a Burkitt tumor cell line, "Raji," has C3 receptors of very high affinity. Binding of C3b to these receptors initiates (in the presence of the later complement components) the killing of these cells. It is thus possible that C3 activation and binding of C3b to B cells may be a tolerance signal, rather than an immunity signal as proposed by Dukor and Hartmann (see Section VIII, A above). The high doses of polymeric antigens needed to activate the complement bypass pathway are consistent with this notion.

However, as Cooper (1973) has pointed out in a recent review, there are too many gaps in our knowledge of tolerance to these various antigens to generalize about *the* mechanism of tolerance, or about whether different pathways may be used with different antigens, or different subpopulation, of cells. It may be that there is a common pathway of tolerance induction at the cellular level, which may for various reasons take different times to become fully expressed. With some antigens, e.g., LPS (Sjöberg, 1972) and SIII (Howard, 1972), the complete pathway to irreversible tolerance does not occur, and tolerance is readily reversed on transfer. With others, e.g., DNP D-GL or POL, tolerance is not reversible upon transfer (Katz *et al.*, 1972; Diener and Feldmann, 1972b), but may be if the cells are trypsinized soon enough. Some factors which may modify the rate of irreversible tolerance induction include heterogeneity of affinity of B-cell receptors, antigens which bind poorly to cells such as those which are hydrophilic or of the same charge as the cell surface (e.g., SIII), the avidity of antigen for the cell surface, which would be related to size, repeating determinants, and epitope density, and adjuvant properties of the antigen (e.g., mitogenicity of LPS).

These considerations emphasize that our knowledge of both immunization and tolerance induction is, at best, rudimentary. The marked resemblances between the conditions for induction and paralysis of B cells emphasize that both problems must be understood together, and indicate that all current theories are approximations. The above discussions have been restricted to B cells, for which data are available. Since there are far fewer data concerning the mechanism of signal discrimination in T cells, an analogous discussion could only be completely speculative. Because there are many differences between T-cell and B-cell recognition and responses to antigen (reviewed by Mitchison, 1971b; McDevitt and Landy, 1972; Greaves *et al.*, 1973) and because of the expression of T-cell function in various competing pathways (Parish, 1972), e.g., cooperation and cell-mediated immunity, it seems very likely that discrimination between immunity and tolerance in T and B cells differs. Thus it is necessary to clearly differentiate between the mechanism of signal discrimination in each of these cell types, a point which tends to be neglected in theoretical discussions of this subject.

IX.   ABBREVIATIONS

ATC	activated thymus cells
ATXBM	adult thymectomized, lethally irradiated, and bone-marrow-injected mice
BSA	bovine serum albumin
Con A	concanavalin A
dansyl	5-(dimethylamino)-1-naphthalenesulfonyl hapten
DNP FγG	DNP fowl gamma globulin
DNP MON	DNP monomeric flagellin
DNP POL	DNP polymeric flagellin
DNP D-GL	dinitrophenylated copolymer of D glutamic acid and lysine
DNP HGG	DNP human gamma globulin
FγG–POL	fowl gamma globulin linked to POL
Ig	immunoglobulin
IgT	immunoglobulin released by T cells
KLH	keyhole limpet hemocyanin
LE	levan
LPS	lipopolysaccharide (endotoxin)
MLR	Mixed lymphocyte reaction
MON	monomeric flagellin This is the subunit (mol. wt. = 40,000) of POL (mol. wt. varies greatly, tends to average about ≃ 300 × MON)

NNP	4-hydroxy-3, 5-dinitrophenyl hapten
PHA	phytohemagglutinin
POL	polymeric flagellin
PVP	polyvinyl pyrrolidone
SRC	sheep red cells
SIII	pneumococcal polysaccharide type III
DNP KLH	dinitrophenylated keyhole limpet hemocyanin
TNP KLH	trinitrophenylated keyhole limpet hemocyanin
TNP KLH– Sepharose	TNP KLH conjugated (covalently) to Sepharose

Cells: B	bursa-equivalent-derived lymphocytes
T	thymus-derived lymphocytes
M	macrophages or equivalent cells

REFERENCES

Aird, J., 1971, *Immunology* **20**: 617.
Andersson, B., and Blomgren, H., 1971, *Cell. Immunol.* **2**: 411.
Andersson, J., Edelman, G.M., Möller, G., and Sjöberg, O., 1972, *Eur. J. Immunol.* **2**: 233.
Basten, A., and Howard, J.G., 1973, In Davies, A.J.S. and Carter, R.L. (eds.) *Contemporary Topics in Immunobiology*, Vol. 2, Plenum Press, New York-London, p. 265.
Basten, A., Miller, J.F.A.P., Sprent, J., and Pye, J., 1972, *J. Exp. Med.* **135**: 610.
Borek, F. (ed.), 1972, *Immunogenicity*, North Holland, Amsterdam.
Borek, F., 1972, Molecular size and shape of antigens. In Borek, F. (ed.), *Immunogencity*, North Holland, Amsterdam, pp. 44–86.
Borel, Y., 1971, *Nature New Biol.* **230**: 180.
Braun, D.L., Kindred, B., Jacobson, E.P., 1972, *Eur. J. Immunol.* **2**: 138.
Bretscher, P., 1972, *Transplant. Rev.* **11**: 217.
Bretscher, P., and Cohn, M., 1968, *Nature (London)* **220**: 444.
Britton, S., 1969, *J. Exp. Med.* **129**: 460.
Bullock, W.W., and Rittenberg, M.H., 1971, *Immunochemistry* **7**: 310.
Byrd, W., Feldmann, M., and Palmer, J., 1974, *Immunology*, in press.
Cheers, C., Breitner, J.C.S., Little, M., and Miller, J.F.A.P., 1971, *Nature New Biol.* **232**: 248.
Chiller, J.M., and Weigle, W.O., 1973, *J. Exp. Med.* **137**: 740.
Claman, H.N., and Chaperon, E.A., 1969, *Transplant. Rev.* **1**: 92.
Cohn, M., 1972, In McDevitt and Landy, M. (eds.) *Genetic Control of Immune Responsiveness*, Academic Press, New York and London, pp. 367–448.
Cone, R.E., Marchalonis, J.T., and Rolley, R., 1971, *J. Exp. Med.* **134**: 1373.
Cone, R.E., Feldmann, M., Marchalonis, J.T., and Nossal, G.J.V., 1974, *Immunology* **26**: 49.
Cooper, M., 1973, In Reisfeld, R.A. and Mandy, W.I. (eds.), *Contemporary Topics in Molecular Immunology*, Vol. 2 Plenum Press, New York, p. 155.
Coutinho, A., and Möller, G., 1973, *Nature New Biol. (London)* **245**: 12.
Davies, A.J.S., Carter, R.L., Leuchars, E., Wallis, V.J., and Dietrich, F.M., 1970, *Immunology* **19**: 945.
del Guercio, P., 1972, *Nature New Biol.* **238**: 213.
del Guercio, P., and Leuchars, E., 1972, *J. Immunol.* **109**: 951.
Dennert, G., and Lennox, E.S., 1973, *Nature New Biol. (London)* **245**: 214.

Desaymard, C., and Feldmann, M. 1974, *Eur. J. Immunol.* in press.
Diener, E., and Armstrong, W.D., 1967, *Lancet* 1: 1281.
Diener, E., and Armstrong, W.D., 1969, *J. Exp. Med.* 129: 591.
Diener, E., and Feldmann, M., 1970, *J. Exp. Med.* 132: 31.
Diener, E., and Feldmann, M., 1972a, *Transplant. Rev.* 8: 76.
Diener, E., and Feldmann, M., 1972b, *Cell. Immunol.* 5: 131.
Diener, E., and Paetkau, V.H., 1972, *Proc. Nat. Acad. Sci. US.* 69: 2364.
Diener, E., and Pernis, B., 1973, *Cold Spring Harbor Symp. Quant. Biol.* in press.
Diener, E., Shortman, K., and Russell, P.J., 1970, *Nature (London)* 225: 731.
Dukor, P., and Hartmann, K. U., 1973, *Cell Immunol.* 7: 349.
Dukor, P., Schumang, G., Gisler, R., Derich, M., Konig, W., Hadding, U., and Bitter Saverman, D., 1974, *J. Exp. Med.* 139: 337.
Fanger, M., 1972, *Immunological Communications* 1: 315.
Feldmann, M., 1972a *J. Exp. Med.* 135: 1049.
Feldmann, M., 1972b, *Eur. J. Immunol.* 2: 130.
Feldmann, M., 1972c, *J. Exp. Med.* 136: 737.
Feldmann, M., 1972d, *J. Exp. Med.* 135: 735.
Feldmann, M., 1972e, *J. Exp. Med.* 136: 532.
Feldmann, M., 1973, *Nature New Biol.* 242: 82.
Feldmann, M., 1974, *Eur. J. Immunol.* in press.
Feldmann, M., and Basten, A., 1971, *J. Exp. Med.* 134: 103.
Feldmann, M., and Basten, A., 1972, *J. Exp. Med.* 136: 722.
Feldmann, M., Boylston, A., and Hogg, N., 1974, *Nature* in press.
Feldmann, M., and Diener, E., 1971a, *Immunology* 21: 389.
Feldmann, M., and Diener, E., 1971b, *Nature New Biol.* 231: 183.
Feldmann, M., Greaves, M.F., Parker, D., and Rittenberg, M., 1974, *Eur. J. Immunol.* in press.
Feldmann, M., and Nossal, G.J.V., 1972, *Transplantant Rev.* 13: 3.
Feldmann, M., and Palmer, J., 1971, *Immunology* 21: 685.
Feldmann, M., and Schrader, J., 1974, *Cell Immunol.* in press.
Feldmann, M., Wagner, H., Basten, A., and Holmes, M.C., 1972, *Aust. J. Exp. Biol. Med. Sci.* 50: 651.
Gershon, R.K., and Kondo, K., 1971, *Immunology* 21: 903.
Gery, I., Gershon, R.K., and Waksman, B.H., 1972, *J. Exp. Med.* 136: 128.
Gery, I., and Waksman, B.H., 1972, *J. Exp. Med.* 136: 143.
Gill, T.J., 1972, in Borek, F. (ed.), *Immunogenicity*, North Holland, Amsterdam, pp. 5–44.
Golub, E.S., and Weigle, W.O., 1967, *J. Immunol.* 98: 1241.
Gorczynski, R., 1973, Ph.D. Thesis, University of Toronto, Toronto, Canada.
Gorczynski, R., and Feldmann, M., 1974, *Eur. J. Immunol.* in press.
Greaves, M.F., and Bauminger, S., 1972, *Nature New Biol.* 235: 67.
Greaves, M.F., and Janossy, G., 1972, *Transplant. Rev.* 11: 87.
Greaves, M.F., Owen, J.J.T., and Raff, M.C., 1973, *Excerpta Med.* in press.
Herzenberg, L.A., Warner, N.L., and Herzenberg, L.A., 1968, *Ann. Rev. Genetics* 2: 209.
Howard, J.G., 1972, *Transplant. Rev.* 8: 50.
Hyslop, N., Dourmashkin, R.R., Green, N.M., and Porter, R.R., 1971, *J. Exp. Med.* 131: 783.
Katz, D.H., and Benacerraf, B., 1972, *Adv. Immunol.* 15: 1.
Katz, D.H., Hamaoka, T., and Benacerraf, B., 1972, *J. Exp. Med.* 136: 1404.
Katz, D.H., and Unanue, E., 1973, *J. Immunol.* 109: 1022.
Kiefer, H., 1973, *Eur. J. Immunol.* 3: 181.
Klinman, N., 1972, *J. Exp. Med.* 136: 241.
Kruger, J., and Gershon, R.K., 1971, *J. Immunol.* 106: 1065.
Lederberg, J., 1959, *Science* 129: 1649.
Leskowitz, S., 1972, in Borek, F. (ed.), *Immunogenicity*, North Holland, Amsterdam, pp. 131–154.
Lesley, T., and Dutton, R.W., 1970, *Science* 169: 487.

Marbrook, K.J., 1967, *Lancet* **1**: 1279.
McDevitt, H.O. and Landy, M. 1972, (eds.), *Genetic Control of Immune Responsiveness*, Academic Press, New York and London.
Miller, J.F.A.P., 1972, *Intern. Rev. Cytol.* **33**: 77.
Miller, J.F.A.P., and Warner, N.L., 1971, *Intern. Arch. Allergy Appl. Immunol.* **40**: 59.
Miranda, J.J., 1972, *Immunology* **23**: 829.
Mishell, R.I., and Dutton, R.W., 1967, *J. Exp. Med.* **126**: 423.
Mitchell, G.F., Humphrey, J., and Williamson, A.R., 1973, *Eur. J. Immunol.* **2**: 460.
Mitchison, N.A., 1971a, Immunopathol. **6**: 56.
Mitchison, N.A., 1971b, in Mäkela, O., Cross, A., and Kosunen, T.U. (eds.), *Cell Interactions and Receptor Antibodies in Immune Responses*, Academic Press, New York and London, pp. 249–260.
Moller, G., Andersson, J., Pohlit, H., and Sjöberg, O., 1972, *Clin. Exp. Immunol.* **13**: 89.
Mosier, D., 1967, *Science* **158**: 1573.
Parish, C.R., 1972, *Transplant. Rev.* **13**: 35.
Pepys, M., 1972, *Nature New Biol.* **237**: 157.
Playfair, J., and Purves, E., 1972, *Nature New Biol.* **235**: 115.
Raff, M.C., Feldmann, M., and dePetris, S., 1973, *J. Exp. Med.* **137**: 1024.
Rittenberg, M., and Bullock, W.W., 1972, *Immunochemistry* **9**: 491.
Roelants, G., and Goodman, J., 1970, *Nature (London)* **227**: 175.
Schrader, J.W., 1973a, *J. Exp. Med.* **138**: 1466.
Schrader, J.W., 1973b, *J. Exp. Med.* **137**: 844.
Schrader, J.W., 1974a, *Cell. Immunol.* in press.
Schrader, J.W., 1974b, *Eur. J. Immunol.* **4**: 14.
Schrader, J.W., and Feldmann, M., 1973a, submitted for publication.
Schrader, J.W., and Feldmann, M., 1973b, *Eur. J. Immunol.* **3**: 711.
Sela, M., 1969, *Science* **166**: 1365.
Sela, M., 1973, *Harvey Lectures (1971-1972), Series 67,* Academic Press, New York, p. 213.
Sjöberg, O., 1972, *J. Exp. Med.* **135**: 850.
Sjöberg, O., and Britton, S., 1972, *Eur. J. Immunol.* **2**: 282.
Shellam, G., 1970, Ph.D. Thesis, University of Melbourne, Melbourne, Australia.
Shortman, K., Diener, E., Russell, P., and Armstrong, W.D., 1971, *J. Exp. Med.* **131**:461.
Shortman, K., and Palmer, J., 1971, *Cell. Immunol.* **2**: 399.
Tada, T., and Okamura, K., 1973, *J. Immunol.* **111**: 952.
Taylor, R., 1969, *Transplant. Rev.* **1**: 114.
Taylor, R., Duffus, W.P.H., Raff, M.C., and de Petris, S., 1971, *Nature New Biol.* **233**: 225.
Unanue, E.R., 1970, *J. Immunol.* **105**: 1339.
Wagner, H., 1972, *J. Immunol.* **109**: 630.
Waldmann, H., and Munro, A., 1973, *Nature (London)* **243**: 356.
Wilson, J.D., and Feldmann, M., 1972, *Nature New Biol.* **237**: 3.
Wilson, J.D., Nossal, G.J.V., and Lewis, H., 1972, *Eur. J. Immunol.* **2**: 225.

mRNA for H and L Chains of Immunoglobulin: Specific Control of H-Chain Production

R. H. Stevens

Division of Biochemistry
National Institute for Medical Research
Mill Hill, London, England

and

A. R. Williamson

Department of Microbiology and Immunology
University of California
Los Angeles, California

I. INTRODUCTION

Messenger RNA (mRNA) was postulated to exist in prokaryotic systems by Jacob and Monod (1961) on the basis of genetic evidence. Extensive studies since that time have proven the universality of the transfer of information from DNA to a messenger RNA which is then translated to give protein. In prokaryotic systems there is a direct coupling of the transcription of the genes into RNA to the translation of that RNA into protein. This elegant and simple coupling provides a regulatory mechanism at several defined stages of protein synthesis. Regulation occurs notably at the level of transcription, via repressor proteins binding directly to the DNA (Ptashne, 1967; Gilbert and Müller-Hill, 1967). It is clear that eukaryotic cells provide more potential sites for control of protein synthesis. The flow of information from the gene (Fig. 1) can be regulated at the following levels: (a) selection of the appropriate genes to be transcribed, (b) processing within the nucleus of the primary RNA transcript, (c) transport of the processed messenger RNA from the nucleus to the cytoplasm, and (d) control of the translation of mRNA in the cytoplasm. Prokaryot-

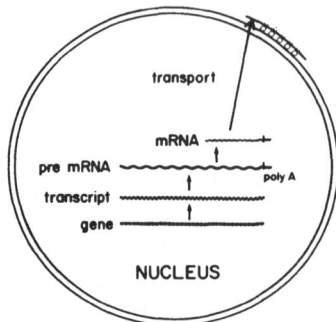

Figure 1. The flow of information from gene to protein. The various steps shown in the processing of mRNA and its transport to the cytoplasm are consistent with the general scheme outlined for eukaryotic cells (Jelinek *et al.*, 1973). The existence of a large pre-mRNA and of its cleavage within the nucleus prior to transport has now been shown for H-chain mRNA. This confirms the general hypothesis for a specific case.

ic mRNA appears to be an ephemeral species which may never exist as a completed molecule since its degradation can start before its completion. By contrast, mRNA in eukaryotic cells is a long-lived species. Following a brief existence in the nucleus in the form of a precursor RNA molecule, functional mRNA is transported to the cytoplasm, where it has a lifetime ranging from hours to days (Greenberg, 1972). During the long lifetime of mRNA in the cytoplasm there is ample scope for variation in the rate of translation.

Differentiation in eukaryotic systems clearly makes use of all of the possible mechanisms of control. The production of antibody in an immune response requires both proliferation and differentiation of cells of the lymphoid line. Study of the control mechanism and the immune response is clearly of fundamental interest to immunology. On the other hand, the immune response with all of the available immunological tools provides an excellent system for basic studies on cell regulation at a molecular level. We will try in this article to illustrate the advances which are being made in a new and exciting approach to studies on the immune system.

The original interest in the isolation of messenger RNA molecules of the heavy and light chains of immunoglobulin stemmed from the need to find a biosynthetic mechanism to explain the variable and constant regions of these chains. It is now accepted on the basis of extensive data reviewed elsewhere that the variable and constant regions of heavy and light chains are coded by separate V and C genes which are integrated at the DNA level (Bevan *et al.*, 1972). The evidence relating to messenger RNA described in this article provides conclusive evidence that the V and C genes are integrated prior to transcription. Investigations of the production and control of mRNA translation in antibody-producing cells have now progressed far beyond the problem which provided the initial stimulus. The results of the investigations are providing a much deeper insight into the control of antibody production and show promise of leading to molecular mechanisms for the immune response.

Recent advances in molecular biology have provided several sensitive techniques for the assay of messenger RNA activity *in vitro*. Such techniques are of prime importance if isolation and purification of specific mRNA is to be achieved. The assay systems for mRNA activity fall into two categories: (a) cell-free protein-synthesizing systems which can be prepared from the subcellular components of a variety of cell types (e.g., rabbit reticulocytes, Krebs ascites cells); (b) a prepackaged, unprogramed, protein-synthesizing system (from amphibian eggs and oocytes) which will translate added exogenous mRNA (Gurdon *et al.*, 1971). These assay systems provide the first essential tool for mRNA purification. Recently it has been discovered that most eukaryotic mRNA molecules are characterized by a stretch of poly(A) up to 200 nucleotides in length at the 3' terminus (Darnell *et al.*, 1971; Edmonds *et al.*, 1971; Lee *et al.*, 1971; Molloy *et al.*, 1972). The hybridization of the poly(A) sequence on mRNA to poly(U) has led to the development of affinity-chromatography methods involving solid-phase-immobilized poly(U) for the rapid isolation of total mRNA. This convenient handle on mRNA does, however, confer an inadventitious degree of similarity on mRNA. This points up the need for novel methods of isolation of specific mRNA species. One such method working directly on the mRNA was used to isolate the silk fibroin mRNA; here density-gradient separation was applied which permitted selection of the desired message on the basis of its high G + C content (Suzuki and Brown, 1972; Suzuki *et al.*, 1972). A possible method would involve the use of specific DNA–RNA hybridization, but this only removes the problem to the level of obtaining specific DNA for use in the hybridization. This method has, however, been successfully applied with DNA viruses, for example, SV40 and adenovirus, where specific mRNA has been isolated (Wall and Darnell, 1971; Wall *et al.*, 1973).

II. L-CHAIN mRNA

Initial attempts to isolate biologically functional mRNA from Ig-synthesizing cells have largely concentrated on the L-chain mRNA. There appear to be several reasons for this: (a) there are available myeloma tumors which synthesize and secrete L chains but not H chains; (b) the expected smaller size of the L-chain mRNA may have seemed more promising, from the viewpoints of both handling without degradation and isolation on the basis of size; (c) complete amino acid sequences are available for a number of mouse L chains, making the L-chain mRNA attractive to those interested in RNA sequence determination; (d) the shorter L-chain mRNA may be more promising for RNA–DNA hybridization studies, especially if reverse transcriptase is to be used to make a DNA copy of the mRNA. At least eight different laboratories have so far attempted to isolate and assay L-chain mRNA. The data are summarized in Table I.

Stavnezer and Huang (1971) first demonstrated that an RNA fraction obtained from an L-chain-synthesizing myeloma tumor could be translated to

Table I. L-Chain mRNA: Isolation and Properties

Source: mouse myeloma tumor	Product	Criteria for isolation	Characterization of RNA	Translation system	Characterization of translation product	Reference
MOPC 21	Kappa	Size, 9–13 S	Translation; (size)	Rabbit reticulocyte cell-free system	Immune precipitation; tryptic peptides	Stavnezer and Huang, 1971
MOPC 21	IgG₁	Size, 10–12 S	Translation; (size)	Krebs II and rabbit reticulocyte cell-free system	SDS–polyacrylamide gel electrophoresis; tryptic peptides	Brownlee, et al., 1972
MOPC 41	Kappa	Membrane-bound ribosomes; poly (A) + (size)	Translation; size (13 S)	Krebs II cell-free system	Immune precipitation; gel electrophoresis; tryptic peptides	Swan, et al., 1972

MOPC 149	Kappa	Immune precipitation of polyribosomes	Size (11–12 S); base composition			Delovitch et al., 1972
5563	IgG$_{2a}$	Poly (A) +	Translation	Xenopus laevis oocyte	Immune precipitation; gel electrophoresis	Stevens and Williamson, 1972
MPC II	Kappa	Membrane-bound ribosomes; size, 12 S	Translation	Krebs II and HeLa cell-free systems	Immune precipitation; gel electrophoresis; tryptic peptides	Delovitch and Baglioni, 1973
MOPC 41	Kappa	Membrane-bound ribosomes; poly (A) +; size	Translation	Rabbit reticulocyte cell-free system	Gel electrophoresis; tryptic peptides	Mach et al., 1973
MOPC 70E	Kappa	Membrane-bound ribosomes; poly (A) +; size	Translation	Rabbit reticulocyte cell-free system	Immune precipitation; gel electrophoresis	Tonegawa and Baldi, 1973

yield L chain in a heterologous cell-free system. Microsomes were prepared from MOPC 41 tumor cells and the total RNA extracted therefrom was fractionated by sucrose-gradient centrifugation. A 9–13 S fraction was collected and assayed for messenger activity in a cell-free system derived from rabbit reticulocytes. Immunoprecipitation in the presence of excess carrier L chain isolated labeled material, which was further characterized by analysis of the tryptic peptides by ion-exchange chromatography and paper electrophoresis. There was a good correspondence between the peptides of the cell-free product and the peptides from authentic L chain with the notable exception of the N-terminal peptide. Thus the 9–13 S RNA fraction contained functional L-chain mRNA, but acrylamide gel analysis of the RNA showed five major bands in addition to 4 S and 5 S RNA and traces of 18 S and 28 S RNA.

Starting with MOPC 21 mouse myeloma cells, Brownlee et al. (1972) were able to repeat Stavnezer and Huang's finding of functional L-chain mRNA in the 10–12 S RNA fraction. These authors scaled up the RNA fractionation by using a zonal rotor. Fractions of RNA were assayed for messenger activity in a cell-free system derived from Krebs II ascites cells. The translation products were analyzed by SDS–acrylamide gel electrophoresis. Two adjacent RNA fractions stimulated incorporation into a component migrating in the position of L chain in both cases; however, another major new component, smaller than L chain, and several minor components were also synthesized. The putative L-chain band was eluted, and fingerprint analysis showed two of the expected three methionine-containing peptides. The active RNA fractions used by these authors were apparently no less heterogeneous than those prepared by Stavnezer and Huang (1971). One interesting development from this study was the finding that the 10–12 S RNA when translated in a rabbit reticulocyte cell-free system yields a polypeptide chain which appears to be a precursor of L chain having an additional 14 or 15 amino acids at the N-terminal end (Milstein et al., 1972).

Two other groups (Swan et al., 1972; Mach et al., 1973) have used a different approach to the purification of L-chain mRNA. Both have used MOPC 41 mouse myeloma and their methods have many similarities (see Table I). Membrane-bound ribosomes were isolated since they are the usual site of synthesis of L and H chains. The poly(A)+ RNA fraction was isolated by chromatography on poly(dT) cellulose.

Swan et al. (1972) assayed this mixed mRNA fraction directly in a Krebs II cell-free system and found that it directed the synthesis of several polypeptide chains. Although one of these products appeared by SDS–polyacrylamide gel electrophoresis to be L chain, the major product was slightly larger than L chain. This was postulated to be an L-chain precursor 6–8 amino acids longer than the final L chain. In addition, two other L-chain-related polypeptides were synthesized in the cell-free system; these products were 20–30 and 40–50 amino acids shorter than L chain. This the authors attributed to incomplete translation.

Because of the selection for poly(A)+ mRNA molecules it would be expected that the 3'-termination signals would be intact. Translation in the cell-free system may be prematurely terminated for other reasons. The size of the L-chain mRNA was indicated by analyzing the mRNA preparation by sucrose-gradient centrifugation and assaying across the gradient for mRNA activity. The major peak was at 13 S; a second peak at 19 S might be attributed to aggregation. The length of 850 nucleotides estimated from the sedimentation coefficient is about 200 nucleotides longer than is needed to code for a single L chain, but most of the excess length could be due to the poly(A) content.

Mach *et al.* (1973) prepared a poly(A)+ RNA from microsomes and then took a 14 S peak from a preparative sucrose gradient. This fraction surprisingly represented 40–50% of the poly(A)+ RNA. A similar major species of mRNA has not been reported by other groups. After a second sucrose-gradient centrifugation of this 14 S RNA, analysis by polyacrylamide gel electrophoresis showed one major peak (estimated to be 1100 nucleotides long) and a few minor components. This is probably the cleanest L-chain mRNA prepared at this time. The major product of translation in a rabbit reticulocyte cell-free system is a polypeptide chain about 20 amino acids longer than L chain and showing all but one of the L-chain tryptic peptides; two additional peptides were found apparently replacing the missing peptide.

Recently Tonegawa and Baldi (1973) obtained a 13.5 S poly(A)+ RNA component from the membrane-bound ribosomes of MOPC 70E. Final purification was by slab polyacrylamide gel electrophoresis. In a cell-free system the major translation product of this 13.5 S RNA was slightly larger than L chain. This RNA fraction is comparable in purity to that prepared by Mach *et al.* (1973).

A 12 S RNA fraction was prepared from MPC 11 microsomes by Delovitch and Baglioni (1973). Three successive sucrose-gradient centrifugations were used, but poly(A)+ RNA was not selected. This 12 S RNA fraction was translated in cell-free systems from Krebs II cells and HeLa cells, and in both cases a portion of the labeled product coelectrophoresed with L chain. In addition, a substantial proportion of the products were smaller than L chain. Paper electrophoresis of a tryptic digest of the product showed only the three methionine-containing peptides of MPC 11 L chain. Other mRNA species present in the 12 S RNA either are not translated in the cell-free system or do not code for polypeptides containing methionine.

In our studies using 5563 mouse myeloma cells in established culture, we initially isolated a poly(A)+ RNA fraction by chromatography on a poly(U) Geon 425 column. This mixture of mRNA molecules was translated by micro-injection into *Xenopus laevis* oocytes. This system, pioneered by Lane *et al.* (1971), is an extremely sensitive and efficient one for assaying heterologous mRNA. Poly(A)+ RNA from either the cytoplasm or nucleus of 5563 cells contained mRNA molecules coding for L chains and also mRNA for H chains. Specific products synthesized in injected oocytes were precipitated with antisera, and the precipitates dissolved in SDS and analyzed by polyacrylamide gel electrophoresis. This showed that L and H chains were made and efficiently assembled to H_2L_2 within the oocyte (Fig. 2). The ratio of H- to L-chain production in oocytes injected with cytoplasmic RNA reflected the ratio in the 5563 cell where an excess of L chain is made (Fig. 2A, C). Nuclear RNA, on the other hand, coded for excess H-chain production in oocytes (Fig. 2B, D). This result suggests a transport imbalance (see discussion in Section IV). Also, this difference between nuclear and cytoplasmic mRNA balance argues against the doubt that nuclear L- and H-chain mRNA's are due to cytoplasmic contamina-

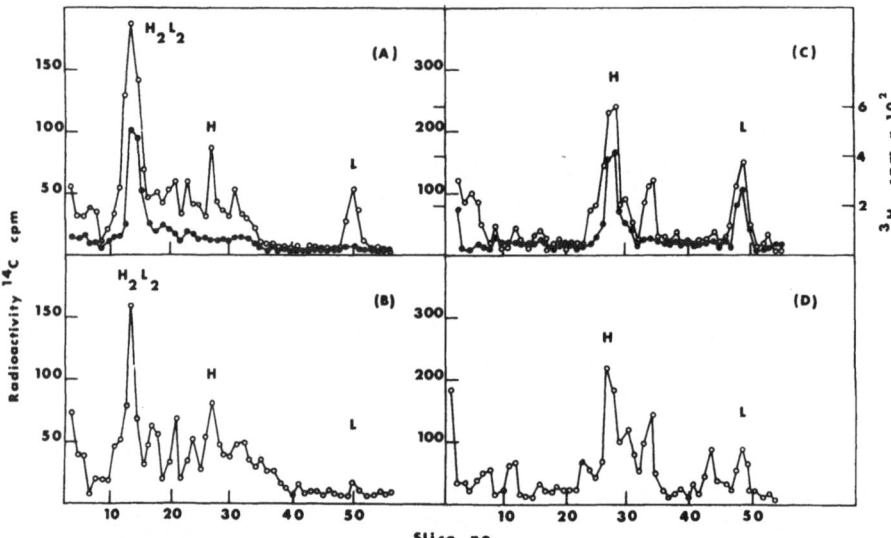

Figure 2. Electrophoretic analysis of the specific antibody-precipitable products of translation of 5563 poly(A)+ RNA in oocytes. Specific products of translation of (A) cytoplasmic RNA, (B) nuclear RNA; specific products after reduction with 0.1 M mercaptoethanol, (C) cytoplasmic RNA, (D) nuclear RNA. ^{14}C, o——o; ^3H, ●——●. Samples of 30 oocytes were injected with either cytoplasmic RNA (15 μg/ml) or nuclear RNA (30 μg/ml) resuspended in injection buffer (88 mM NaCl, 1.0 mM tris–HCl, pH 7.6) containing 1.25 mCi/ml ^{14}C-amino acid mixture. Incubation (6 hr) was performed in 66% Hanks BSS containing the above concentration of ^{14}C-amino acid mixture. The eggs were homogenized, ^3H-5563 protein was added and the indirect antibody precipitation was performed using rabbit anti-5563 and goat antirabbit antisera. The washed immunoglobin precipitates were dissolved in 2% SDS and heated to 100°C for 1 min. A portion of nuclear- and cytoplasmic-RNA-injected samples was alkylated with iodoacetamide (0.1 M) and loaded onto a 7.5% acylamide gel (A and B). Another portion of each sample was reduced by mercaptoethanol (to 0.1 M) (C and D). Following incubation at room temperature for 1 hr, a 50% molar excess of iodoacetamide was added; the solution was heated to 100°C for 1 min and then layered on a 7.5% acrylamide gel. Electrophoresis was performed as described by Summers et al. (1965).

tion. Although some doubt about contamination still remained in this study, our subsequent results on H-chain mRNA clearly show a large nuclear precursor form of that mRNA.

Only one attempt at the specific isolation of L-chain mRNA has been reported to date. Delovitch *et al.* (1972) used the F(ab')₂ fragment of rabbit antibody raised against MOPC 149 L chain to precipitate polyribosomes from MOPC 149 cells. The RNA was labeled for 30 min *in vivo* with ³²P, and polyribosomes were isolated from the solid tumor and fractionated by sucrose-gradient centrifugation. The specifically precipitated fraction of the polyribosomes yielded one major peak of ³²P-labeled RNA. This RNA peaked at 11–12 S and had a G + C content of 47 mol. %. These properties are consistent with those expected of L-chain mRNA, but unfortunately no translation has been attempted. This approach should prove useful despite technical difficulties. The immune precipitation methods have been described recently (Delovitch *et al.*, 1973).

In summary, it has been shown that an RNA species containing poly(A) and having a size in the range 9–14 S can be isolated from membrane-bound polyribosomes and can be translated to give either L chain or a precursor of L chain in an *in vitro* protein-synthesizing system. In all cases where translation was attempted, there was evidence for the presence of mRNA species other than L-chain mRNA. This is really not surprising, since none of the procedures used in those studies involved any step specific for L-chain mRNA. Although the evidence varies, even for the same tumor source, L-chain mRNA is apparently longer than the necessary coding length, and some portion of this extra length (18–60 nucleotides, probably at the 5' terminus) is translated with subsequent proteolytic cleavage of the longer precursor of L chain.

III. H-CHAIN mRNA

In contrast to the extensive attention that has been paid to the L-chain mRNA, the H-chain mRNA has received virtually no attention. This is perhaps surprising, since the early data on the precipitation of specific polysomes by antiserum directed to the nascent H and L chains showed much better results with heavy-chain- than with light-chain-synthesizing polyribosomes (Williamson and Askonas, 1967). Moreover, the discrete large size of the H-chain-synthesizing polyribosomes makes them good candidates for separation from the bulk of the cellular polyribosomes. There are difficulties to the methodology of isolating polyribosomes by using specific antibody, but it is surprising that this methodology should have been applied to light-chain polyribosomes and not to heavy-chain polyribosomes.

The synthesis of H chain has been demonstrated in cell-free systems derived from immunoglobulin-producing tissue. Using polyribosomes or microsomes derived from hyperimmune rat lymph node tissue, Vassalli *et al.* (1971) showed the complete synthesis of H chains labeled from the N terminus to the C terminus. They showed that in the system using intact microsomes, assembly of the H and L chains into $H_2 L_2$ molecules took place, in contrast to the polysome system where single chains were the final products. Using a cell-free system derived from rabbit lymph nodes, Ralph and Rich (1971) showed synthesis of both heavy and light chains, although most of the synthesis was the completion of chains already initiated on the polyribosome. These authors did, however, make use of the size difference in H-chain- and L-chain-synthesizing polyribosomes to select fractions of the polyribosomes enriched for H chain or L chain message; this enrichment was demonstrated in the cell-free system. No attempt was made in either of these two studies to further purify the H-chain mRNA.

In initial studies on the messenger RNA for both heavy and light chains in mouse myeloma cells, we showed that the poly(A)+ RNA from these cells contained both heavy and light chain mRNA as demonstrated by microinjection into *Xenopus laevis* oocytes (Stevens and Williamson, 1972). In this case, complete heavy and light chains were synthesized, and the large majority of the chains were found in completely assembled $H_2 L_2$ molecules (Fig. 2). These initial studies on the translation of total mRNA from myeloma cells using the oocyte system laid the basis for further studies on the purification of individual mRNA molecules.

We have obtained a highly purified preparation of H-chain mRNA from mouse plasmacytoma cells, using a purification procedure which takes advantage of a binding site on the H-chain mRNA for 5563 7 S immunoglobulin (Stevens and Williamson, 1973a). An interaction between $H_2 L_2$ and H-chain mRNA was postulated from experiments in which the synthesis of H chain appeared to be regulated by the intracellular level of $H_2 L_2$ immunoglobulin. Following an increase in the intercellular level of $H_2 L_2$, H-chain synthesis was shown to be selectively decreased with respect to L-chain and total protein synthesis. This feedback repression of H-chain synthesis is further discussed in Section V.

The binding of $H_2 L_2$ to myeloma mRNA was initially demonstrated by two experiments designed to measure the specific binding of mRNA molecules to the 7 S immunoglobulin protein and the binding of 7 S protein to mRNA. In the former experiment, a population of RNA molecules was shown to specifically bind to 5563 $H_2 L_2$ protein at ionic strengths between 75 and 150 mM Na^+; the resulting protein–RNA complex could then be precipitated by anti-5563 antiserum. RNA from chicken fibroblasts which produce no immunoglobulin served as a control and showed only nonspecific binding to the precipitate at low ionic strength. In the second experiment, binding of $H_2 L_2$ to mRNA was investigated by adding increasing amounts of 5563 protein labeled with ^{35}S-methionine to a controlled amount of myeloma mRNA. The mixtures were passed through a poly(U) filter which recovered mRNA by hybridization with the $3'$ poly(A) sequences thought to be present on most mRNA molecules. With increasing 5563 protein added per unit of RNA, there was increased binding to mRNA, apparently approaching but not reaching saturation (Fig. 3). The lack of saturation may reflect the equilibrium nature of the protein–RNA interaction. These two experiments showed that there exists within myeloma cells a population of mRNA molecules, each of which has the capacity to bind to and be bound by 5563 H_2L_2.

The size of RNA molecules bound to the antigen–antibody complex can conveniently be measured by polyacrylamide gel electrophoresis; under denaturing conditions the mobility of an RNA molecule is related to the logarithm of the molecular weight. The cytoplasmic RNA which is bound to 5563 H_2L_2 and subsequently precipitated by anti-5563 antiserum can be resolved into two distinct species by electrophoresis on 4% polyacrylamide gels. These RNA molecules have molecular weights of 6×10^5 (Band II) and 3×10^5 (Band III) with respect to mRNA marker molecules (Fig. 4). The RNA in Band III was shown to be enriched in poly(A) by its ability to bind to poly(U) filters, and by resistance of 8% of the RNA to digestion by T1 and pancreatic RNase. Band II fails to bind to poly(U) filters and shows less than 2% RNase resistance and, therefore, contains shortened sequences of poly(A).

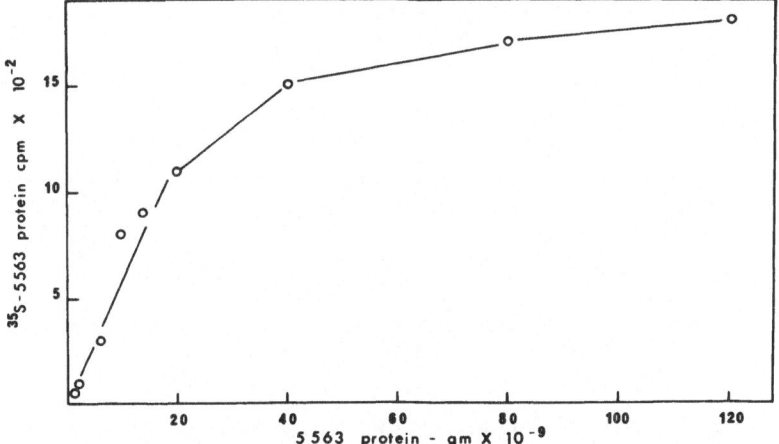

Figure 3. Binding of 5563 myeloma protein to myeloma RNA containing A-rich sequences, isolated from 5563 cells. Aliquots of ^{3}H-adenosine labeled myeloma RNA (2.0×10^4 cpm/μg) were mixed with increasing amounts of ^{35}S-methionine labeled myeloma protein (2.2×10^6 cpm/μg) under conditions described previously (Stevens and Williamson, 1973b). The samples were filtered through fiberglass filters containing bound poly(U), and the radioactivity was determined. Each point is corrected to 0.8 g of RNA bound and represents triplicate samples.

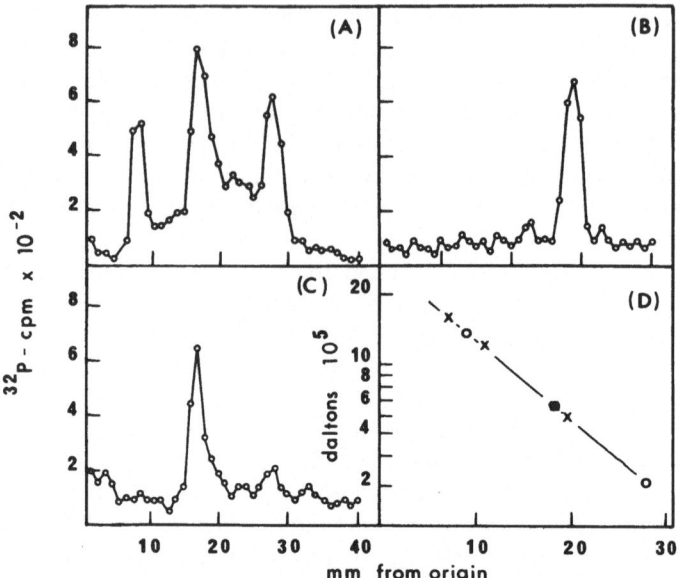

Figure 4. Acrylamide gel analysis of antibody-bound RNA. 5563 myeloma cells (10^7/ml) were labeled for 6 hr with ^{32}P-orthophosphate (100 μCi/ml) and total and cytoplasmic RNA isolated (Stevens and Williamson, 1973a). Total cellular RNA (A), cytoplasmic RNA enriched in mRNA (B), and cytoplasmic RNA enriched in rRNA (C) were treated 5 min at 0°C with 5563 myeloma protein and anti-5563 antiserum, and the precipitates were washed twice with solution A. ^{3}H-labeled 28 S and 18 S ribosomal RNA from myeloma cells and 23 S and 16 S ribosomal RNA from *E. coli* were added to the precipitates which were then made 2% with respect to SDS. The mixtures were layered upon 4% polyacrylamide gels containing SDS and electrophoresis was conducted at 10 mA/gel for 90 min at room temperature. The gels were sliced into 1-mm sections, hydrolyzed with concentrated NH₄OH, and the radioactivity was determined by scintillation counting. The relationship between mobility and molecular weight for the four ribosomal RNA species (X) is shown in (D). The mobilities of the three RNA bands (I, II, and III respectively from the top of the gel) are plotted on this line (o) to estimate apparent molecular weights.

Both cytoplasmic RNA molecules (Bands II and III) removed by antibody precipitation are able to code for complete H chain. Each RNA species was electrophoretically eluted from the polyacrylamide gel and injected into *Xenopus laevis* oocytes. The only antibody-precipitable protein formed by either of the RNA species was H chain, L chain being undetectable (Fig. 5). The identity of the product was confirmed as H chain by tryptic digest analysis. The fact that both Bands II and III code for H chain is paradoxical. The mRNA coding for H chain containing 450 amino acids should have a molecular weight of 4.5–5.0 X

10^5. The RNA in Band III, with an apparent molecular weight of 3×10^5, would be expected to contain an insufficient number of nucleotides to code for a complete H chain. The RNA in Band II, on the other hand, contains an excess number of nucleotides. The resolution of the paradox is probably to be found in the increased mobility of H-chain mRNA containing poly(A) sequences. The RNA in Band II appears to arise from the RNA in Band III by cleavage of poly(A) sequences during phenol extraction.

Messenger RNA has been shown to exist in eukaryotic cells as a complex of RNA and protein (Blobel, 1972). Total messenger RNP particles can be isolated by treatment of mammalian polyribosomes with EDTA or puromycin, both of which cause disassociation of ribosomal subunits and release of the messenger RNP. Fractionation of the RNP can be achieved by sucrose-gradient analysis.

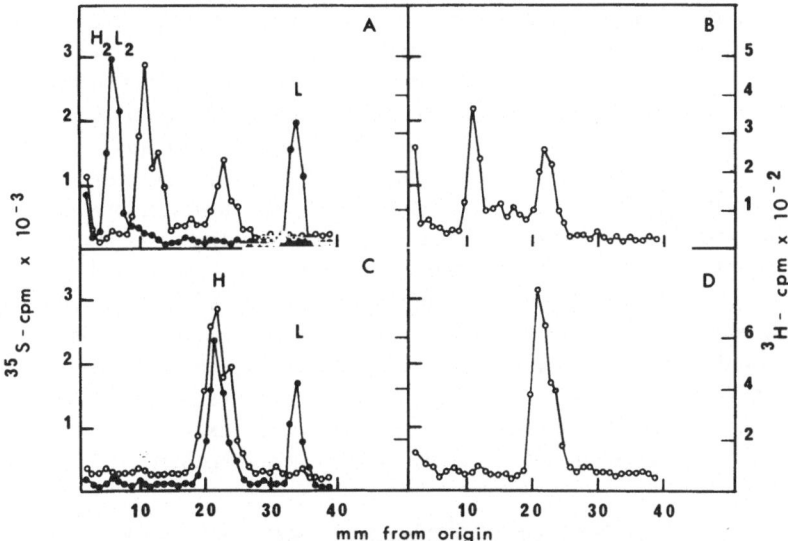

Figure 5. Translation products of RNA specifically purified from 5563 myeloma cells. Oocytes from *Xenopus laevis* were injected with purified RNA from Bands II or III. (Fig. 4) The oocytes were homogenized following 24 hr incubation at room temperature, and synthesized 5563 protein was precipitated by direct antibody precipitation with anti-5563 antiserum. The precipitates were washed four times with PBS, ^{3}H-labeled 5563 marker protein added, and the precipitates dissolved in 2% SDS. The samples were divided into two portions, one portion being alkylated with iodoacetamide (0.15 M) and the other portion being reduced with mercapto-ethanol (0.1 M) prior to alkylation. Unreduced and reduced samples from oocytes injected with RNA from band II (A and C respectively), or from oocytes injected with RNA from band III (B and D respectively), were analyzed by electrophoresis on 7.5% polyacrylamide gels containing SDS. Following electrophoresis the gels were sliced into 1-mm sections, hydrolyzed and the radioactivity determined. ^{35}S, o—o; ^{3}H •—•.

The specificity of binding of H-chain mRNA to H_2L_2 has been shown to extend to H-chain mRNP. The majority of the RNA which can be isolated from the RNP particles binding to H_2L_2 coelectrophoreses on 4% acrylamide gels with the RNA in Band III isolated from total cellular RNA. When the RNA isolated from specifically purified RNP particles is analyzed by sucrose-gradient centrifugation, it sediments with a value of 16–18 S, equivalent to the apparent size of Band II RNA. This result further suggests that the rapid mobility of the mRNA in Band III is an artifact of electrophoresis.

The H-chain mRNP particle contains 3 or 4 proteins bound to the mRNA. Two of the proteins appear to be similar in size to the proteins isolated from RNP particles containing globin mRNA (Blobel, 1972; Morel et al., 1971). Little is known about the function of these proteins on mRNA. Several proteins have been shown to be associated with the poly(A) sequences on the mRNA and perhaps function in the transport of mRNA from the nucleus (Kwan and Brawerman, 1972). It is interesting to speculate about specific binding sites for protein on mRNA in light of the apparent excess of nucleotides over those which are needed to code for either α or β chain, with excess sequences being found on both the 3′ and 5′ ends of the mRNA. Similarly, several of the L-chain mRNA preparations appear to contain a 20–40% excess of nucleotide bases. H-chain mRNA isolated in our laboratory is 20% larger than needed to code for H chain. The excess nucleotide bases on mRNA may, however, serve as specific sites for binding of proteins serving regulatory functions. As stated above, H-chain mRNP isolated from polyribosomes actively synthesizing H chain contains three or four different proteins. Furthermore, we have shown that a binding site exists on the mRNA for at least one additional protein, H_2L_2, which binds only under certain conditions. It would appear unlikely that these proteins would be associated with the RNA sequences coding for H chain. Regulatory nucleic acid–protein interactions exist in eukaryotic cells and have been well documented in microbial systems (Kozak and Nathans, 1972).

IV. NUCLEAR PRECURSOR OF H-CHAIN mRNA

Nuclei of eukaryotic cells contain nonribosomal RNA of high molecular weight which has been termed heterogeneous nuclear RNA (HnRNA) (Penman et al., 1968; Melli and Pemberton, 1972). This RNA has a DNA-like base composition and is metabolically very active with a lifetime in the nucleus of between five and fifteen minutes (Soeiro et al., 1968). Within recent years, a large amount of evidence has accumulated which suggests that part of the HnRNA molecules serves as a precursor to cytoplasmic mRNA molecules. This evidence has come from several sources. Direct demonstration of a precursor–product relationship between HnRNA and cytoplasmic mRNA has been difficult to obtain, and more refined techniques have been needed. The first such refined technique to be applied to this problem was that of RNA–DNA hybridization. Using this technique, Wall and Darnell (1971) demonstrated that in the nuclei of SV40-transformed cells a population of RNA molecules exist which can be specifically hybridized with SV40 DNA. Subsequent experiments have shown that this RNA is larger than the messenger RNA found in the cytoplasm and contains host sequences integrated with the SV40-specific RNA (Aloni, 1973).

More recently, it has been shown that most mRNA molecules contain poly(A) sequences at the 3′ hydroxy terminus. The association of the poly(A) sequences with HnRNA provides further evidence of a precursor–product relationship between these molecules and cytoplasmic mRNA (Jelinek *et al.*, 1973; Mendecki *et al.*, 1972). Direct demonstration of RNA sequences in the nucleus

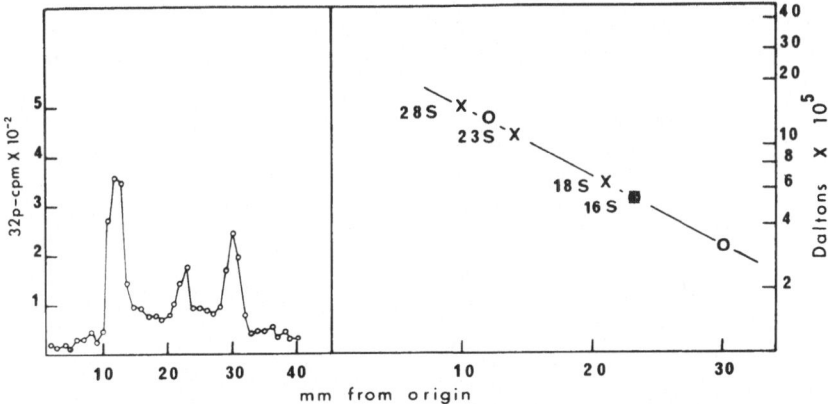

Figure 6. Electrophoretic pattern of nuclear RNA isolated from 5563 myeloma cells by specific precipitation with 5563 protein and anti-5563 antibody. On the right the mobilities of the specific RNA bands are compared to rRNA markers for estimation of apparent molecular weights. Cultured murine myeloma cells (5563), maintained in exponential growth, were concentrated to 7×10^6 cells/ml and incubated for 5 hr in phosphate-free L-15 medium containing 250 μCi/ml ^{32}P-orthophosphate. Nuclei and cytoplasm were then separated after a 15 min incubation with 1% NP-40 at 4°C and the RNA prepared by the method of Lee *et al.* (1971). The *p*H 7.6 and 9.0 RNA fractions were combined and precipitated overnight at −20°C by the addition of two volumes of ethanol. The RNA precipitate was collected by centrifugation (30,000*g* for 15 min) and the excess ethanol evaporated. All subsequent steps were conducted at 0°C. The RNA was resuspended in 0.5 ml solution A (0.5 mM MgCl$_2$, 75 mM NaCl, 20 mM phosphate buffer, *p*H 7.5), and the mixture centrifuged at 3000*g* for 3 min to remove any aggregated RNA. 50 μg DEAE-purified 5563 protein was added to the supernatant fluid and the mixture incubated 1 min. Purified immunoglobulin fraction of anti-5563 antiserum was then added to equivalence and incubation was continued an additional 2 min. The precipitate was collected by centrifugation (3000*g* for 5 min) and washed twice with solution A. The precipitate was made to 2% with sodium dodecylsulfate (SDS), ^{3}H-labeled marker rRNA was added, and the RNA analyzed by electrophoresis on a 4% polyacrylamide gel (10 mA/gel for 2 hr). Gels were sliced into 1-mm sections, hydrolyzed with concentrated NH$_4$OH, and the radioactivity determined in a Beckman liquid scintillation counter model.

coding specifically for hemoglobin (Williamson *et al.,* 1973) or mouse immuno-globulin H and L chains (Stevens and Williamson, 1972) has been obtained using the sensitive oocyte assay system. In both of these studies, the criticism could be leveled that the oocyte system, being so sensitive, was in fact measuring cyto-plasmic contamination in the nucleus. Our experiments on immunoglobulin mRNA have been much further refined, using the technique for isolating H-chain mRNA by direct binding to immunoglobulin. This technique has now been extended to the isolation of nuclear pre-mRNA. Total RNA was isolated from the nuclei of myeloma cells after labeling briefly with ^{32}P-orthophosphate, and treated with anti-5563 antibody; three distinct RNA peaks were obtained (Fig. 6). Two of these peaks correspond in size to the H-chain mRNA molecules with and without poly(A) which were found in the cytoplasm. The presence of these molecules does not seem to be caused by cytoplasmic contamination of the nuclear preparations; the completed cytoplasmic H-chain mRNA is apparently

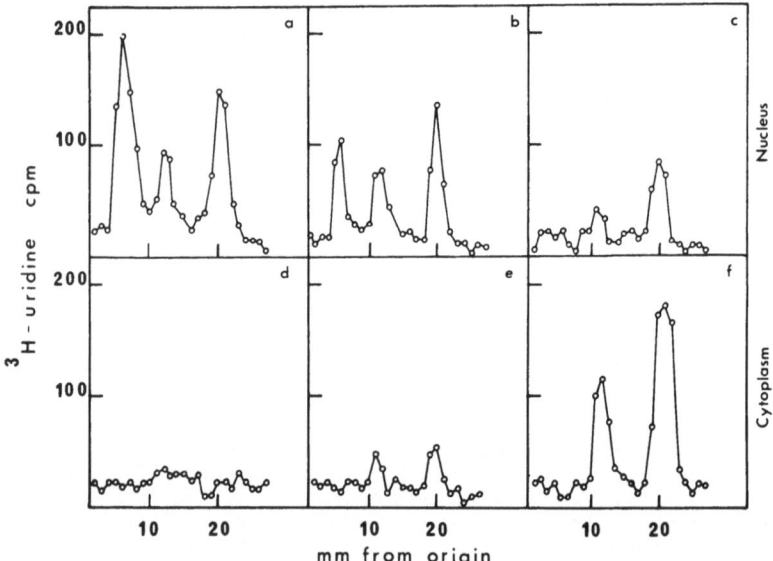

Figure 7. Synthesis and transport of H-chain pre-mRNA. 5563 myeloma cells (5 X 10⁵ cells/ml) were incubated at 37°C for 20 min with ³H-uridine (200 μCi/ml, 26 mCi/mmole). Actinomycin D (10 μg/ml) was added and incubation continued an additional 30 min. Equal samples of cells were removed immediately prior to the addition of the actinomycin D, and 15 min and 30 min thereafter. The nuclear and cytoplasmic RNA were prepared and each RNA sample was treated with 5563 protein–anti-5563 antibody as described under Fig. 6. Electrophoretic analysis of the specific RNA in the precipitates was performed on 4% polyacryl-amide gels. a,b, and c represent nuclear RNA samples at 0, 15, and 30 min following addition of actinomycin D; d,e, and f represent corresponding cyto-plasmic RNA samples.

formed within the nucleus and exists there for a short time prior to transport into the cytoplasm. The largest component, Band I, is confined to the nucleus. Following a brief labeling of myeloma cells with ^{3}H-uridine, the majority of the radioactive nuclear RNA precipitating with the antibody—antigen complex is found in Band I (Fig. 7a). At the same time, no labeled H-chain mRNA is present in the cytoplasm (Fig. 7d). In a chase experiment in which incubation was continued in the presence of actinomycin-D to inhibit further RNA synthesis, the radioactivity in Band I was found to be reduced with the concomitant appearance of radioactivity in the RNA of Bands II and III; these cytoplasmic mRNA species still remained in the nucleus (Fig. 7b). With further incubation, these two mRNA species appear within the cytoplasm (Fig. 7f). The existence within Band I of sequences coding for 5563 H chain was conclusively demonstrated by direct injection into oocytes of RNA electrophoretically eluted from Band I.

These experiments provide a direct demonstration of the existence in the nucleus of a large RNA precursor to H-chain mRNA. We do not yet know whether this H-chain pre-mRNA is the original RNA transcript of the H-chain gene or whether it is an early cleavage product of the transcript. The precursor mRNA is subsequently cleaved, within the nucleus, to the size of the cytoplasmic H-chain mRNA, which, following a short lag, is transported into the cytoplasm. This evidence confirms the hypothetical scheme shown in Fig. 1. The ability to isolate the nuclear precursor as well as the cytoplasmic mRNA paves the way for intensive investigations into the processes regulating messenger RNA selection and transport into the cytoplasm.

V. TRANSLATIONAL CONTROL OF H-CHAIN SYNTHESIS

The segregation of the genetic information contained in DNA from the machinery for translating this information into functional protein is accomplished in eukaryotic cells by a nuclear membrane. The process of information transfer from DNA to functional protein involves several intermediate steps within the nucleus, followed by transport of informational RNA across the nuclear membrane (Fig. 1). This is a lengthy process and can respond only sluggishly to environmental changes or specific stimuli.

The need for a differentiated cell to continually perform given functions implies that select classes of mRNA have either rapid rates of synthesis compensating for degradation or, more economically, a reduced rate of synthesis combined with a much longer lifetime within the cytoplasm. Evidence has been reported recently suggesting that the latter of the two possibilities is the case, i.e., mRNA molecules in the cytoplasm of eukaryotic cells have lifetimes of more than one cell generation (Greenberg, 1972). This mRNA stability requires a further cytoplasmic regulatory mechanism to modulate the rate of protein synthesis in general, and of specific proteins in particular, in response to small changes in the external environment of the cell. Such regulatory mechanisms have been termed translational control. One of the best-characterized examples of a general translational control mechanism is found in dividing cells where a specific block on initiation results in a 70% reduction of protein synthesis during the period of mitosis (Fan and Penman, 1970).

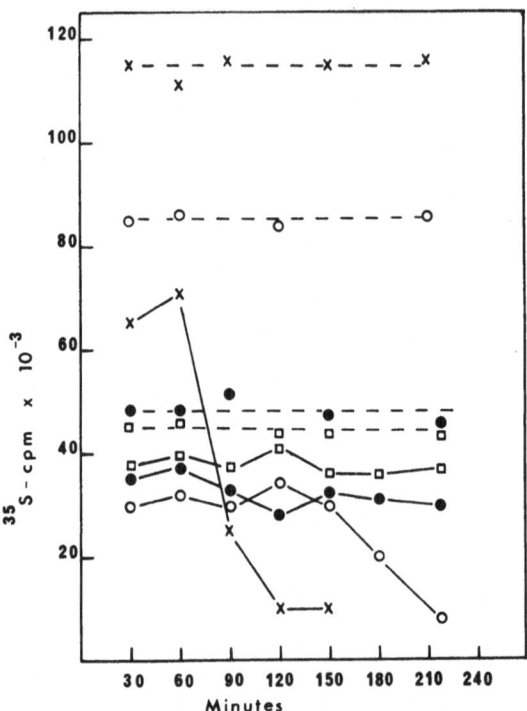

Figure 8. Effect of increased intracellular 5563 protein on H- and L-chain synthesis. Cultures of stationary and exponential growing cells were resuspended in medium lacking methionine and divided into two aliquots, one aliquot being incubated at $37°C$ and one at $25°C$. Samples were removed at intervals and incubated with ^{35}S-methionine for 30 min. Total 5563 protein was precipitated from each sample, and the radioactivity in H and L chains was determined by acrylamide gel electrophoresis following reduction and alkylation. The key to the figure is as follows: X--------X, exponential cells, H chain, $37°C$; X———X, exponential cells, H chain, $25°C$; ●--------●, exponential cells, L chain, $37°C$; ●———●, exponential cells, L chain, $25°C$; ○--------○, stationary cells, H chain, $37°C$; ○———○, stationary cells, H chain, $25°C$; □--------□, stationary cells, L chain, $37°C$; □———□, stationary cells, L chain, $25°C$.

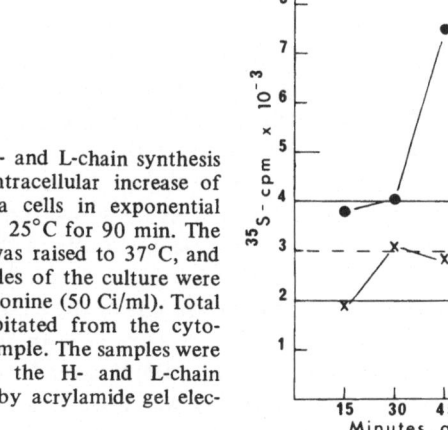

Figure 9. Recovery of H- and L-chain synthesis at 37°C following an intracellular increase of $H_2 L_2$ at 25°C. Myeloma cells in exponential growth were incubated at 25°C for 90 min. The incubation temperature was raised to 37°C, and at 15 min intervals samples of the culture were incubated with ^{35}S-methionine (50 Ci/ml). Total 5563 protein was precipitated from the cytoplasmic extract of each sample. The samples were reduced, alkylated, and the H- and L-chain radioactivity determined by acrylamide gel electrophoresis.

More specific translational control mechanisms are found in the synthesis of hemoglobin (Lodish, 1971; Hunt *et al.*, 1969), chicken ovalbumin (Palmiter, 1972), and immunoglobulin (Stevens and Williamson, 1973b, c)

We have recently demonstrated in 5563 myeloma cells a form of translational control in which an increased intracellular pool of $H_2 L_2$ results in a specific decrease in the synthesis of H chain. Secretion of $H_2 L_2$ from 5563 cells can be stopped by incubation at 27°C. At this temperature the synthesis and assembly of H and L chains continues at 40–50% of the rate at 37°C. This continued synthesis results in an increased intracellular level of $H_2 L_2$. When cells containing a naturally large intracellular pool of $H_2 L_2$ (exponetially growing cells) and cells containing a reduced intracellular $H_2 L_2$ pool (cells in stationary phase) are incubated at 27°C, expansion of the intracellular pools continues in both cases. If the rates of synthesis of H and L chains are measured at various times following temperature reduction, it can be shown that the reduction of H-chain synthesis is effected nearly an hour sooner in cells containing a larger $H_2 L_2$ intracellular pool than in those with a smaller $H_2 L_2$ pool (Fig. 8). Thus, there appears to be a correlation between the level of $H_2 L_2$ and H-chain synthesis. This correlation can be extended to 37°C. An increase in $H_2 L_2$ can be effected by low-temperature incubation, and upon raising the temperature to 37°C, the synthesis of H chain takes over 60 min to return to the normal rate, whereas L-chain synthesis returns much more rapidly to the preincubation rate (Fig. 9).

These and similar experiments (Stevens and Williamson, 1973b,c) led us to postulate that a specific binding site for $H_2 L_2$ on H chain mRNA was involved in a feedback mechanism for controlling the level of H_2L_2 with 5563 plasma cells. This hypothesis has been greatly strengthened by the direct demonstration of H_2L_2 binding to H-chain mRNA (discussed above) and the measurement of the strength of this interaction (see Section VI). In line with other forms of translational control, this mechanism would appear to function at the level of initiation, as polyribosomes synthesizing H chain exhibit a specific decrease in polyribosome size following the increase of the H_2L_2 pool (Stevens, 1973).

The nature of the H_2L_2 interaction with H-chain mRNA within the cell is difficult to envisage. Translation of H-chain mRNA takes place on membrane-bound ribosomes, and the nascent H chain grows into the cisternae of the endoplasmic reticulum. Electron microscopy confirms that the assembled H_2L_2 is thereby confined to the cisternae so that it is formally separated from the H-chain mRNA which is on the opposite side of the endoplasmic reticulum. It is unlikely that the H_2L_2 pool is in equilibrium with the cytoplasm, but it is equally unlikely that portions of the mRNA extend into the cisternae of the endoplasmic reticulum. The hypothesis which we now favor, and which is being tested experimentally, is that during conditions of an increased H_2L_2 pool, a portion of the H_2L_2, possibly part of the Fc region (see Section VI), extends through the membrane leading to interaction with H-chain mRNA and the resultant reduction in H-chain synthesis (Fig. 10).

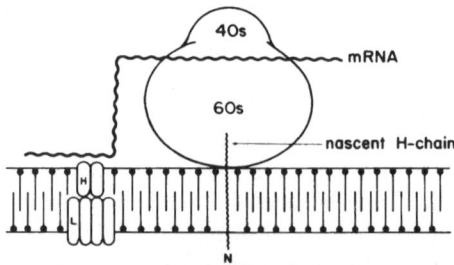

Figure 10. A model to explain the interaction between H_2L_2 and H-chain mRNA *in vivo*. An immunoglobulin molecule is shown inserted into the membrane carrying H-chain-synthesizing polyribosomes. The diagram is drawn approximately to scale. Clearly the C-terminal portion of the H chains can contact the H-chain mRNA on one side of the membrane while the antibody-combining site is exposed on the other side of the membrane. This orientation would be consistent with biosynthetic data (Bevan *et al.*, 1972) and the production of surface immunoglobulin receptors. The H_2L_2 binding site is assumed to be near the initiation site for translation of the H-chain mRNA, which is shown running 5' to 3' across the ribosome.

Table II. Isolation of H-Chain mRNA by Interaction with Immunoglobulin (H_2L_2) and Antiimmunoglobulin

Cells	H_2L_2	Rabbit anti-body raised against	H-chain mRNA precipitated		Product of translation of precipitated RNA (cytoplasm) in oocyte
			nucleus	cytoplasm	
MOPC 315	315	315	+	+	α chain
MOPC 104E	104E	104E	N.D.	+	μ chain
P3 (MOPC 21)	21	21	+	+	γ chain
MOPC 315	Human IgG	Human IgG	N.D.	+	α chain

N.D. signifies no determination. In each case the mRNA precipitated from the cytoplasmic poly (A) + RNA was equivalent to Band III RNA isolated from 5563 cells. In the cases where nuclear HnRNA has been examined, a component comparable to Band I was present (Premkumar et al., 1973).

VI. SPECIFICITY AND NATURE OF H_2L_2 INTERACTION WITH H-CHAIN mRNA

There is probably a conserved binding site for any H_2L_2 molecule on mRNA molecules coding for any H chain. This sweeping generalization is made on the basis of qualitative experiments using mouse myeloma cells synthesizing various classes and subclasses of immunoglobulin (Table II). In each case the homologous myeloma protein was used together with rabbit antibody against the myeloma protein to precipitate an RNA fraction which was shown to be H-chain mRNA by translation in oocytes (Premkumar et al., 1973). Cross-specificity experiments showed that the myeloma protein used to precipitate the H-chain mRNA did not need to be homologous. Moreover, mouse H-chain mRNA can also bind to rabbit immunoglobulin (see below). This cross-specificity between different classes of immunoglobulin and immunoglobulins of different species indicates a high degree of evolutionary conservation. An amino acid sequence must be conserved in the immunoglobulin molecules, and a presumably nontranslated nucleotide sequence must be conserved on all H-chain mRNA molecules.

The data collected so far are not sufficient to prove the opening statement of this section. However, we would be surprised if it were not justified by subsequent studies. Several fascinating questions are raised by this hypothesis. Among these are the nature of the RNA–protein interaction and the main function of the specific binding between H_2L_2 and H-chain mRNA. Experimentally we have shown that this interaction can play a role in translational control under conditions of a perturbed system in vitro. It may well be that translational control of H-chain production is also effected that way in vivo. The nature of the specificity of the binding site leads us to think of other possible roles for the interaction.

The initial experiments demonstrating the interaction between 5563 H_2L_2 and H-chain mRNA (Stevens and Williamson, 1973c) led us to think that the binding was relatively weak. More recently, however, we have measured the equilibrium binding constant for the interaction between rabbit IgG and 5563 H-chain mRNA using the method developed for studying lac repressor–operator interaction (Riggs et al., 1970a). The binding was found to be very tight ($K_{equilibrium} = 2 \times 10^{-13}$ M at 20°C and 150 mM Na$^+$). This protein–RNA interaction is therefore within the range of the lac and λ phage repressor–DNA interactions (10^{-13} M and 3×10^{-14} M respectively) (Riggs et al., 1970a,b; Chadwick et al., 1970).

An analogous translational control involving a protein–RNA interaction occurs with RNA coliphage. The phage coat protein binds at or near the initiation site for the RNA synthetase, thus limiting translation of that message (Kozak and Nathans, 1972). Sugiyama (1969) showed that MS2 coat protein at 6×10^{-7} M exerted its full repressor function on MS2 RNA (10^{-7} M). Although the complete sequence of MS2 coat protein gene and the initiation site for RNA synthetase are now available (Min Jou *et al.*, 1972), a model for the coat protein–RNA interaction has not been postulated.

A detailed model has been proposed for the binding of *lac* repressor to DNA (Adler *et al.*, 1972). This model makes the reasonable prediction that a linear sequence of amino acids in *lac* repressor interacts with a linear sequence of the operator DNA region. Following this prediction we scanned the currently available sequences of immunoglobulin H chains for linear peptide sequences that remain constant through all species. The longest stretch showing the required degree of invariance is one starting from Cys 425. The prototype sequence for this region is

$$(425)\ \text{Cys Ser Val Met His Glu Ala Leu His Asn }\genfrac{}{}{0pt}{}{\text{His}}{\text{Arg}}$$

The known variations in this sequence are shown in Table III. The occurrence of this highly conserved sequence at the C terminus of H chains is consistent with

Table III. Conservation of Amino Acid Sequence in Various H Chains

Species	H Chain	\- 425					430					435
	γ_1	C	S	V	M	H	E	A	L	H	N	H
	γ_2	–	–	–	–	–	–	–	–	–	–	–
Human	γ_3	–	–	–	–	–	–	–	–	–	–	R
	γ_4	–	–	–	–	–	–	–	–	–	–	–
	μ	–	V	–	A	–	–	–	–	P	B	R
Rabbit	γ	–	–	–	–	–	–	–	–	–	–	–
Guinea pig	γ_2	–	–	–	–	–	–	–	–	–	–	–
Dog	$\gamma_{A,B}$				–	–	–	–	–	–	B	–
	γ_D				–	–	–	–	–	Q	–	–
Horse	γ				–	–	–	–	–	–	–	–
	γ_T				–	–	–	–	V	E	–	–
Bovine	γ_1				–	–	–	–	–	–	–	–
	γ_2				–	–	Z	–	–	–	B	–

The prototype sequence is shown for human γ_1, and dashes indicate identity with this sequence. Variation is apparently permitted at position 433. Otherwise only isolated conservative changes have occurred. Sequence data is taken from Dayhoff (1969) with the addition that the sequence of human μ chain has been corrected from the data of Shimizu *et al.* (1971).

our model (Fig. 10) for $H_2 L_2$–H-chain mRNA interaction *in vivo*. This sequence would be exposed twice at the end of the Fc region to make contact with the mRNA. As with the tetrameric *lac* repressor, the availability of more than one binding site would be advantageous. This might require the existence of two identical repeating sequences in the mRNA. For an unambiguous binding site in mammalian DNA, about 16 nucleotides would be required. This could be (a) a unique single-stranded stretch of 16 nucleotides, (b) two identical repeats of single-stranded sequences of 8 nucleotides, (c) a double-stranded sequence of 8 base pairs, or (d) two identical repeats of double-stranded sequences of 4 base pairs each. Shorter double-stranded sequences are acceptable, because the complementary bases in an RNA hairpin loop are independently transcribed from DNA sequences. In view of the rather short region of H-chain amino acid sequence identified above as a possible binding site, the short double-stranded RNA sequences would provide a more suitably sized combining site on H-chain mRNA.

VII. CONCLUDING REMARKS

Myeloma cells have proven to be a most profitable system for the study of control mechanisms. The interaction between $H_2 L_2$ and H-chain mRNA has no precedent in eukaryotic cells.

These studies can be regarded in three different ways: (a) as a model for the flow of information from gene to protein in eukaryotic cells; (b) as a model for antibody-producing cells which must have specific controls on gene expression; and (c) as a model for a neoplastic cell in which controls may be found to vary in subtle ways when compared to normal cells.

The present information on the processing of the nuclear precursor of H-chain mRNA and the transport of the mRNA to the cytoplasm confirms and enhances the schemes devised from ingenious experiments on total mRNA (Jelinek *et al.*, 1973). Detailed studies are more easily performed on the specific mRNA since it can be identified at various stages either by the $H_2 L_2$ binding site and/or by translation in oocytes.

As a model for the immune response, myeloma cells may appear uninviting. However, the specific control of H-chain synthesis operating in myeloma cells could well play a role in the mechanism of antibody induction. In any case, the method afforded for the specific isolation and assay of H-chain mRNA should prove to be an invaluable tool in studies on the immune response. Because of the nature and specificity of H-chain mRNA–$H_2 L_2$ interaction, it can be used to probe either specific antigen-induced responses or broad-specificity mitogen-induced responses in immunocompetent cells.

The wealth of systems and methodologies now available for study of immune phenomena at a molecular level should place immunological research at the forefront of expanding knowledge of the molecular biology of eukaryotic cells.

REFERENCES

Adler, K., Beyreuther, E., Fanning, E., Geisler, N., Gronenborn, B., Klemm, A., Müller-Hill, B., Pfahl, M., and Schmitz, A., 1972, *Nature* 237: 322.
Aloni, Y., 1973, *Nature New Biol.* 243: 2.
Bevan, M. J., Parkhouse, R. M. E., Williamson, A. R., and Askonas, B. A., 1972 *Progr. Biophys. Mol. Biol.* 25: 131.
Blobel, G., 1972, *Biochem. Biophys. Res. Comm.* 47: 88.
Brownlee, G. G., Harrison, T. M., Mathews, M. B., and Milstein, C., 1972, *FEBS Lett.* 23: 244.
Chadwick, P., Pirrotta, V., Steinberg, R., Hopkins, N., and Ptashne, M., 1970, *Cold Spring Harbor Symp. Quant. Biol.* 34: 283.
Darnell, J., Wall, R., and Tushinski, R., 1971, *Proc. Nat. Acad. Sci. US* 68: 1321.
Dayhoff, M. O., 1969, *The Atlas of Protein Sequence and Structures,* Vol. 4, National Biomedical Research Foundation, Silver Spring, Md.
Delovitch, T. L., and Baglioni, C., 1973, *Proc. Nat. Acad. Sci. US* 70: 173.
Delovitch, T. L., David, B. K., Holme, G., and Sehon, A. J., 1972, *J. Mol. Biol.* 69: 373.
Delovitch, T. L., Boyd, S. L., Tsay, H. M., Holme, G., and Sehon, A. J., 1973, *Biochim. Biophys. Acta* 299: 621.
Edmonds, M., Vaughan, M. J., and Nakazato, H., 1971, *Proc. Nat. Acad. Sci. US* 68: 1336.
Fan, H., and Penman, S., 1970, *J. Mol. Biol.* 50: 655.
Gilbert, M., and Müller-Hill, B., 1967, *Proc. Nat. Acad. Sci. US* 58: 2415.
Greenberg, J. R., 1972, *Nature* 240: 102.
Gurdon, J., Lane, C., Woodland, H., and Marbaix, G., 1971, *Nature* 233: 177.
Hunt, T., Hunter, T., and Munro, A., 1969, *J. Mol. Biol.* 43: 123.
Jacob, F., and Monod, J., 1961, *J. Mol. Biol.* 3: 318.
Jelinek, W., Adesnik, M., Salditt, M., Sheiness, D., Wall, R., Molloy, G., Philipson, L., and Darnell, J. E., 1973, *J. Mol. Biol.* 73: 515.
Kozak, M., and Nathans, D., 1972, *Bacteriol. Rev.* 36: 109.
Kwan, S., and Brawerman, G., 1972, *Proc. Nat. Acad. Sci. US* 69: 3247.
Lane, C. D., Marbaix, G., and Gurdon, J. B., 1971, *J. Mol. Biol.* 61: 73.
Lee, S., Mendecki, J., and Brawerman, G., 1971, *Proc. Nat. Acad. Sci. US* 68: 1331.
Lodish, H., 1971, *J. Biol. Chem.* 246: 7131.
Mach, B., Faust, C. H., and Vassalli, P., 1973, *Proc. Nat. Acad. Sci. US* 70: 451.
Melli, M., and Pemberton, R., 1972, *Nature New Biol.* 236: 172.
Mendecki, J., Lee, Y., and Brawerman, G., 1972, *Biochemistry* 11: 792.
Milstein, C., Brownlee, G. G., Harrison, T. M., and Mathews, M. B., 1972, *Nature New Biol.* 239: 117.
Min Jou, W., Haegeman, M., Ysebaert, T., and Fiers,W., 1972, *Nature* 237: 82.
Molloy, G., Sporn, M. B., Kelley, D. E., and Perry, R. P., 1972, *Biochemistry* 11: 3256.
Morel, C., Kayibanda, B., and Scherrer, K., 1971, *FEBS Lett.* 18: 84.
Palmiter, R., 1972, *J. Biol. Chem.* 247: 6770.
Penman, S., Vesco, C., and Penman, M., 1968, *J. Mol. Biol.* 34: 49.
Premkumar, E., Stevens, R. H., and Williamson, A. R., 1973, in preparation.
Ptashne, M., 1967, *Nature* 214: 232.
Ralph, P., and Rich, A., 1971, *Biochemistry* 10: 4717.
Riggs, A. D., Suzuki, H., and Bourgeois, S., 1970a, *J. Mol. Biol.* 48: 67.
Riggs, A. D., Bourgeois, S. and Cohn, M., 1970b, *J. Mol. Biol.* 53: 401.
Shimizu, A., Paul, C., Köhler, H., Shinoda, T., and Putnam, F. W., 1971, *Science* 173: 629.
Soeiro, R., Vaughan, M. H., and Darnell, J. E., 1968, *J. Cell Biol.* 39: 112.
Stavnezer, J., and Huang, R-C. C., 1971 *Nature New Biol.* 230: 172.

Stevens, R. H., 1973, *Europ. J. Biochem.* **42:** 553.
Stevens, R. H., and Williamson, A. R., 1972 *Nature* **239:** 143.
Stevens, R. H., and Williamson, A. R., 1973a *Proc. Nat. Acad. Sci. US* **70:** 1127.
Stevens, R. H., and Williamson, A. R., 1973b, *J. Mol. Biol.* **78:** 505.
Stevens, R. H., and Williamson, A. R., 1973c, *J. Mol. Biol.* **78:** 516.
Sugiyama, T., 1969, *Cold Spring Harbor Symp. Quant. Biol.* **34:** 687.
Summers, D., Maizel, J., and Darnell, J., 1965, *Proc. Nat. Acad. Sci. US* **54:** 505.
Suzuki, Y., and Brown, D., 1972, *J. Mol. Biol.* **63:** 409.
Suzuki, Y., Gage, L., and Brown, D., 1972, *J. Mol. Biol.* **70:** 637.
Swan, D., Aviv, H., and Leder, P., 1972, *Proc. Nat. Acad. Sci. US* **69:** 1967.
Tonegawa, S., and Baldi, I., 1973, *Biochem. Biophys. Res. Commun.* **51:** 81.
Vassalli, P., Lisowska-Bernstein, B., and Lamm, M. E., 1971, *J. Mol. Biol.* **56:** 1.
Wall, R., and Darnell, J. E., 1971, *Nature New Biol.* **232:** 73.
Wall, R., Weber, J., Gage, Z., and Darnell, J. E., 1973, *J. Virol.* **11:** in press.
Williamson, A. R., and Askonas, B. A., 1967, *J. Mol. Biol.* **23:** 201.
Williamson, R., Drewienkiewicz, C. E., and Paul, J., 1973, *Nature New Biol.* **241:** 66.

The J Chain of Polymeric Immunoglobulins

F. P. Inman

Department of Microbiology
University of Georgia
Athens, Georgia

and

J. Mestecky

Department of Microbiology
Institute for Dental Research
University of Alabama Medical Center
Birmingham, Alabama

I. INTRODUCTION

The polypeptide chain structures and properties of immunoglobulins from both human serum and colostrum were compared in 1966 by Rejnek *et al.* and by Cederblad *et al.* After cleavage of disulfide bonds and subsequent analysis of isolated heavy (H) and light (L) chain fractions, an electrophoretically fast, anodally moving polypeptide became detectable in the light chain fraction of immunoglobulin derived from colostrum. When these fractions were analyzed by starch-block gel electrophoresis in urea at alkaline *p*H, the polypeptide appeared as a sharp, intensely stained band that preceded the electrophoresis banding pattern typical of L chains. Further characteristics of this polypeptide were not determined, and for a time its origin remained obscure. In 1967 Cebra and Small detected a similar polypeptide in secretory IgA isolated from rabbit milk. Because of the earlier findings of Tomasi *et al.* (1965), this polypeptide was termed T chain and was assumed to represent a part of an additional entity of S-IgA, a secretory component (SC). At this stage, human and rabbit S-IgA molecules were thought to consist of two 7 S molecules, each containing two α and two L chains, connected by SC that was composed of two T chains (Cebra,

111

1969; Small *et al.*, 1971). The reasoning behind this hypothesis was obvious: The research methods used revealed only H, L, and T chains, and the total molecular weights of the individual components corresponded to the molecular weight of the S-IgA molecule. The presence of T chain in serum myeloma IgA (Poulik, 1967) was assumed to result from the possible binding of SC to that type of IgA.

The findings of Halpern and Koshland (1970a,b) and Mestecky *et al.* (1971a,b) introduced a new conception of the structure of secretory and other polymeric immunoglobulins. Analysis of reduced rabbit S-IgA made it apparent that T chain (renamed J chain) was not a constituent of SC and that these chains are actually two different polypeptides. This fact was verified by the following observations: Both free and reduced SC had the same molecular weight and yielded no J chain after disulfide bond cleavage. J chain was present in serum polymeric immunoglobulins that contained no SC. The antigenic determinants, electroporetic mobility, and amino acid analysis of secretory component and J chain were different.

When the constituents of reduced and alkylated S-IgA were separated by gel filtration in the presence of dissociating agents, SC eluted with the α chains and J chain with the L chains (O'Daly and Cebra, 1971a; Mestecky *et al.*, 1972b). The common elution position of SC and α chain led to the erroneous assumption that only α, L, and J chains were components of S-IgA molecules. Further, a similarity in charge made it difficult to distinguish between SC and α chain when they were examined by disc electrophoresis at pH 9, or by immunoelectrophoresis at the same pH.

Halpern and Koshland (1970b) suggested that J chain is a component of polymeric but not monomeric IgA proteins and, therefore, might be involved in joining monomeric IgA molecules to form the corresponding polymers. J chain later was found in IgM molecules (Mestecky *et al.*, 1971b).

II. CLASS DISTRIBUTION

Of five human immunoglobulin classes, J chain has been detected by disc electrophoresis and/or by other immunochemical means in colostral, salivary, and serum polymeric IgA (Rejnek *et al.*, 1966; Cederblad *et al.*, 1966; Halpern and Koshland, 1970a, b; Metstecky *et al.*, 1971b; Mestecky *et al.*, 1972b; Poulik, 1967) and in macroglobulinemic IgM (Mestecky *et al.*, 1971a, b; Meinke and Spiegelberg, 1971; Morrison and Koshland, 1972; Kownatzki, 1971; Frangione *et al.*, 1971; Ricardo and Inman, 1973; Raam and Inman, 1973). Monomeric serum IgA (Halpern and Koshland, 1970a, b; Mestecky *et al.*, 1971b), IgG (Rejnek *et al.*, 1966; Cederblad *et al.*, 1966; Mestecky *et al.*, 1971b; Halpern and Koshland, 1970b), myeloma IgD (Mestecky *et al.*, 1972a) and IgE (Tomasi and Grey, 1972) were devoid of J chain. Unlike L chain, free J chain has not been detected in serum and urine of patients with Bence Jones protein (Mestecky *et al.*, 1972a). Meinke (1973) recently reported that from patients with multiple myeloma, two out of 100 urine samples exhibited trace amounts (1–5 μg/ml) of free J chain.

III. SPECIES DISTRIBUTION

A polypeptide which is released from polymeric IgA or IgM after cleavage of disulfide bonds and which has at least the electrophoretic characteristic of J chain has been detected in the following animals: rabbit (Cebra and Small, 1967; O'Daly and Cebra, 1971a,b; Halpern and Koshland, 1970a,b), dog (Kehoe *et al.* 1972), sheep (Heimer *et al.*, 1969), pig (Zikan, 1973), mouse (Underdown *et al.*, 1971; Halpern and Coffman, 1972; Parkhouse, 1972; Raam and Inman, 1973), pheasant (Weinheimer *et al.*, 1971), marine toad (Weinheimer *et al.*, 1971), catfish (Weinheimer *et al.*, 1971), and leopard shark (Klaus *et al.*, 1971). Although the electrophoretic characteristic strongly suggested its presence, more definite proof of J chain's association with these immunoglobulins was based on the demonstration of antigenic and chemical similarities between human J chain and that of other animals.

Kobayashi *et al.* (1973d) used rabbit antibodies to human J chain for detecting the polypeptide in completely reduced and alkylated polymeric immunoglobulins prepared from the following animals: dog (IgA and IgM), cat (mixture of IgA and IgM), cow (S-IgA and IgM), goat (S-IgA and IgM), sheep (mixture of S-IgA + IgM, and purified IgM), pig (S-IgA), horse (S-IgA and IgM), guinea pig (S-IgA and IgM), rat (IgA and IgM), mouse (IgA and IgM), hedgehog (mixture of IgA + IgM), and chicken (mixture of S-IgA + IgM). These investigations demonstrated that a protein which is antigenically related to human J chain is present in many mammals as well as in phylogenetically distant species.

Structural studies of J chains of animal origin are limited to the polypeptide isolated from rabbit (O'Daly and Cebra, 1971a), dog (Kehoe *et al.*, 1972), pig (Zikan, 1973), and mouse (Rosenstein and Jackson, 1973) polymeric immunoglobulins. The amino acid compositions of these J chains and their comparison with a human counterpart are presented in Table I. Most striking is that the composition of mouse J chain bears little resemblance to that of human J chain. This is surprising since the polyacrylamide gel electrophoretic migration of mouse and human J chains is similar (Parkhouse, 1972; Raam and Inman, 1973) and mouse J chain cross-reacts with antiserum to human J chain (Kobayashi *et al.*, 1973d). Additional amino acid composition analyses of mouse J chain are needed in order to verify this one.

Considerably less notable are the differences in amino acid composition of pig, dog, or rabbit J chain as compared to human J chain (Table I). These dissimilarities perhaps are more easily visualized by reference to the statistical

Table I. Comparative Amino Acid Compositions
(in residues per 1000) of J Chains

Amino acid	Human[a]	Pig[b]	Rabbit[c]	Dog[d]	Mouse[e]
Lys	45.6	56.9	43.4	24	76.9
His	8.3	18.2	13.8	8	29.6
Arg	73.6	49.4	56.6	68	35.5
Asp	165.8	168.4	144.1	168	88.8
Thr	99.3	83.2	97.9	84	59.2
Ser	66.8	64.7	84.5	76	82.8
Glu	116.3	127.2	99.8	128	142.0
Pro	63.9	40.9	70.5	60	53.3
Gly	19.3	19.7	47.7	40	82.8
Ala	46.8	45.4	44.5	48	88.8
Val	74.0	61.3	58.0	88	53.3
Met	7.2	8.4	7.4	20	11.8
Ile	51.1	62.4	53.4	48	29.6
Leu	60.1	80.9	70.4	60	88.8
Tyr	42.7	36.3	40.6	28	35.5
Phe	8.8	22.1	22.7	8	41.4
Cys	50.3	53.6	47.1	44	N.D.
Trp	0.0	N.D.[f]	N.D.	N.D.	N.D.

[a]Myeloma IgA (Mestecky et al., 1973a).
[b]Colostral IgA (Zikan, 1973).
[c]Colostral IgA (O'Daly and Cebra, 1971a).
[d]Myeloma IgA (Kehoe et al., 1972).
[e]Myeloma IgA (Rosenstein and Jackson, 1973).
[f]Not done.

analysis of the composition of human J_α chains given in Table IV. The most distinct variances from human J chain are pig (Arg, Glu, Val, and Leu), rabbit (Arg, Asp, Ser, Gly, and Val), and dog (Lys, Ser, Glu, Gly, and Tyr). In these animals' J chains, the characteristic composition of human J chain obviously is reflected.

It appears that J chains from various sources are highly similar polypeptides. The correspondence of electrophoretic mobility, antigenic cross-reactivity, and the equable content of amino acids indicates that few differences exist even between such phylogenetically distant species as man and shark (antigenic cross-reactivity; Koshland and Wilde, 1974). Primary sequence studies are necessary to support these extraordinary findings.

IV. DETECTION OF J CHAIN

The net charge difference between J and L chains allowed the detection of J chain by starch-block electrophoresis at alkaline pH (Rejnek et al., 1966;

Cederblad *et al.*, 1966). Samples of purified polymeric immunoglobulins had to be treated with agents that produced cleavage of disulfide bonds by reduction or oxidative sulfitolysis before J chain could be unmasked. This suggested that J chain is attached by disulfide bonds to the immunoglobulin molecules.

The same conclusions were reached when disc electrophoresis in polyacrylamide gel at alkaline *p*H was used in the presence of urea (Reisfeld and Small, 1966); J chain was seen as an intensely stained band(s) with fast anodic electrophoretic mobility (Fig. 1). The polypeptide could not be released solely by exposing immunoglobulin samples to dissociating agents such as urea, guanidine, or acetic acid.

Monospecific antisera to isolated J chain have been produced in several laboratories. For the preparation of anti-J-chain antiserum, the J-chain region of polyacrylamide gels may be homogenized in complete Freund's adjuvant and injected into animals (Mestecky *et al.*, 1971b; Raam and Inman, 1973). Alternatively, the antigen may be prepared by various chromatographic methods. The antisera obtained are often weak, probably because of the low molecular weight (*vide infra*) and the limited availability of the protein injected into the animals. Rabbits usually are used for immunization. They have their own J chain, however, that apparently is structurally similar to human J chain; there-

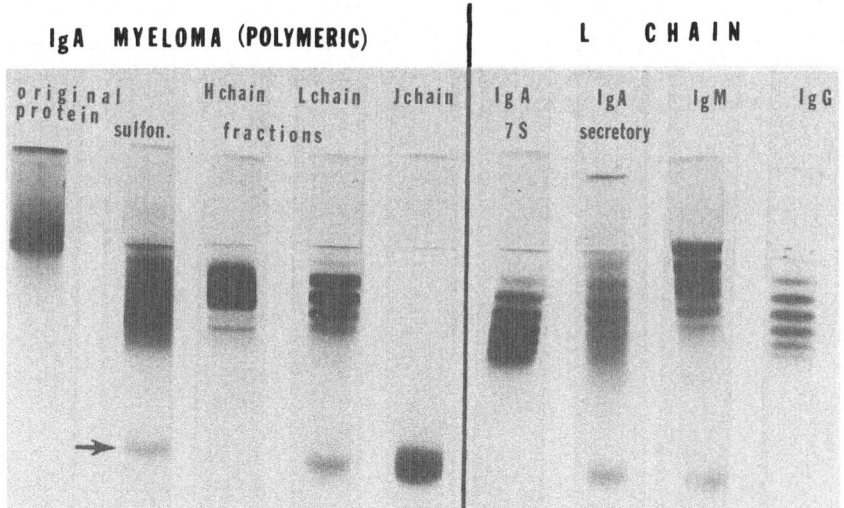

Figure 1. The detection of J chain by polyacrylamide disc electrophoresis (Reisfeld and Small, 1966) in 10 M urea, *p*H 9.4. J chain is not released from untreated polymeric IgA molecules (first gel), but becomes detectable as a protein with a fast electrophoretic mobility (arrow) when disulfide bonds are cleaved (second gel). After separation of heavy (H) and light (L) chains by gel filtration, J chain is coeluted with the latter fraction. L-chain fractions of monomeric IgA (7 S) and IgG lack J chain. It is present in secretory (colostrum) IgA and IgM.

fore, the injected J chain seems to be poorly immunogenic. Although easily detectable in reduced and alkylated or sulfonated immunoglobulins (Fig. 2), J chain is only rarely detectable in untreated immunoglobulins when examined by these antisera (Meinke, 1973; Mestecky *et al.*, 1972a; Morrison and Koshland, 1972; Kobayashi *et al.*, 1973b; Kownatzki, 1973a,b). Kobayashi *et al.* (1973b) reported that after the treatment of polymeric immunoglobulins with 8 M urea, 5 M guanidine, or 1 M propionic acid, the J-chain determinants became accessible. Moreover, presently available antibodies are directed against heavily denatured human J chain. The failure of antisera to give a precipitin reaction with native polymeric immunoglobulins might be explained by the inaccessibility of J chain epitopes, which are concealed in native unfolded molecules.

Kownatzki (1973b) has noted that the precipitation of J chain with certain antisera was dependent on alkylation with iodacetamide. A possibility that iodacetamide might act as a haptenic group in J chain alkylated with this agent and be responsible for production of antibodies that will cross-react with J chains from other sources was discussed by Kunkel (1974).

Morrison and Koshland (1972) and Kobayashi *et al.* (1973b) reported that untreated myeloma polymeric IgA and IgM from serum were able to inhibit the reaction between J chain and its antisera. No inhibition of precipitation was seen when human secretory IgA, bovine gamma globulin, IgGκ and IgGλ myeloma proteins, isolated α chain, and secretory component were substituted for intact polymeric IgA and IgM. These results indicated that most of the J-chain antigenic determinants are buried within the polymeric IgA and IgM molecules and are revealed after denaturation.

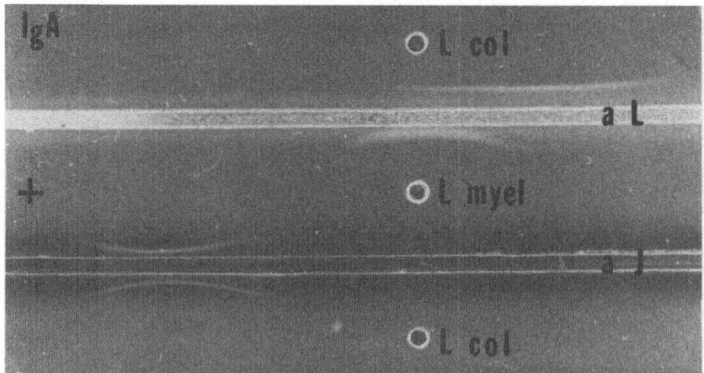

Figure 2. The detection of J chain by a monospecific anti-J chain (aJ) serum. Light-chain fractions of colostral IgA (L col) and polymeric myeloma IgA (L myel) were analyzed by immunoelectrophoresis. J chain is detected as an arc in the anodal portion of the slide. Antiserum to L chain (aL) does not react with J chain indicating the different antigenic determinants of L and J chains.

The antigenic identity of J chain derived from IgA and IgM has been documented (Mestecky *et al.*, 1971b; Morrison and Koshland, 1972; Meinke, 1973; Kobayashi *et al.*, 1973b; Raam and Inman, 1973). A rabbit antiserum to human J chain cross-reacted with both mouse and dog J chains (Meinke, 1973).

V. ISOLATION OF J CHAIN

Since J chain is covalently attached to polymeric IgA molecules and to IgM molecules by disulfide bridges, the first step leading to its isolation is treatment of the immunoglobulin with a disulfide-bond-cleaving agent. The reagents most frequently used are Na_2SO_3 and mercaptans.

When immunoglobulins are treated with Na_2SO_3, the disulfides are converted into S-sulfocysteine residues. Below pH 9, proteins with net negative charges react slowly, and those with net positive charges react rapidly (Cecil, 1963). Charged residues near a disulfide bond influence the rate of its reaction with the $SO_3^=$ ion. Sulfitolysis has been done in the presence of Cu^{++} which is an oxidizing agent. The overall reaction is

$$P-S-S-P' + 2SO_3^= + 2Cu^{++} \rightarrow P-S-SO_3^- + P'-S-SO_3^- + 2Cu^+$$

The S-sulfocysteine residues are stable products in neutral solution and the reaction is not readily reversible in the absence of mercaptans. Thus, a protein with an increased negative charge and in a form convenient to handle, results from sulfonation. In the procedure frequently used for sulfonation of IgM and IgA as a step in the preparation of J chains (Edelman and Marchalonis, 1967), the sulfite concentration is 0.25 M and the reaction is allowed to proceed for 24 hours. This probably is an excessively harsh procedure since a concentration of 0.014 M Na_2SO_3 permitted to react with human IgM (Gra) for 30 minutes caused release of all the J chain (Ricardo and Inman, 1973).

Mercaptans, especially dithiothreitol and 2-mercaptoethanol, also have been used to dissociate J chain from immunoglobulins. A concentration of dithiothreitol as low as 0.001 M was just sufficient to release J chains from a small portion of a population of IgA molecules, but 0.005 M resulted in a better yield (Mendez *et al.*, 1973). Higher concentrations frequently are used. When 2-mercaptoethanol is utilized to reduce IgA, the concentration of mercaptan usually is 0.1 M or 0.2 M (Kobayashi *et al.*, 1973a,b,c; Morrison and Koshland, 1972). Dithiothreitol (0.02 M) and 2-mercaptoethanol (0.2 M) were used by Kownatzki (1971) for reduction of IgM, and alkylation was with iodoacetamide. In these cases, each carboxamidomethylcysteine residue added a positive charge to the protein. Mercaptoethylamine also has been used to free the J chain from IgM (Ricardo and Inman, 1973). In this work, 0.024 M mercaptoethylamine was enough to allow dissociation of all J chains from the population of IgM (Gra) molecules.

The release of J chain after cleavage of disulfide bridges may be demon-strated by polyacrylamide gel electrophoresis at alkaline pH (Fig. 1), or by serological techniques (Fig. 2). In the former case, the high net negative charge which is attributed primarily to its amino acid composition (Table IV) allows the J chain to migrate electrophoretically much more rapidly anodally than the other components of treated immunoglobulin molecules. In the latter method, it has been found that specific anti-J-chain antiserum will precipitate J chain in treated IgM or IgA preparations.

A. Electrophoretic Methods

Small amounts of J chain can be eluted from sliced alkaline-urea polyacryla-mide gels by dialysis against distilled water or volatile buffers (Meinke and Spiegelberg, 1972a). The location of J chain is determined first by the compari-son with a stained gel from the parallel run. O'Daly and Cebra (1971a,b) used preparative acrylamide electrophoresis to separate rabbit J chain from the other components of totally reduced and alkylated S-IgA. The yield of J chain is restricted by the size of the acrylamide column. Some 50 mg of S-IgA was applied to the gels and the theoretical yield would not exceed 2–3 mg of J chain.

Kownatzki (1971) purified J chain from human IgM by use of zone electrophoresis on Pevikon in a barbital buffer at pH 8.6 and 0.05 ionic strength. The protein also has been prepared by polyacrylamide gel block electrophoresis (Ricardo and Inman, 1973). Tomasi and Hauptman (1974) pointed out that since α_1 antitrypsin and albumin have a similar electrophoretic mobility, J-chain preparations might be contaminated by them.

B. Ion-Exchange Chromatography

J chain can be isolated in somewhat larger quantities by DEAE-cellulose (or Sephadex) chromatography. The first isolation of J chain was achieved on DEAE-Sephadex equilibrated in 0.01 M phosphate buffer (pH 9) in the presence of 8 M urea. A linear gradient of 0.7 M NaCl was used for the elution of J chain (Mestecky et al., 1971b) (Fig. 3). S-sulfonated secretory IgA, or its L-chain fraction which contained J chain, was used as a starting material (Mestecky et al., 1971b, 1972a). J chain was eluted with approximately 0.4 M NaCl, whereas α and L chains and SC were eluted earlier.

Stepwise elution from DEAE-cellulose equilibrated in 0.01 M Tris-acetate buffer and 8 M urea was used by O'Daly and Cebra (1971a) to separate rabbit J chain from L chains. In these experiments, too, most of the J chain was eluted with a 0.4 M solution of NaCl. The initial concentration of salt can, therefore, be increased to eliminate the retention of polypeptides other than J chain. The chromatographic approach also was used successfully by Mendez et al. (1973)

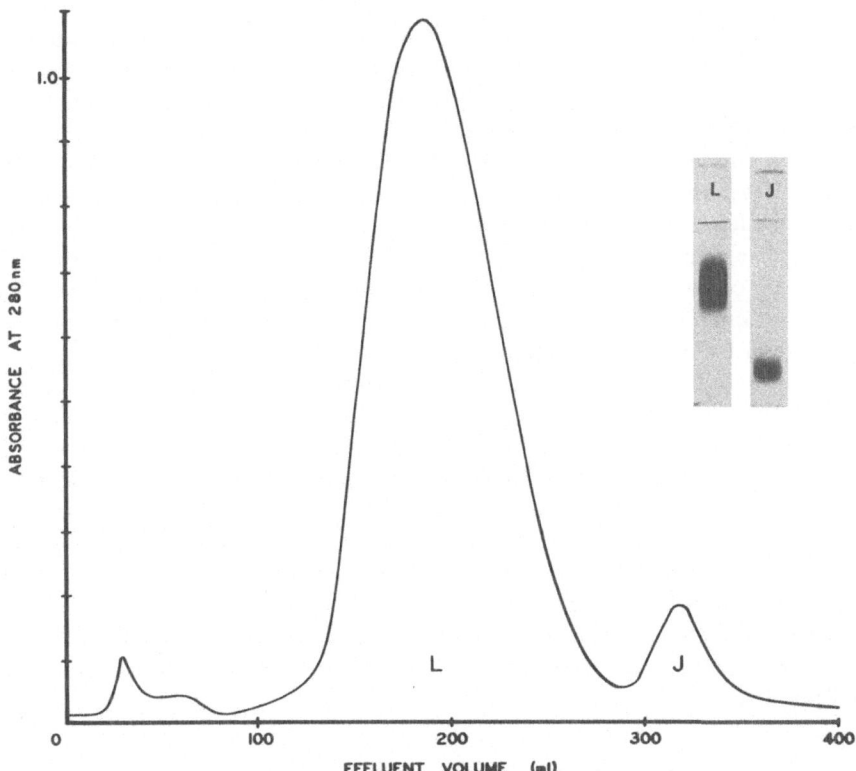

Figure 3. The separation of L and J chain by ion-exchange chromatography (Mestecky *et al.*, 1972a). The purity of both chains was examined by polyacrylamide disc electrophoresis (upper right corner).

and Zikan (1973) to isolate human and pig J chains. QAE-Sephadex equilibrated in carbonate-bicarbonate buffer with 6 M urea was employed for the purification of dog J chain (Kehoe *et al.*, 1972).

Although urea frequently is used during purifications of J chains, its presence is not always necessary. Kobayashi *et al.* (1973a) obtained J chain, by gel filtration and DEAE-cellulose chromatography of S-sulfonated serum IgA of both subclasses, S-IgA, and IgM in the absence of dissociating agents. Rosenstein and Jackson (1973) purified mouse J chain in the absence of urea also.

C. Other Methods

Morrison and Koshland (1972) separated J chain from L and α chains by use of immunosorbent columns of Sepharose 4B to which antisera to κ, λ, and α chains were conjugated. The mixture of polypeptide chains obtained after the reduction and alkylation of polymeric immunoglobulins was passed through the columns in a sequence that was dependent on the immunoglobulin source. Differences in the antigenic determinants of individual chains prevented the retention of J chain which was collected in the eluate.

A simplified procedure for J-chain preparation was reported by Kobayashi *et al.* (1974). Human polymeric IgA and IgM were totally reduced and alkylated and then dialyzed against aqueous solvents such as neutral buffers, saline, and distilled water. It was found that J chain remained soluble, whereas the major part of the H and L chains became insoluble and could be removed by centrifugation. Pure J chain was obtained after subsequent gel filtration on Sephadex G-100 in aqueous solvent.

The methods of preparation of J chain, both from IgA and IgM, have made it clear that there are no noncovalent associations of significance between J chain and the free 7 S immunoglobulin subunits (IgMs or IgA). When IgM is sulfonated or reduced, the molecule dissociates into IgMs molecules (Deutsch and Morton, 1957; Morris and Inman, 1968; Ricardo and Inman, 1973). Simultaneously, J chain is freed from its covalent attachment to the subunits. At low concentrations of Na_2SO_3 or mercaptoethylamine where not all the IgM is dissociated to IgMs, however, some of the J chain may remain covalently attached to IgMs (Ricardo and Inman, 1973). The amount of the attached polypeptide depends on reagent concentration but is less than 20% of the total available J chain.

VI. PHYSICAL-CHEMICAL PROPERTIES

A. Partial Specific Volume

The apparent partial specific volume of J chain was determined in 5 M guanidine-HCl using the polypeptide derived from the human IgM. The value was reported to be 0.710 ml/g (Table II). When the experiments were done on protein suspended in borate-saline (0.001 M sodium borate, 0.16 M NaCl) solution, *p*H 8, the partial specific volume was 0.719 ml/g. The value obtained from the amino acid and carbohydrate (assumed to be the same as that in J_α) compositions was 0.714 ml/g (Ricardo *et al.*, 1974). The partial specific volumes calculated from the chemical composition of human J_α chains were 0.705 ml/g (Schrohenloher *et al.*, 1973) and 0.710 ml/g (Wilde and Koshland, 1973) (Table II). For the rabbit J_α chain a value of 0.716 ml/g was calculated (O'Daly and Cebra, 1971a).

B. Molecular Weight

Of the several techniques used to determine the molecular weight of J chain from different sources, the paucity of the polypeptide has necessitated that the

TABLE II. Physical Properties of J Chains

Parameter	Value	Source	Reference
Partial specific volume			
$\bar{v}$	0.710 ml/g	human Waldenström IgM	Ricardo et al. (1974)
	0.714 ml/g	human Waldenström IgM	Ricardo et al. (1974)
	0.719 ml/g	human Waldenström IgM	Ricardo et al. (1974)
	0.705 ml/g	human myeloma IgA	Schrohenloher et al. (1973)
	0.710 ml/g	human myeloma IgA	Wilde and Koshland (1973)
	0.716 ml/g	rabbit colostral IgA	O'Daly and Cebra (1971a)
Molecular weight[a]	15,000	rabbit S-IgA	O'Daly and Cebra (1971a)
	15,600 ± 200	human myeloma IgA	Schrohenloher et al. (1973)
	15,000 ± 500	human myeloma IgA	Wilde and Koshland (1973)
	15,000	human myeloma IgA and IgM	Tomasi and Hauptman (1974)
	29,200[b]	human Waldenström IgM	Ricardo et al. (1974)
	15,200[b]	human Waldenström IgM	Ricardo et al. (1974)
Sedimentation velocity			
$S_{20,\,W}$	1.28×10^{-13} sec^{-1}	human myeloma IgA	Wilde and Koshland (1973)
$S_{20,\,W}^{0}$	2.49×10^{-14} sec^{-1}	human Waldenström IgM	Ricardo and Inman (unpublished)[c]
Axial ratio (minimum)	17.9	human myeloma IgA	Wilde and Koshland (1973)
Diffusion coefficient			
$D_{20,\,W}$	6.96×10^{-7} sec^{-1}	human myeloma IgA	Wilde and Koshland (1973)
Extinction coefficient			
$E_{275\ nm(max)}^{1\%\ 1\ cm}$	6.5	human myeloma IgA	Mestecky et al. (1973a)
$E_{278\ nm}^{1\%}$	7.0	human myeloma IgA	Wilde and Koshland (1973)

[a] Determined by ultracentrifugal methods.
[b] See Table III.
[c] See text.

majority of determinations be performed on polyacrylamide gels in the presence of sodium dodecylsulfate (SDS) (Weber and Osborn, 1969). Values obtained by this method have varied slightly according to the standards used. For human J_α chain, Morrison and Koshland (1972) reported 24,500 ± 1000, Kobayashi et al. (1973a) 24,000 ± 1200, Mestecky et al. (1973a) 25,700, and Mendez et al. (1973) 24,500.

By gel filtration through Sephadex G-100 or G-200, the molecular weight of J chain is dependent on the solvent used. Kobayashi et al. (1973a) confirmed the molecular weight of 48,000 for J_μ chains calculated by Kownatzki (1971) in Tris-buffers and in propionic acid. However, in the presence of 5 M guanidine or urea, J chain eluted in the L-chain fraction and the molecular weight was calculated to be 22,000 (Mestecky et al., 1973a).

With gel electrophoresis in SDS, O'Daly and Cebra (1971a) examined J chain isolated from rabbit S-IgA and reported the value of 22,500. When determined by equilibrium-sedimentation ultracentrifugation, however, the molecular weight of the identical protein in 5 M guanidine was estimated to be 15,000 (Table II). Human J_α chain analyzed under similar conditions exhibited an average molecular weight of 15,600 ± 200 (Schrohenloher et al., 1973) (Table II). The value was extrapolated to zero protein concentration and corrected according to the amino acid and carbohydrate analyses of this J chain. No lipids were detectable in the molecule (Tomana, unpublished observation). Wilde and Koshland (1973) used sedimentation analysis to determine the molecular weight of human J chain isolated from myeloma IgA. Under the conditions of their experiments, the molecular weight of 15,000 ± 500 was determined (Table II). The same preparation of J chain was examined by SDS disc electrophoresis and values previously reported (approximately 25,000) were obtained. The anomalous behavior of J chain in polyacrylamide gel and during gel filtration was explained by its elongated configuration (vide infra).

Molecular weight determinations have been done on J chains extracted from IgM. Mestecky et al. (1971b) treated Waldenström's IgM with Na_2SO_3 and isolated the light-chain component by filtration through Sephadex G-200 equilibrated in 5 M guanidine-HCl. They noted that J chains coeluted with light chains. By polyacrylamide gel electrophoresis in SDS, the molecular weight of the J chains was about 26,000.

Kownatzki (1971) treated Waldenström's IgM with 2-mercaptoethanol, and filtered the alkylated protein through Sephadex G-200 in a Tris-NaCl buffer to obtain J chain. The molecular weight determined by molecular sieving on Sephadex G-200 was approximately 48,000. When the weight was ascertained by SDS-polyacrylamide gel electrophoresis, however, it was 25,400.

Ricardo et al. (1974) prepared J chains from sulfonated Waldenström's IgM. The molecular weight of the purified protein was 27,000 when determined by

SDS-polyacrylamide gel electrophoresis. Some samples of J chain were suspended in 5 M guanidine-HCl for 2–21 days and the molecular weight was determined again. The protein in guanidine-HCl for two days still had a high molecular weight by the SDS-polyacrylamide gel electrophoretic method. Most of the protein suspended in guanidine-HCl for 21 days, however, dissociated into three rapidly migrating bands of apparent molecular weights 14,900, 14,500, and 14,300. The remainder of the protein appeared as a slowly migrating triplet, the component molecular weights of which were about 28,600, 26,200, and 24,000.

These data were substantiated by the determination of the molecular weight by sedimentation-equlibrium measurements (Ricardo *et al.*, 1974). The results are given in Table III. In borate-saline solution, the molecular weight was about 29,000. For protein suspended in 5 M guanidine-HCl for two or seven days (Table III, Experiments 3 and 4) the trend was for the molecular weight to decrease as the rotor speed increased. At higher rotor speeds the calculated

Table III. The Molecular Weights of J Chains as Determined by Ultracentrifugation[ab]

Experiment	Rotor speed (rev/min)	Solvent	pH of solvent	Period in solvent (days)	Minimum mol. wt.	Average mol. wt.
1	10,000	Borate-saline	8.0	2		29,766
2	36,000	Borate-saline	8.0	2		28,543
3	10,000	Gd · HCl	6.1	2	27,279	30,267
		Gd · HCl	6.1	7	22,467	26,714
4	14,125	Gd · HCl	6.1	2	25,017	28,308
		Gd · HCl	6.1	7	18,375	22,605
		Gd · HCl	6.1	14	15,410	21,301
5	16,130	Gd · HCl	5.6	2	23,083	26,543
		Gd · HCl	5.6	14	14,828	19,893
		Gd · HCl	8.0	14	15,132	19,945
6	20,060	Gd · HCl	5.6	2	22,165	24,636
		Gd · HCl	5.6	21	15,699	17,365
		Gd · HCl	8.0	2	21,318	23,973
		Gd · HCl	8.0	21	15,067	17,618
7	24,350	Gd · HCl	5.6	21	14,990	17,190
		Gd · HCl	8.0	28	15,320	17,248

[a] Ricardo *et al.*, 1974.

[b] J chains prepared from sulfonated human IgM were suspended for the periods indicated in borate-saline solution or in 5 M guanidine-HCl (Gd–HCl) solution. All molecular weight determinations of a given experiment were done with the same J-chain preparation and at the same rotor speed.

molecular weight increasingly reflects that of the smaller entities (Table III, Experiments 3–7). The lowest minimum molecular weights were first found in samples suspended in guanidine-HCl for 14 days (Table III, Experiments 4 and 5). The average of the lowest minimum molecular weights was 15,200, a value very close to that obtained by SDS-polyacrylamide gel electrophoresis.

It appears that human J chains have a tendency toward polymer formation in nondissociating buffers. The basic unit seems to have a molecular weight of about 15,000. Dimeric forms are apparently held strongly since complete dissociation does not occur in SDS (Mestecky *et al.*, 1971b; Kownatzki, 1971; Ricardo *et al.*, 1974), or even in guanidine-HCl (Ricardo *et al.*, 1974).

The sedimentation constant ($S_{20, w}^0$) of J_μ chains in a nondissociating solution was found to be $2.49S$ (Ricardo and Inman, unpublished data; Table II). As discussed above, the molecular weight of this protein in the same solution was 29,000 even though the minimum molecular weight of the dissociated protein was about 15,000 (Tables II and III). The sedimentation constant, then, must represent the dimeric form. A sedimentation coefficient ($S_{20,w}$) of 1.28 $\times 10^{-13}$ sec^{-1} was reported for J_α chains (Wilde and Koshland, 1973) (Table II). The concentration of the latter protein was so low that this coefficient must approach the sedimentation constant for J_α chains. The molecular weight of the J_α chains in nondissociating solvent, as determined by sedimentation-equilibrium analysis, was about 15,000 and therefore 1.28 S must be close to the sedimentation constant of the monomeric form of J_α chain. Because of the tendency for both J_α and J_μ chains to polymerize, this may be an unusual form of J_α chain. Considering their similar amino acid compositions alone (Table IV; *vide infra*), there seems to be no overt reason to expect physical differences between J_α and J_μ chains.

C. Shape

The minimum axial ratio of J_α chains was reported to be 17.9 (Wilde and Koshland, 1973) (Table II). This indicates an unusually linear molecule. Its content of aspartic acid, glutamic acid, threonine, arginine, and proline reduces the likelihood of extensive stabile α-helix conformation. If the protein were totally α-helical. however, its length could be about 180 Å.

It also was concluded that J_μ chains, in the dimeric form (*vide supra*), are more linear than globular in shape (Inman, 1974). The circumference of the Fc5μ region is approximately 270 Å (Metzger, 1970). Thus the J_μ chains could not function as the bracelet in the model of Wilde and Koshland (1973). In a form containing only a limited amount of α-helical configuration, however, the influence of J chain on the noncovalent association of IgMs molecules may be greater than is currently recognized.

There are no published data which allow one to describe the folding of J chain. How the cysteine residues function will have an influence on this. For example, if the clasp model (Wilde and Koshland, 1973) is correct, only two of the cysteine molecules are needed for covalent attachment of J_μ to the rest of the IgM molecule. The other cysteines probably are engaged in intrachain disulfide bonds which would force some rigidity and folding on the protein.

Some additional physical-chemical data are given in Table II. The diffusion coefficient of J_α chains was reported to be 6.96×10^{-7} sec^{-1} (Wilde and Koshland, 1973). The extinction coefficient was given as 7.0 (Wilde and Koshland, 1973) or 6.53 (Mestecky *et al.*, 1973a; Barth *et al.*, 1972).

VII. CHEMICAL COMPOSITION

Halpern and Koshland (1970b) reported the first indication of the unique amino acid composition of J chain. The comparison of L-chain fractions from rabbit IgG and S-IgA indicated differences in the amount of arginine, aspartic acid, serine, glycine, alanine, valine, and isoleucine. This was confirmed after the isolation of J chain from human S-IgA and IgM proteins (Mestecky *et al.*, 1971b; Kownatzki, 1971; Morrison and Koshland, 1972; Mestecky *et al.*, 1973a). A contrasting of the amino acid compositions (expressed in residues per 1000) of H, L, and J chain indicated a higher content of aspartic acid, cysteine, isoleucine, and arginine in J chain, whereas the content of serine, glycine, alanine, leucine, and phenylalanine is lower. A comparison of the amino acid contents of J_α chain from various species' proteins is given in Table I.

Although there are several published analyses of J_α chains, similar analyses of J_μ chains are limited. Enough data are available on J_μ chains, however, that one may compare the contents of J chains derived from human IgA and IgM (Table IV). It is evident that the two chains have very similar compositions in terms of amino acid residues per 1000 residues. Based on a molecular weight of 15,000, Wilde and Koshland (1973) found the J_α chain comprised 119 amino acids, excluding tryptophan. The amount of the latter amino acid in J chains was reported as zero (Barth *et al.*, 1972). Assuming for convenience that the number of residues per mole is 120 (refer to end of this section), the compositions may be converted from residues per thousand to residues per mole as shown in Table IV. From these computations, the similarities in composition are clearly evident. The cysteine content is especially important, the apparent number being six. Also, there is one methionine residue.

The utilization of the cysteine residues for interchain and intrachain disulfide bridges is an especially important question. A good argument for the union of one J chain by two disulfide bridges, one to each of two IgMs molecules or 7 S IgA molecules, has been given (Wilde and Koshland, 1973). The information responsible for this concept was derived from J_α chains in which all disulfide bonds had been broken during preparation. The critical experiment with IgM

Table IV. Amino Acid Composition of J_α and J_μ Chains

Amino acid	$J_\alpha{}^a$ Average residues per 1000 residues[c]	$J_\alpha{}^a$ Average residues per 120 residues	$J_\mu{}^b$ Average residues per 1000 residues	$J_\mu{}^b$ Range	$J_\mu{}^b$ Average residues per 120 residues
Lys	46.2 ± 2.8	5.5	45.2	8.2	5.4
His	10.0 ± 2.4	1.2	8.9	1.6	1.1
Arg	71.0 ± 4.3	8.5	75.4	5.9	9.1
Asp (asx)	159.5 ± 8.2	19.1	165.3	7.8	19.8
Thr	90.9 ± 6.3	10.9	90.1	6.3	10.8
Ser	60.9 ± 10.2	7.3	57.7	13.9	6.9
Glu (glx)	110.3 ± 4.9	13.2	115.7	13.7	13.9
Pro	69.7 ± 4.4	8.4	66.3	9.9	8.0
Gly	24.3 ± 8.5	2.9	21.8	2.3	2.6
Ala	43.6 ± 5.6	5.2	46.6	6.0	5.6
Val	72.7 ± 5.0	8.7	71.1	21.7	8.5
Met	6.1 ± 1.7	0.7	6.7	2.4	0.8
Ile	62.5 ± 4.6	7.5	59.3	22.6	7.1
Leu	64.1 ± 2.3	7.7	65.4	4.5	7.9
Tyr	42.2 ± 2.7	5.1	42.2	6.0	5.1
Phe	15.1 ± 4.0	1.8	11.8	3.9	1.4
CM-C² total[d]	53.2 ± 7.9	6.4	49.3[e]	11.7[e]	5.9[e]
Cysteine	50.7 ± 1.2[f]	6.1[f]	50.6[g]		6.1[g]

[a] A total of 8 amino acid compositions reported for J_α were corrected to number of residues per 1000 residues and averaged. The sources of the original data were Wilde and Koshland (1973), O'Daly and Cebra (1971a), Mestecky et al. (1971b), Schrohenloher et al. (1973), Mestecky et al. (1972a), and Morrison and Koshland (1972).

[b] A total of 3 amino acid compositions reported for J_μ chains were used for the compilations. The sources of the original data were Mestecky et al. (1971b), Kownatzki (1971), and Morrison and Koshland (1972).

[c] Confidence limits (95%) were calculated from the range according to Dean and Dixon (1951).

[d] Carboxamidomethylcysteine or carboxymethylcysteine. Reduction was stated or was assumed to be complete. The data were calculated from five reported determinations.

[e] Only two analyses reported.

[f] Only three analyses reported.

[g] Only one analysis reported.

molecules, which remains to be reported, is one in which disulfide bond disruption is restricted to the postulated J–μ bonds. Alternatively one might attempt the isolation of the hypothetical IgMs dimer ([IgMs]$_2$J). It may be possible to satisfy one or both of these suggestions by utilizing the technique of limited reduction of IgM with mercaptoethylamine to prepare the J_μ chains (Ricardo and Inman, 1973). The number of labeled cysteine residues in those J_μ chains probably would be less than the six residues (Table IV) of completely reduced J_μ chains. Judicious use of mercaptoethylamine (Morris and Inman, 1968) might enable one to produce and isolate the IgMs dimer. Although present evidence favors a "clasp" model (Wilde and Koshland, 1973), additional investigations are needed to help allay any doubts as to its correctness.

Thus far, information concerning the primary structure of J chain is limited to analyses of cysteine-containing peptides and knowledge of the N- and C-terminal amino acids. By enzymatic fractionation of reduced and alkylated J chain, eight cysteine-containing peptides were obtained by Mendez *et al.* (1973). After purification, amino acid analysis, and partial sequencing, these peptides were found to differ from those derived from H and L chains. The apparent number of cysteine residues (8) was higher by one or two than those found in previously analyzed J chains (Mendez *et al.*, 1972; Mestecky *et al.*, 1973a; Koshland and Wilde, 1974) (Table IV). This discrepancy might be attributed to association of polymeric serum myeloma IgA with some other proteins (Tomasi and Hauptman, 1974) that coeluted with J chain during its purification. The intra-J-chain distribution of the cysteine-containing peptides is unknown except for one that contains an unreactive N-terminal group (PCA—pyrrolidonecarboxylic acid). The blocked N terminus for J chains isolated from human IgA and IgM previously was reported by Meinke and Spiegelberg (1972a,b). These investigators also isolated a glycopeptide following subtilin digestion of J chain derived from either class of immunoglobulin. The amino acid composition of this glycopeptide differed from glycopeptides originating from α_1 and μ chains. The C-terminal amino acid was determined by Zikan (unpublished results) as aspartic acid.

One methionine residue is present near the C-terminal end (Mestecky *et al.*, 1973b; 1974a). Cyanogen bromide cleavage does not appreciably diminish the molecular weight of J chain, and a homoserine residue which results from methionine conversion is associated with the main peptide. A small C-terminal peptide released by cyanogen bromide treatment of J chain contained 13–18 amino acids, namely 2–3 aspartic acid, 2–3 threonine, 1–2 glutamic acid, 2–3 proline, 2–3 alanine, 1 valine, 1 leucine, 1 tyrosine, and 1 cysteine residues. The cysteine residue evidently is involved in an intra-J-chain disulfide bridge, because the C-terminal peptide was released only after disulfide bond disruption subsequent to treatment with cyanogen bromide (Mestecky *et al.*, 1974a).

Analyses of human J chain isolated from S-IgA and serum IgA have revealed that both chains contain approximately 7.6% carbohydrate (Table V). Fucose, mannose, galactose, glucosamine, and sialic acid were detected in the amounts indicated in Table V(Niedermeier *et al.*, 1972; Tomana *et al.*, 1972).

When the results of amino acid and carbohydrate analyses are related to the molecular weight, it follows that human J chain is composed of 118–125 amino

Table V. Carbohydrate Composition J_α Chain[a]

Carbohydrate	Percentage	Residues per chain[b]
Fucose	0.34 − 0.38	1
Mannose	2.13 − 2.27	2
Galactose	1.27 − 1.61	1−2
Glucosamine	1.93 − 2.72	2−3
Galactosamine	0.00	0
Sialic acid	1.11 − 1.42	1
Total	7.6 (average)	7−9

[a] Human myeloma and colostral IgA (Niedermeier et al., 1972).
[b] Based on molecular weight 15,600 (Schrohenloher et al., 1973) and corrected for losses due to fractionation procedures (Tomana et al., 1972).

acid residues (Mestecky et al., 1973a; Wilde and Koshland, 1973) and 7−8 carbohydrate residues (Mestecky et al., 1973a).

VIII. STOICHIOMETRY

It was important from a structural point of view to determine the number of J chains in different polymeric immunoglobulins. Quantitation of the amount of J chain has been attempted by several methods that were based on ascertaining the proportion of J to L chains, differential amino acid analyses, and yield of J chain. When polypeptide chains of totally sulfonated or reduced and alkylated secretory IgA, serum IgA, and IgM were separated on a Sephadex G-200 column equilibrated in 5 M guanidine-HCl, J chains eluted together with L chains. After this, J chains separated from L chains during polyacrylamide gel disc electrophoresis at alkaline pH. By scanning the stained gels, one could roughly estimate the proportions of both chains. When it was assumed that an 11 S S-IgA contained 4 L chains and 19 S IgM contained 10 L chains per molecule, scanning experiments revealed the presence of one molecule of J in both IgA and IgM (Mestecky et al., 1972a,b).

In another case, human IgM was dissociated with Na_2SO_3 and subjected to polyacrylamide gel electrophoresis (Ricardo and Inman, 1974). The gels were stained with Coomassie Blue and then scanned. The J-chain band accounted for 3.3% of the total absorbance. Although the molecular weight of these J_μ chains was 15,000, they existed as dimers in nondissociating solvent (Table II) (Ricardo et al., 1974). Taking the molecular weight of IgM as 900,000 (Miller and Metzger, 1965), and the amount of J chain as 3.3%, the data suggested the possibility that there may be two J chains per IgM molecule.

Data derived from quantitative analyses of stained proteins may be criticized, because it has not been shown that α and μ chains, light chains, and J chains absorb the dye proportionally. The slower migrating proteins (α chain, μ chain, and light chain forms) also are less well separated and more compact than the J chain, and this may interfere with absorption of the dye.

O'Daly and Cebra (1971a) made a more precise determination of the proportion of individual polypeptides in rabbit S-IgA. Totally reduced and radioalkylated chains of S-IgA were separated by analytical polyacrylamide gel electrophoresis. Relative concentrations of S-carboxymethyl cysteine in J and L chains were then related to the molecular weight and amino acid composition of the respective chains. It appeared that no more than one J chain could occur in each S-IgA molecule.

Koshland and Wilde (1974) based their calculations of the stoichiometry of J chain on the large differences in the amount of seven amino acids that appeared in J and L chains. A single J chain was found in both dimeric and tetrameric forms of S-IgA. By alkylating totally reduced IgM with radioactively labeled iodoacetic acid, the amount of J chain was calculated from the ^{3}H-carboxymethylcysteine contents in μ, L, and J chains. One J chain per pentameric molecule was discerned. It should be pointed out that in all methods used thus far, determination of J-chain stoichiometry requires the assumption of an even distribution of J chain in the population of the molecules of polymeric immunoglobulins.

IX. SITE OF J-CHAIN ATTACHMENT

To substantiate the hypothesis that J chain joins 7 S subunits of polymeric immunoglobulins, it was necessary to establish the site of its attachment. To obtain this information, human polymeric immunoglobulins were enzymatically cleaved by trypsin at temperatures of 50–60°C (Plaut and Tomasi, 1970). Secretory IgA (Mestecky et al., 1971a; Zikan et al., 1972) and serum IgM (Meinke and Spielgelberg, 1971; Mestecky et al., 1971a; Putnam et al., 1972; Inman and Ricardo, 1974) have been hydrolyzed by this method. Fab, F(ab)₂, and polymeric Fc fragments were produced and subsequently isolated. It was reported that J chain was absent from the Fab and F(ab)₂ fragments and present in Fc fragments. Satisfactory proteolytic digestion of S-IgA is more difficult to achieve because this type of immunoglobulin is highly resistant to enzymatic cleavage. At the elevated temperature, however, sufficient amounts of F(ab)₂ and Fab fragments were produced so that they could be analyzed for J chain.

Further information as to the approximate site of J-chain attachment was obtained through studies of proteins that were isolated from patients who had α-chain disease or aberrant IgA myeloma proteins with the deletion in the C-terminal part of the α chain (Seligman and Mihaesco, 1974; Grey et al., 1974).

The α-chain proteins, composed of the Fc portion of the α chain and a variable length of the Fd fragment, were found to be associated with J chain. On the contrary, human IgA1 myeloma protein with the deletion in the C-terminal portion of the α chain (100 amino acids) was found exclusively in a monomeric form and was devoid of J chain. These data indirectly imply that J chain is covalently attached to the C-terminal end of the α chain (Grey et al., 1974).

A precise localization of J-chain attachment to the α chain was ascertained by cyanogen bromide cleavage of different myeloma proteins that contained J chain (Mestecky et al., 1974a,b; Franklin, 1974). Peptides released by this treatment exhibited characteristics by which it was established that J chain is attached by disulfide bonds to the penultimate cysteine residue(s) of the α chain. This portion of α chain has been sequenced by Prahl et al. (1971) and by Chuang et al. (1973). It has not yet been definitely resolved whether J chain is connected to one or two α chains of each 7 S IgA in the polymer.

The disulfide bonds involved in linkage of the IgMs molecules in IgM are located on the μ chains in the Fc region (Putnam et al., 1972). The sites of attachment of J chain in IgM molecules have not been defined clearly. It has not been proven, for example, that J chains are attached to each of the ten μ chains of IgM. Indeed, Wilde and Koshland (1973) have offered an alternative model where J chain is attached only to two μ chains and each of these derives from separate IgMs subunits. The best one has done is to define the region of IgM with which J chains are associated.

Highly purified Fc5μ fragments were prepared from human IgM by digestion with trypsin (Inman and Ricardo, 1974). The Fcμ units were covalently attached in the high-molecular-weight fragment. J chain was not detected by polyacrylamide gel electrophoresis of the fragment. When treated with mercaptoethylamine, however, the 11.7 S fragment dissociated to 3.4 S particles and J chains were then disclosed by polyacrylamide gel electrophoresis. These data indicated that the J chain is covalently attached to the IgM molecule in the Fc5μ region. The cysteine residues most likely to be involved are those associated with pentamer formation.

X. THE REQUIREMENT FOR J CHAIN BY IgM MOLECULES

To ask if J chain is a required component of the IgM molecule is a cogitative question. The examined 19 S immunoglobulin of most species has contained a polypeptide which seemed to be similar to J chain of human IgA molecules. The macroglobulin of the paddlefish and the gar, however, reportedly did not contain J chain (Weinheimer et al., 1971). Additionally, J chain was absent in the macroglobulin of the nurse shark (Weinheimer et al., 1971) but it was associated with the 19 S immunoglobulin of the leopard shark (Klaus et al., 1971).

A similar situation may be found among human IgM molecules, too. For example, in a population of Waldenström's IgM, a portion appeared not to contain J chain, while the remainder did (Kownatzki, 1973d). Furthermore, J chains were reported to be totally lacking in the monoclonal IgM purified from one patient (Eskeland and Brandtzaeg, 1974). Until these discrepancies are resolved, one cannot state that all human IgM molecules have an obligatory requirement for J chain.

It has been postulated that the J chain may influence the polymerization of IgMs molecules to IgM (Morrison and Koshland, 1972; Ricardo and Inman, 1973). Several investigators have attempted to study polymerization with experiments done *in vitro*. It recently was demonstrated that 0.024 M mercapto-ethylamine was sufficient to dissociate a Waldenström's IgM 100% to IgMs (Ricardo and Inman, 1973). Molecules treated in this way seemed to retain most of their intrasubunit interchain disulfide bridges. When the protein was allowed to reoxidize, about 40% sedimented in a manner characteristic of the native IgM (Ricardo and Inman, 1974). Most (75%) of the reassembled IgM did not dissociate when suspended in guanidine-HCl solution.

Nondissociable reassembled IgM was treated with trypsin to produce Fc5μ fragments. After reduction of the purified fragment, J chain was detected by polyacrylamide gel electrophoresis. Further, J chain was similarly detected in the reassembled IgM, and based on densitometric measurements of stained gels, the amount was nearly the same as that found in the native IgM (Ricardo and Inman, 1974).

These data testify that J chain will reassociate with IgMs molecules during *in vitro* assembly of IgM apparently to the same extent that it is in native IgM. In addition, the J chain reincorporates covalently in the Fc5μ region (Inman and Ricardo, 1974). It is not known if the J chain reattaches to the 7 S subunits exactly in the same way it is bound in the native protein.

The results of these experiments do not answer the basic query of whether J chain is required for reassembly of IgMs molecules into native-like IgM. Additional attempts to investigate its role, however, have been made (Kownatzki, 1972, 1973c; Wilde and Koshland, 1972; Schrohenloher and Mestecky, 1973). In one report, Waldenström's IgM was treated with 0.02 M dithiothreitol, and virtually all intersubunit and interchain disulfide bonds were disrupted (Kownatzki, 1973c). J chains were separated from the noncovalently associated IgMs molecules by gel filtration. Reassociation of IgMs molecules in the absence or in the presence of J chains was then permitted. Large polymers were formed in both experimental systems. No data were given to establish that J chain, when present in the experimental system, was incorporated into the polymers. Further, it was not proven that any polymers were constructed like native IgM. The implication of the first criticism is self-evident. The latter point is important because higher polymers produced by reoxidation of IgMs in which there is considerable loss of intrasubunit interchain disulfide bond fidelity may not be structurally like native IgM (Mukkur and Inman, 1971).

Eskeland and Harboe (1973) prepared 7 S IgM from the serum of a patient whose 19 S IgM lacked J chain (Eskeland and Brandtzaeg, 1974). After reduction of 19 S IgM a substantial amount of repolymerization occurred but when the 7 S IgM was treated similarly there was little polymerization. Reassociation of the 7 S IgM did take place when 7 S and 19 S IgM were mixed together, reduced, and reassociated. The authors concluded that the presence of J chain should not be regarded as a requirement for the polymerization of IgM.

Some very elegant experiments were recently reported by Della Corte and Parkhouse (1973b). IgM secreted by mouse tumor cells was depolymerized by reduction. Complete covalent reassociation took place only in the presence of added J chains and disulfide-exchanging enzyme. Further, after reduction in the presence of added J chain, secreted 7 S IgM completely polymerized to 19 S IgM when the enzyme was added to the mixture. Both enzyme and J chain were essential for polymerization. J chain did become associated with repolymerized IgMs to the same extent that it was found in the native IgM.

At this time there are so few reports of human IgM molecules lacking J chains that their significance is difficult to assess. The molecules studied may be unique in not reflecting true IgM structure. Alternatively, there may be two classes of IgM, only one of which may require J chain for polymerization. It seems advisable, therefore, to screen many preparations of IgM, normal as well as paraprotein, for the presence or absence of J chain.

XI. CELLULAR ORIGIN OF J CHAIN

The basic components of all immunoglobulins (H and L chains) are produced and assembled in lymphoid cells distributed throughout the body. The only exception seems to be the molecule of secretory IgA that is a product of two different cell types: the polymeric IgA molecule is a product of subepithelial plasma cells, whereas the secretory component is produced and acquired during the passage of IgA between and/or through epithelial cells that line mucosal surfaces (Tomasi and Bienenstock, 1968; Tourville et al., 1969). The SC is attached by disulfide bonds. It was, therefore, pertinent to investigate the possibility that J chain is added to the molecules of polymeric immunoglobulins during intracellular biosynthesis. Alternatively, its incorporation could be similar to that of SC and occur after the cells have secreted the immunoglobulin.

O'Daly and Cebra (1971b) stained rabbit lymph nodes, spleen, and intestinal tissue with fluorochrome-labeled anti-J-chain serum. J chain was found in plasma cells of these organs and its distribution in the small intestine was similar to that of the α chain. Radl et al. (1974) studied doubly labeled bone marrow cells from patients with multiple myeloma and Waldenström's macroglobulinemia. J chain was present in the same cell that secreted IgA or IgM, and in two cases L chains only were present. No J chain was detectable in cells that produced IgG, monomeric IgA, or IgD. The fluorescence was most pronounced at the rim of these cells and also in the Golgi apparatus. These results may indicate that J chain is incorporated into the polymeric immunoglobulin molecules either at the time of the secretion or during the assembly in the Golgi apparatus. No J-chain determinants were found on the membrane of IgA-producing cells (Hijmans *et al.*, 1974).

Conclusive evidence of the cellular origin of J chain was obtained by biosynthetic studies on murine plasmacytomas (Parkhouse, 1972; Halpern and Coffman, 1972; Raam and Inman, 1973). MOPC 104E cells or TEPC 183 cells were incubated with radioactive leucine and the purified secreted IgM was examined for J chains. In both cases, labeled J chains were found associated with the secreted IgM. The intracellular IgMs from TEPC 183 cells was devoid of J chains (Parkhouse, 1972). These observations showed that J chain is made by the cells which synthesized the μ and light chains, but they did not provide information on the mechanism or site of polymerization.

A direct demonstration of the intracellular presence of J chains was made with cells of the murine plasmacytomas HPC 76 (Raam and Inman, 1973). The detected J chains existed free of covalent attachment to other proteins. The results of these experiments established that J chains are to be found intracellularly and that they are not all attached to membranes or to other protein molecules.

XII. THE ASSEMBLY OF POLYMERIC IMMUNOGLOBULINS

A. Assembly of IgA

The synthesis and assembly of different immunoglobulins has been studied extensively in several laboratories (Askonas and Scharff, 1971; Askonas and Williamson, 1968; Melchers, 1972; Sherr *et al.*, 1971; Scharff and Laskov, 1970). Most of the studies were performed on human and murine plasma cell tumors.

The immunoglobulin molecules are assembled intracellularly from separately produced H and L chains. Several pathways of construction have been described that precede the appearance of a product consisting of a covalently bonded H_2L_2 molecule with carbohydrate attached (Baumal *et al.*, 1971a). Intermediates of assembly are composed of either dimerized H chains (H_2) or of H and L chains (HL). Schematically expressed, the pathway of covalent assembly would be as follows: $H + H \rightarrow H_2$; $H_2 + L \rightarrow H_2L$; $H_2L + L \rightarrow H_2L_2$. Alternatively, $H + L \rightarrow HL$; $HL + HL \rightarrow H_2L_2$ (Baumal *et al.*, 1971a,b; Askonas and Williamson, 1968; Parkhouse, 1971a; Bargellesi *et al.*, 1972; Sutherland *et al.*, 1970).

Carbohydrate moieties are appended to the molecules at the different stages of immunoglobulin biosynthesis. Glucosamine and mannose are added at an early stage of intracellular transport, whereas fucose and galactose are attached at the time when immunoglobulin leaves the cell (Sherr *et al.*, 1971; Melchers, 1971).

Immunoglobulins that occur in a polymeric form outside of the cell are present intracellularly in a prevalently monomeric form, although a small proportion of intracellular immunoglobulin also occurs in a polymeric form (Parkhouse and Askonas, 1969; Matsuoka *et al.*, 1970; Buxbaum *et al.*, 1971; Parkhouse, 1971b; Askonas and Parkhouse, 1971; Grey *et al.*, 1971; Bargellesi *et al.*, 1972; Melchers, 1972; Radl *et al.*, 1974). The final assembly of IgA into the polymeric form must take place just before or during the secretion of the immunoglobulin from the cell rather than occurring extracellularly in body fluids. This point was clarified by studies on secretory IgA (Lawton and Mage, 1969; Bienenstock and Strauss, 1970). Several factors that include carbohydrates, J chain, and an enzyme that catalyzes disulfide bond interchange reactions have been considered as essential for final polymerization of these immunoglobulins.

The most recent results from Parkhouse's laboratory (Parkhouse and Della Corte, 1973, 1974; Della Corte and Parkhouse, 1973a,b; Parkhouse, 1973) indicated that the J chain is essential to and plays a controlling role in polymerization. Mouse tumor cells secreting either IgA or IgM were employed in this research. These investigations examined the rate of incorporation and the content of radioactively labeled leucine, mannose, galactose, and fucose into extracellular and intracellular IgA and concluded that the polymerization was unlikely to be controlled by the carbohydrate content and composition. However, the polymerization of both intracellular and extracellular monomeric IgA, as well as repolymerization of reduced polymeric IgA, was achieved in the presence of J chain and of the disulfide-exchanging enzyme obtained from liver. The specificity of polymerization was demonstrated by futile attempts to polymerize IgG or albumin in this system. During the *in vitro* polymerization of IgA and IgM, J chain was incorporated into the reassembled polymers.

To explain a relatively uniform secretion of pentameric IgM on the one hand and monomeric, as well as polymeric, secretion of IgA on the other hand, the determinations of intracellular J chain were performed in corresponding cells. There was a balanced synthesis of 7 S subunits and J chain in cells producing IgM, but after a time the IgA-synthesizing cells appeared to produce decreasing quantities of J chain. In these cells, the size of the intracellular pool of J chain seemed to determine whether an intracellular monomer molecule is secreted in this form or polymerized with J chain. When the availability of intracellular J chain is limited, monomers will be secreted.

B. Assembly of IgM

IgM assembly from μ and light chains has been investigated using cells from several sources. The building of the IgM molecule is accomplished methodically like that of other classes of immunoglobulins. The distinguishing difference is that 7 S subunits must undergo a polymerization process. Since five subunits become covalently associated, the process is even more complex than that usually required for polymerization of IgA molecules.

The cellular formation of IgMs is through a covalently associated μ-L-chain intermediate with subsequent dimerization to IgMs $(\mu L)_2$. This route of assembly has been demonstrated in murine tumor (plasmacytoma) cells (Parkhouse, 1971a), human bone marrow cells (Buxbaum et al., 1971), and concanavalin A-stimulated murine bone marrow-derived lymphocytes (Andersson and Melchers, 1973). The μ-μ disulfide bonds in IgMs molecules appear to be formed prior to polymerization (Parkhouse, 1971a; Buxbaum et al., 1971).

The immunoglobulin content of the intracellular fluid of murine tumor cells and mitogen-treated spleen cells making IgM is primarily in the IgMs form. The cells apparently accumulate IgMs. About 10% or less of the immunoglobulin is in the 19 S form (Parkhouse and Askonas, 1969; Andersson and Melchers, 1973). It is questionable whether the IgM is really intracellular protein or if it is extracytoplasmic IgM sticking to cells after its secretion (Andersson and Melchers, 1973).

Bone marrow and lymph node cells from humans with gammopathies also were found to contain relatively large amounts of IgMs. In contrast to the mouse system, cells from most patients seemed to accumulate fully assembled IgM (Buxbaum et al., 1971). In many instances, the sera of patients with IgM abnormalities contained IgMs in substantial quantities (Eskeland and Harboe, 1973), indicating that the polymerization process is possibly not fully functional.

Intracellular IgMs is apparently a covalently assembled molecule with its interchain disulfide bridges intact. What then, has become of the sulfhydryl groups that normally are involved in intersubunit linkage? In the MOPC 104E tumor line, the IgMs molecules' sulfhydryl groups appear to be blocked (Askonas and Parkhouse, 1971). The nature of the blocking agent is not known. Mixed disulfides of cysteine or glutathione are possible explanations. It may also be possible for the sulfhydryl groups to form an intrasubunit inter-μ-chain bridge. An interesting point to be made is that intracellular IgMs molecules did not spontaneously polymerize unless they first were treated with a reducing agent in the presence of extraneous IgM (Askonas and Parkhouse, 1971). Thus, the block on the potential intersubunit disulfide-bond-forming cysteine is a reversible one. It was suggested that polymerization is controlled by removal of this block and that an enzyme catalyzing disulfide exchange might participate.

Melchers (1972) also found that intracellular IgMs did not tend to polymerize in vitro. The data were interpreted, however, in terms of the differences in carbohydrate content of intracellular IgMs as compared to fully assembled IgM. The addition of galactose, fucose, and neuraminic acid to sites near the cysteines destined to become involved in intersubunit bridges was postulated to cause conformational changes in the Fcμ region which then would allow disulfide-bridge formation. These three sugars were absent from intracellular IgMs, but were present on the extracellular 19 S IgM molecules.

In the same report (Melchers, 1972), ^{3}H-leucine-labeled intracellular IgMs was mixed with increasingly large amounts of reduced, extracellularly derived IgM. After mild reduction, repolymerization of the mixture was encouraged. As the molar ratio of intracellular IgMs to IgMs prepared from extracellular IgM decreased (by factors up to 10^4), an increasing proportion of available labeled intracellular IgMs appeared in the 19 S material. These data seem inconsistent with a role for J chain in the polymerization process. The theoretical molecular ratio of J chain to IgMs molecules remained essentially unchanged over most of the experiment, yet radioactivity incorporation into repolymerized 19 S material increased.

Strong evidence of a requirement of J chain for polymerization of intracellular 7 S IgM was given recently (Della Corte and Parkhouse, 1973b). In *in vitro* experiments intracellular 7 S IgM could be made to polymerize completely only in the presence of added J chain. An enzyme which catalyzed disulfide exchange also was required. The specificity of the system for polymeric IgA and IgM assembly was extraordinary. A mixture of IgM and IgA was reduced and reassembled without the formation of hybrid molecules. In the experiments the J chain was prepared only from serum IgA.

Since no one has established unambiguously a reason for the necessity of J chain in IgM molecules, it is difficult to propose a mechanism for its hypothetical function during assembly. A few possibilities, nevertheless, will be discussed in the hope that fruits of new ideas will be harvested.

An obvious role for the J chain would be to serve as a template upon which a limited number (usually five) of IgMs molecules would attach. To make a symmetrical molecule, ten cysteine residues would have to be available for J–μ interchain disulfide bond formation. There are several rebuttals to this hypothesis: (1) The cysteine content of J chains seems to be less than ten residues (Table IV). and the experimentally determined number of J–μ disulfide bridges is not available. If it should be that there are two J chains per IgM molecule (*vida supra*), sufficient cysteine residues would reside in the J-chain dimer to form ten bonds. Its conformation might not allow such bond formation, however. (2) In order to achieve the symmetrical arrangement shown by electron microscopy for IgM molecules (Metzger, 1970), the cysteine residues would have to be periodically located in J chains. Such precise spacing might also imply that J_μ chains consist of repeating homologous regions but there is no evidence for this. (3) Unless there were an intrachain disulfide bond linking the two end regions of the J_μ chains, it is difficult to understand how the circular shape of IgM would be maintained. Perhaps one way to achieve this shape would lie in the existence of strong noncovalent forces in overlapping N-terminal and C-terminal regions.

A second idea suggests that intracellular J chain initiates polymerization by binding to one μ chain through a disulfide bridge. This somehow induces polymerization between the other subunits. After five IgMs molecules are covalently joined, the sulfhydryl group on the one remaining unbound μ chain joins to another sulfhydryl on the same J chain, which initially was attached to the first IgMs molecule. The final product (IgM) would structurally resemble the "clasp" model (Wilde and Koshland, 1973). The function of J chain in this hypothetical scheme could be to initiate disulfide interchange by presenting a sulfhydryl group to the blocked cysteine on the μ chain. It would seem easier to explain if the appropriate μ-chain cysteines were in the form of an inter-μ-chain disulfide bond.

Several questions can be raised regarding this mechanism. One asks how polymerization continues after the initial contact. Disulfide interchange occurs among physically close residues. Since the cells accumulate IgMs (Parkhouse and Askonas, 1969), this closeness could be the result of physical crowding in the cisterna. The blocked thiol residues must be at the surface of the subunits so as to enhance *their* becoming involved, rather than one of the many other disulfide bridges in IgMs molecules. As a consequence of disulfide interchange, one is left with a free sulfhydryl on one μ chain of the final IgMs molecule and possibly on the J chain also. Are these joined by an enzyme? Alternatively the thiol on the J chain could be blocked, and the last step in interchange could result in removal of the block and formation of a μ–J disulfide bridge. An esthetic objection to this mechanism is that it results in an unsymmetrical IgM molecule. A similar final product would be the result of initial union between two IgMs molecules and a J chain (IgMs–J–IgMs). This event would be followed by addition of three IgMs molecules to complete the pentamer.

In either mechanism, any molecule or system which presented a free sulfhydryl group or alternative disulfide-bond-reducing scheme in catalytic quantity could conceivably initiate the polymerization process just as effectively as J chain. Why, then, must the cell produce a polypeptide to initiate the process? Is it probable that there is a covert role for J chain, one that makes the polypeptide an essential structural component of IgM molecules?

One can also ask why polymerization terminates at five IgMs molecules. An answer to this question might be that thermodynamic stability dictates the pentameric structure.

Regardless of which mechanism is more nearly correct, careful experimental work should allow detection of polymers of two, three, or four IgMs molecules which contain covalently attached J chain, provided the secreted IgM does normally contain J chain.

In addition to the IgM assembly processes discussed above, there is one in which the polymerization step is omitted. IgM is a class of immunoglobulin which frequently is present on mouse, human, and rabbit lymphocytes which carry immunoglobulins on their membranes (Unanue *et al.*, 1973). On the surface of Daudi cells (human Burkitt's lymphoma cells) and normal small splenic lymphocytes of the mouse, the surface immunoglobulin is in the mono-mer form (Uhr and Vitetta, 1973). These cells are not nearly so active in immunoglobulin secretion as plasma cells, and that which is secreted apparently is structurally equivalent to IgMs. It is assumed that when normal B lymphocytes undergo differentiation they will be capable of secreting 19 S IgM or other classes of immunoglobulin.

In undifferentiated lymphocytes do the IgMs molecules bear blocked thiols which prevent polymerization? Or, are the appropriate cysteine residues absent? Of these two choices the former would be a more reasonable one since the latter would invoke an unacceptable genetic change required for later synthesis of normal μ chains. A more likely explanation for a 7 S IgM would be the absence of J chain synthesis by lymphocytes or the lack of an appropriate enzyme. Thus, if J chain is an obligatory requirement for the polymerization step, then its absence would result in the lack of 19 S IgM. What is needed, then, is evidence for the absence or presence of intracellular J chain in lymphocytes carrying membrane-bound IgM.

An experiment could be done using bone-marrow-derived lymphocytes from athymic mice. One would examine the cells for the presence of J chains intracellularly. The cells would not secrete 19 S IgM, but should carry mem-brane-bound IgMs. Upon treatment with concanavalin A, however, they should begin to secrete IgM (Andersson and Melchers, 1973). The mitogen-treated cells would then be examined for the presence of intracellular J chains. If J chains were found only in the latter treated cells, a probable relationship between J chain and polymerization or secretion of IgMs would be suggested.

It appears that lymphocytes can switch heavy-chain synthesis from μ to γ chains (Nisonoff et al., 1971). The manufacture of J chain by μ-chain-synthesizing lymphocytes might pose problems for those cells which switch to γ-chain synthesis. Hence, the possibility that J chain is not made by lympho-cytes may be a cellular method of permitting a μ-to-γ chain switch without the problems posed by the turning on and off of the J chain gene. Additionally, if J chain synthesis is found only in differentiated lymphocytes, a new avenue of research into control of protein synthesis would be opened.

ACKNOWLEDGMENT

The work done under the supervision of F.P. Inman was supported by grants from the National Science Foundation (GB-8449) and the National Institutes of Health (5-tol-GB 01968-02). The research performed by J. Me-stecky received support from National Institutes of Health grants AI-10854 and DE-02670.

REFERENCES

Andersson, J., and Melchers, F., 1973, *Proc. Natl. Acad. Sci. U.S.* **70**:416.
Askonas, B. A., and Parkhouse, R. M. E., 1971, *Biochem. J.* **123**:629.
Askonas, B. A., and Schariff, M. D., 1971, in Amos, B. (ed.), *Progress in Immunology,* Academic Press, New York, p. 1333.
Askonas, B. A., and Williamson, A. R., 1968, *Biochem. J.* **109**:637.
Bargellesi, A., Periman, P., and Scharff, M. D., 1972, *J. Immunol.* **108**:126.
Barth, G., Bunnenberg, E., and Djerassi, C., 1972, *Anal. Biochem.* **48**:471.
Baumal, R., Coffino, P., Bargellesi, A., Buxbaum, J., Laskov, R., and Scharff, M. D., 1971a, *Ann. N.Y. Acad. Sci.* **190**:235.
Baumal, R., Potter, M., and Scharff, M. D., 1971b, *J. Exptl. Med.* **134**:1316.
Bienenstock, J., and Strauss, H., 1970, *J. Immunol.* **105**:274.
Buxbaum, J., Zolla, S., Scharff, M. D., and Franklin, E. C., 1971, *J. Exptl. Med.* **133**:1118.
Cebra, J. J., 1969, *Bacteriol. Rev.* **33**:159.
Cebra, J. J., and Small, P. A. Jr., 1967, *Biochemistry* **6**:503.
Cecil, R., 1963, in Neurath, H. (ed.), *The Proteins,* Academic Press, New York, p. 380.
Cederblad, G., Johansson, B. G., and Rymo, L., 1966, *Acta Chem. Scand.* **20**:2349.
Chuang, C.-Y., Capra, J. D., and Kehoe, J. M., 1973, *Nature.* **244**:158.
Dean, R. B., and Dixon, W. J., 1951, *Anal. Chem.* **23**:636.
Della Corte, E., and Parkhouse, R. M. E., 1973a, *Biochem. J.,* **136**:589.
Della Corte, E., and Parkhouse, R. M. E., 1973b, *Biochem. J.,* **136**:597.
Deutsch, H., and Morton, J., 1957, *Science.* **125**:600.
Edelman, G. M., and Marchalonis, J. J., 1967, in Williams, C. A., and Chase, M. W. (eds.), *Methods in Immunology and Immunochemistry,* Academic Press, New York, p. 405.
Eskeland, T., and Brandtzaeg, P., 1974, *Immunochemistry,* in press.
Eskeland, T., and Harboe, M., 1973, *Scand. J. Immunol.,* **2**:511.
Frangione, B., Prelli, F., Mihaesco, C., and Franklin, E. C., 1971, *Proc. Natl. Acad. Sci. U.S.* **68**:1547.
Franklin, E. C., 1974, in Mestecky, J., and Lawton, A. R. (eds), *The Immunoglobulin A System,* Plenum Press, New York, in press.
Grey, H. M., Abel, C. A., and Zimmerman, B., 1971, *Ann. N.Y. Acad. Sci.* **190**:37.
Grey, H. M., Despont, J.-P. J., Abel, C. A., and Penn, G. M., 1974, in Mestecky, J., and Lawton, A. R. (eds.), *The Immunoglobulin A System,* Plenum Press, New York, in press.
Halpern, M. S., and Coffman, R. L., 1972, *J. Immunol.* **109**:674.
Halpern, M. S., and Koshland, M. E., 1970a, *Federation Proc.* **29**:#2228 (Abstract).
Halpern, M. S., and Koshland, M. E., 1970b, *Nature* **228**:1276.
Heimer, R., Jones, D. W., and Maurer, P. H., 1969, *Biochemistry* **8**:3937.
Hijmans, W., Schuit, H. R. E., Radl, J., and Vossen, J. M. J. J., 1974, in Mestecky, J., and Lawton, A. R. (eds.), *The Immunoglobulin A System,* Plenum Press, New York, in press.
Inman, F. P., 1974, in Mestecky, J., and Lawton, A. R. (eds.), *The Immunoglobulin A System,* Plenum Press, New York, in press.
Inman, F. P., and Ricardo, M. J., 1974, *J. Immunol.,* **112**:229.
Kehoe, J. M., Tomasi, T. B. Jr., Ellouz, F., and Capra, J. D., 1972, *J. Immunol.* **1**:59.
Klaus, G. G. B., Halpern, M. S., Koshland, M. E., and Goodman, J. W., 1971, *J. Immunol.* **107**:1785.
Kobayashi, K., Vaerman, J.-P., and Heremans, J. F., 1973a, *Biochim. Biophys. Acta,* **303**:105.
Kobayashi, K., Vaerman, J.-P., and Heremans, J. F., 1973b, *Eur. J. Immunol.* **3**:185.
Kobayashi, K., Vaerman, J.-P., and Heremans, J. F., 1974, *Immunochemistry,* in press.
Kobayashi, K., Vaerman, J.-P., Bazin, H., Lebacq-Verheyden, A.-M., and Heremans, J. F., 1973d, *J. Immunol.* **111**:1590.

Koshland, M. E., and Wilde, C. E., 1974, in Mestecky, J., and Lawton, A. R. (eds.), *The Immunoglobulin A System,* Plenum Press, New York, in press.
Kownatzki, E., 1971, *Eur. J. Immunol.* 1:486.
Kownatzki, E., 1972, *Federation Proc.* 31:#3034 (Abstract).
Kownatzki, E., 1973a, *Z. Immunitaetsforsch.* 145:333.
Kownatzki, E., 1973b, *Z. Immunitaetsforsch.* 145:342.
Kownatzki, E., 1973c, *Immunol. Commun.,* 2:105.
Kownatzki, E., 1973d, *9th Intern. Congress Biochem. Abstract* p. 316.
Kunkel, H. G., 1974, in Mestecky, J., and Lawton, A. R. (eds.), *The Immunoglobulin A System,* Plenum Press, New York, in press.
Lawton, A. R. III, and Mage, R. G., 1969, *J. Immunol.* 102:693.
Matsuoka, Y., Yagi, Y., Moore, G. E., and Pressman, D., 1970, *J. Immunol.* 104:1.
Meinke, G. C., 1973, *Federation Proc.* 32:#4206 (Abstract).
Meinke, G. C., and Spiegelberg, H. L., 1971, *Federation Proc.* 30:#1526 (Abstract).
Meinke, G. C., and Spiegelberg, H. L., 1972a, *J. Immunol.* 109:903.
Meinke, G. C., and Spiegelberg, H. L., 1972b, *Federation Proc.* 31:#3044 (Abstract).
Melchers, F., 1971, *Histochem. J.* 3:389.
Melchers, F., 1972, *Biochemistry* 11:2204.
Mendez, E., Frangione, B., and Franklin, E. C., 1972, *Federation Proc.* 31:#3045 (Abstract).
Mendez, E., Frangione, B., and Franklin, E. C., 1973, *Biochemistry* 12:1119.
Mestecky, J., Kulhavy, R., and Kraus, F. W., 1971a, *Federation Proc.* 30:#1527 (Abstract).
Mestecky, J., Zikan, J., and Butler, W. T., 1971b, *Science* 171:1163.
Mestecky, J., Zikan, J., Butler, W. T., and Kulhavy, R., 1972a, *Immunochemistry,* 9:883.
Mestecky, J., Kulhavy, R., and Kraus, F. W., 1972b, *J. Immunol.* 108:738.
Mestecky, J., Hammack, W. J., Schrohenloher, R. E., and Bennett, J. C., 1973a, *Protides of the Biological Fluids,* 20:279.
Mestecky, J., Kulhavy, R., Stanton, T. H., Wright, G. P., and Bennett, J. C., 1973b, *Federation Proc.* 32:#4203 (Abstract).
Mestecky, J., Schrohenloher, R. E., Kulhavy, R., Wright, G. P., and Tomana, M., 1974a, *Proc. Natl. Acad. Sci. U.S.,* 71:544.
Mestecky, J., Schrohenloher, R. E., Kulhavy, R., Wright, G. P., and Tomana, M., 1974b, in Mestecky, J., and Lawton, A. R. (eds.), *The Immunoglobulin A System,* Plenum Press, New York, in press.
Metzger, H., 1970, *Adv. Immunol.* 12:57.
Miller, F., and Metzger, H., 1965, *J. Biol. Chem.* 240:3325.
Morris, J. E., and Inman, F. P., 1968, *Biochemistry* 7:2851.
Morrison, S. L., and Koshland, M. E., 1972, *Proc. Natl. Acad. Sci. U.S.* 69:124.
Mukkur, T. K., and Inman, F. P., 1971, *J. Immunol.* 107:705.
Niedermeier, W., Tomana, M., and Mestecky, J., 1972, *Biochim. Biophys. Acta* 257:527.
Nisonoff, A., Wilson, S. K., Wang, A. C., Fudenberg, H. H., and Hopper, J. E., 1971, in Amos, B. (ed.), *Progress in Immunology,* Academic Press, New York, p. 61.
O'Daly, J. A., and Cebra, J. J., 1971a, *Biochemistry* 10:3843.
O'Daly, J. A., and Cebra, J. J., 1971b, *J. Immunol.* 107:436.
Parkhouse, R. M. E., 1971a, *Biochem. J.,* 123:635.
Parkhouse, R. M. E., 1971b, *FEBS Lett.* 16:71.
Parkhouse, R. M. E., 1972, *Nature New Biol.* 236:9.
Parkhouse, R. M. E., 1973, *Transplant. Rev.* 14:131.
Parkhouse, R. M. E., and Askonas, B. A., 1969, *Biochem. J.* 115:163.
Parkhouse, R. M. E., and Della Corte, E., 1973, *Biochem. J.,* 136:607.
Parkhouse, R. M. E., and Della Corte, E., 1974, in Mestecky, J., and Lawton, A. R. (eds.), *The Immunoglobulin A System,* Plenum Press, New York, in press.
Plaut, A. G., and Tomasi, T. B. Jr., 1970, *Proc. Natl. Acad. Sci. U.S.* 65:318.
Poulik, M. D., 1967, in Greenwalt, T. J. (ed.), *Advances in Immunogenetics,* Lippincot, Philadelphia.

Prahl, J. W., Abel, C. A., and Grey, H. M., 1971, *Biochemistry* **10**:1808.
Putnam, F. W., Shimizu, A., Paul, C., and Shinoda, T., 1972, *Federation Proc.* **31**:193.
Raam, S. V., and Inman, F. P., 1973, *J. Immunol.* **110**:1044.
Radl, J., Schuit, H. R. E., Mestecky, J., and Hijmans, W., 1974, in Mestecky, J., and Lawton, A. R. (eds.), *The Immunoglobulin A System,* Plenum Press, New York, in press.
Reisfeld, R. A., and Small, P. A. Jr., 1966, *Science* **152**:1253.
Rejnek, J., Kostka, J., and Kotynek, O., 1966, *Nature* **209**:926.
Ricardo, M. J., and Inman, F. P., 1973, *Biochem. J.* **131**:677.
Ricardo, M. J., and Inman, F. P., 1974, *Biochem. J.,* **137**:79.
Ricardo, M. J., Brewer, J. M., and Inman, F. P., 1974, *Biochem. J.,* **137**:71.
Rosenstein, R. W., and Jackson, P., 1973, *Biochemistry* **12**:1659.
Scharff, M. D., and Laskov, R., 1970, *Prog. Allergy* **14**:37.
Schrohenloher, R. E., and Mestecky, J., 1973, *J. Immunol.,* **111**:1699.
Schrohenloher, R. E., Mestecky, J., and Stanton, T. H., 1973, *Biochim. Biophys. Acta* **295**:576.
Seligman, M., and Mihaesco, E., 1974, in Mestecky, J., and Lawton, A. R. (eds.), *The Immunoglobulin A System,* Plenum Press, New York, in press.
Sherr, C. J., Schenkein, I., and Uhr, J. W., 1971, *Ann. N.Y. Acad. Sci.* **190**:250.
Small, P. A. Jr., Curry, J. H., and Waldman, R. H., 1971, in Dayton, D. H., Small, P. A., Chanock, R. M., Kaufman, H. E., and Tomasi, T. B. (eds), *The Secretory Immunologic System,* Government Printing Office, Washington.
Sutherland, E. W. III, Zimmerman, D. H., and Kern, M. 1970, *Proc. Natl. Acad. Sci. U.S.* **66**:987.
Tomana, M., Mestecky, J., and Niedermeier, W., 1972, *J. Immunol.* **108**:1631.
Tomasi, T. B. Jr., and Bienenstock, J., 1968, *Adv. Immunol.* **9**:1.
Tomasi, T. B. Jr., and Grey, H. M., 1972, *Prog. Allergy* **16**:81.
Tomasi, T. B. Jr., and Hauptman, S., 1974, in Mestecky, J., and Lawton, A. R. (eds.), *The Immunoglobulin A System,* Plenum Press, New York, in press.
Tomasi, T. B., Tan, E. M. Solomon, A., and Prendercast, R. A., 1965, *J. Exp. Med.* **121**:101.
Tourville, D. R., Adler, R. H., Bienenstock, J., and Tomasi, T. B., Jr., 1969, *J. Exp. Med.* **129**:411.
Uhr, J. W., and Vitetta, Ellen S., 1973, *Federation Proc.* **32**:35.
Unanue, E. R., Engers, H. D., and Karnovsky, M. J., 1973, *Federation Proc.* **32**:44.
Underdown, B. J., Simms, E. S., and Eisen, N. H., 1971, *Biochemistry* **10**:4359.
Weber, K., and Osborn, M. 1969, *J. Biol. Chem.* **244**:4406.
Weinheimer, P. F., Mestecky, J., and Acton, R. T., 1971, *J. Immunol.* **107**:1211.
Wilde, C. E. III, and Koshland, M. E., 1973, *Biochemistry* **12**:3218.
Zikan, J., 1973, *Immunochemistry* **10**:351.
Zikan, J., Mestecky, J., Schrohenloher, R. E., Tomana, M., and Kulhavy, R., 1972, *Immunochemistry* **9**:1185.

Phylogenetic Aspects of Immunoglobulin Variable Region Diversity

J. Michael Kehoe and J. Donald Capra

Department of Microbiology
Mount Sinai School of Medicine
City University of New York
New York, New York

I. INTRODUCTION

There is now widespread agreement that the antigen-binding function of immunoglobulin molecules is mediated by the variable regions of their heavy and light polypeptide chains. Studies from a number of laboratories have shown that many general features of antibodies, such as the capacity to interact with a given antigen (e.g., dinitrophenyl), susceptibility to proteolytic cleavage, and mediation of biological properties (e.g., complement fixation), are shared across a wide phylogenetic spectrum of animal species. From a broad biological standpoint, an important question arises. To what extent do these various animal species produce similar immunoglobulin proteins to fulfill the functional requirements of the humoral response system? One approach to answering this question is to study the molecular products of the humoral response in a wide variety of species, especially including amino acid sequence analyses. Unfortunately, such studies have been impeded by the difficulty of obtaining sufficient quantities of pure material from the different species, in large part because of the restriction of the availability, until recently, of homogeneous myeloma proteins to man and the mouse. However, the discovery and sequence analysis of myeloma proteins

J.M.K. is an Established Investigator of the American Heart Association and J.D.C. is the recipient of National Institutes of Health Career Development Award 6-K4-GM-35,190. The work reported herein from our own laboratory was aided by grants from the National Science Foundation (GB 17046) and the U.S. Public Health Service (AI 09810) and by a grant-in-aid from the New York Heart Association.

from dogs and cats (Kehoe and Capra, 1972), progress in amino acid sequence studies of murine myeloma proteins (Bourgois and Fougereau, 1970; Hood and Talmage, 1970; Rudikoff *et al.*, 1973), the recent discovery of myeloma proteins in rats (Bazin *et al.*, 1972; Querinjean *et al.*, 1974), and the remarkable complete sequence analyses performed by Cebra *et al.* (1971) on pools of immuno-globulins from inbred guinea pigs has considerably widened the scope of the available sequence data on the characteristics of antibody proteins from various species.

The intent of this review, which will emphasize heavy chains in particular, is to collate these and other related data and to offer an interpretation of how it speaks to one aspect of the question posed above; that is, what is the nature and extent of the array of variable region sequences utilized in the humoral immune response by the various species?

II. VARIABLE REGION SUBGROUPS

A. Definition

It is a curious and unanticipated fact that the orderly cataloging of immuno-globulin variable regions has been aided greatly by the discovery that it is possible to subdivide variable region sequences from heavy chains, kappa chains, and lambda chains into *subgroups* of variability (Milstein, 1967; Cunningham *et al.*, 1969). The exact definition of a subgroup depends to some extent on one's belief in the rules that determine the origin of antibody variability, but its essence can be stated as follows: members of a given variable region subgroup are more related to one another by the criterion of amino acid sequence homology than they are to members of other subgroups. There is general acceptance of the concept that at least one gene must exist in the genome for each subgroup, since no known genetic mechanisms would be likely to generate a protein of one subgroup from a gene coding for a different subgroup. Representative partial sequences of human heavy chains belonging to three different subgroups are presented in Figure 1.

B. Distribution of Variable Region Subgroups Among Various Species

1. Myeloma Proteins

Two general approaches to the determination of the distribution of variable region subgroups are possible. One involves the classification of all myeloma proteins that have been studied for a given species. Since more human myeloma proteins have been sequenced than those of any other species, this type of data is most complete for man. With the exception of a very few proteins classified as $V_H IV$ (Kohler *et al.*, 1970), all human myeloma heavy chains studied to date have been classifiable into one of the subgroups illustrated in Fig. 1.

V_H I   10   20   30

Eu (γ1) PCA VAL GLN LEU VAL GLU SER GLY **ALA** GLU VAL LYS LYS PRO GLY SER SER VAL **LYS** VAL SER CYS **LYS** ALA SER GLY GLY THR PHE SER

Ca (γ1) PCA _____ ARG _____ ALA _____ ILE _____ THR _____ THR _____

V_H II

Daw (γ1) PCA VAL THR LEU ARG GLU SER GLY **PRO** ALA LEU VAL ARG PRO THR GLN THR LEU **THR** LEU THR CYS **THR** PHE SER GLY PHE SER LEU SER

Ou (μ) PCA _____ THR _____ LYS ___ PRO _____

V_H III

Tei (γ1) GLU VAL GLN LEU VAL GLU SER GLY **GLY** GLY LEU VAL GLN PRO GLY GLY SER LEU **ARG** LEU SER CYS **ALA** ALA SER GLY PHE THR PHE SER

Was (γ1) _____ LEU _____ SER _____

Figure 1. Amino terminal sequences of various human heavy chains illustrating the principle of subgroups of amino acid sequence variability. Subgroup-specific residues are indicated in bold-faced type.

Among 10 rat myeloma protein heavy chains that have been analyzed in our laboratory by automated sequencing (Querinjean et al., 1974), five were found to belong to the V_H III subgroup. The other five may ultimately be assignable to the V_H I or V_H II subgroups, but additional experimentation will be required to definitively establish this point.

In the mouse, the myeloma proteins whose heavy chains have been sequenced to date have been nearly 100% V_H III (Bourgois and Fougereau, 1970; Potter, 1972; Rudikoff et al., 1973; Capra, J. D., and Kehoe, J. M., unpublished results; Hood, L., personal communication). However, there is some reason to believe that these results may be skewed to some extent either because of the induced nature of the murine myelomas (Potter and Boyce, 1962) or because a disproportionate share of all IgA proteins are of the V_H III subgroup (Capra et al., 1973a).

The discovery and sequence analysis of myeloma proteins in dogs and cats (Kehoe and Capra, 1972) has shown that 10 of 10 heavy chains from such proteins are assignable to the V_H III subgroup. This result, admittedly still a low sample number, implied that most, if not all, canine and feline heavy chain variable regions might be of the V_H III subgroup, a result which was confirmed by the study of pooled immunoglobulins, as described below (Capra et al., 1973b).

As far as is known to the authors at present, man, mouse, rat, dog, and cat are the only species which have produced myeloma proteins which have been studied by amino acid sequence analysis.

2. Pools of Immunoglobulins

The second approach to analyzing subgroup distributions involves the study of nonmyeloma immunoglobulins. The unanticipated results with the dog and cat heavy chains from myeloma proteins led to the determination of the distribution of this subgroup in *pools* of immunoglobulins from these species, and later, to similar analyses for other species (Capra *et al.*, 1973b).

The approach to such analyses depended upon a useful characteristic of most proteins of the $V_H III$ subgroup, namely, the presence of an unblocked amino terminal amino acid rather than the cyclized pyrollidone-2-carboxylic acid which is characteristic of most members of the other heavy chain subgroups. This means that the $V_H III$ members of a mixture will be selectively sequenced when automated sequencing methodology is used on the pool. This can be monitored by searching for the characteristic linked residues which define the different subgroups (Fig. 1). If the stoichiometry is carefully controlled by providing a carefully quantitated sample at the start of the degradation, then the yield of the protein actually sequenced will be an index of the quantity of $V_H III$ protein present in the mixture. A convenient probe for this yield is a residue that is readily quantitatible as the phenylthiohydantoin (PTH) derivative. The valine at position 2 or the leucine at position 4 have proven to be useful residues for this purpose. As previously mentioned, the definitive assignment of such a pool sequence to the $V_H III$ subgroup depends upon obtaining an adequate stretch (10–25 residues) which corresponds to the $V_H III$ prototype.

This approach was used to quantitate the $V_H III$ heavy chains in IgG pools from the dog, the cat, and a wide variety of other species (Capra *et al.*, 1973b). Table I shows the results obtained from these various preparations. As shown here, many different animal species showed a different content of $V_H III$ heavy chains in their pool. The value for man (20%) corresponded to the value previously determined for man in another laboratory (Wang *et al.*, 1971) and, as anticipated from the results with the dog and cat myeloma proteins discussed above, these two species had over 90% $V_H III$ proteins in their normal pool. Of greater interest, however, was the observation that the distribution of the $V_H III$ subgroups among these various species correlated directly with their phylogenetic status. That is, animals with an established close phylogenetic relationship such as dog and cat, man and monkey, or cow and sheep also shared the same proportion of $V_H III$ proteins in their IgG heavy chain pools. This correlation is best displayed in diagrammatic form as shown in Fig. 2. This pattern implies that, for the $V_H III$ subgroup at least, some degree of variable region selection has occurred during phylogenetic development and that different species possess, or choose to utilize, different levels of the variable region pool that is known to be available in the biological world as a whole. In other words, by the criterion of heavy chain subgroup distribution at least, the potentiality pool for building antibody-combining sites seems to differ throughout the animal kingdom in a manner that is correlated with phylogeny. Unfortunately, the distribution of other heavy chain subgroups among the various species is more difficult to determine for methodological reasons, so it is not presently

Table I. Determination of Proportion of $V_H III$ Subgroup in Pools[a,b]

Pool	A Load (nmol)	B Valine step 2 (nmol)	C^c Yield at step 2 (%)	D^d Unblocked (%)
MOPC 173	152	128	84	
MOPC 21A	131	121	92	87 100
Tei IgG1	153	132	86	
Lev IgG3	148	7	5	
Taf IgG2	149	9	6	5 0
MOPC 40	166	7	4	
Opossum	155	131[e]	85	97
Dog	152	122	80	91
Mink	80	68	85	97
Cat	161	130	81	92
Sea lion	95	80	84	96
Seal	85	74	87	100
Guinea pig	157	38	24	23
Mouse	154	36	23	22
Rat	102	22	22	20
Monkey (African Green)	103	30	29	29
Monkey (cynomolgus)	161	42	26	26
Monkey (rhesus)	144	30	21	19
Man	156	34	22	20
Rabbit	107	8	7	2
Pig	144	6	4	28[f]
Cow	137	7	5	0
Sheep	137	7	5	0
Goat	176	9	5	0
Moose	160	7	4	0
Horse	129	7	5	0
White whale	164	8	4	0
Fin whale	141	6	4	0

[a] Determination of the proportion of unblocked, $V_H III$, polypeptide chains in a mixture of heavy chains isolated from pooled IgG from various species (Reproduced with permission from the *Journal of Experimental Medicine*). The data on the pig were determined in collaboration with Dr. F. Franek and Dr. J. Novotny of the Institute for Organic Chemistry, Prague.

[b] Data used in determining percentage of unblocked residues. Column A indicates the molar quantity sequenced, column B the yield of valine measured at step 2 of the degradation, and column C the percentage yield of valine at step 2. The percentage of unblocked chains is given in column D, determined as described in the text.

[c] Column B divided by column A × 100.

[d] Considering 87% as 100% unblocked and 5% as 100% blocked; thus, for the cat 100(81−5)/(87−5) = 92.

[e] Measured as isoleucine in position 2.

[f] Pig unblocked percentage calculated from leucine in position 4.

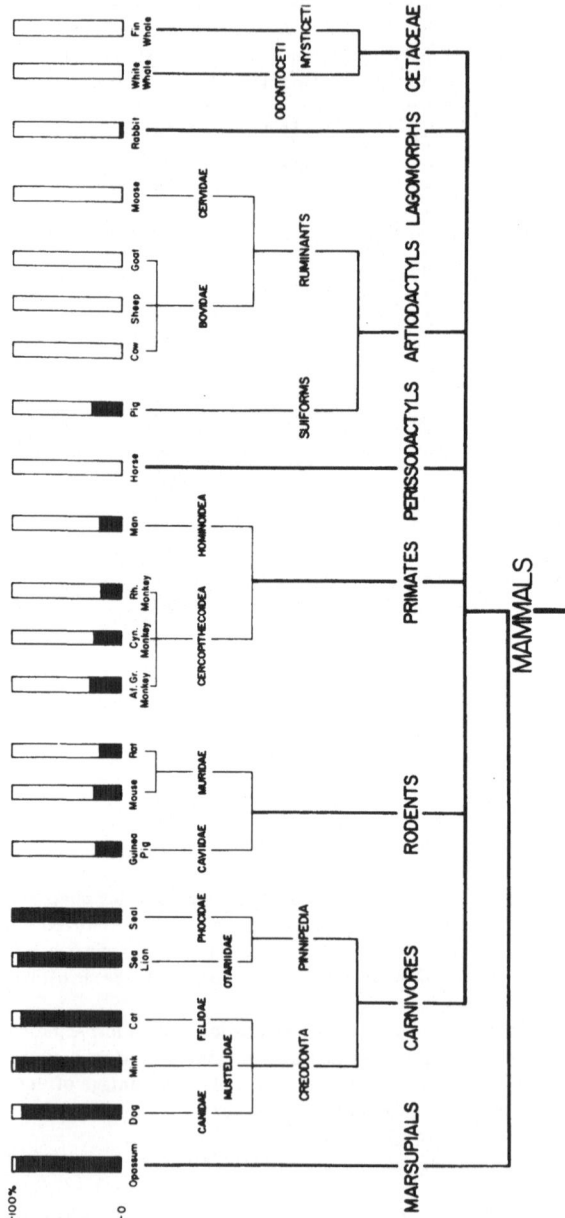

Figure 2. Distribution of $V_H III$ subgroup among various mammalian species. The percentage of the unblocked $V_H III$ subgroup is depicted in black. (Reproduced with permission, and slight modification, from the *Journal of Experimental Medicine*.)

possible to make the same kinds of analyses for them. Hopefully this will be possible in the near future. In view of the nonallelic character of subgroups, however, similar principles of distribution might well be anticipated for the others.

C. Limitations on Sequence Variability in the V Region

1. Myeloma Proteins

As more and more sequence data on immunoglobulins has accrued, a curious irony has developed with regard to the concepts of *variable* region and *constant* region as originally enunciated by Hilschmann and Craig (1965). This irony is a consequence of the observations that certain stretches of variable regions show more homology among various species than do the constant regions of such proteins (Bourgois and Fougereau, 1970; Kehoe and Capra, 1972). In such considerations the so-called hypervariable regions (Kabat and Wu, 1971; Kehoe and Capra, 1971; Capra and Kehoe, 1973) are not taken into account since such regions *may* have a unique genetic origin (Wu and Kabat, 1970). The interspecies *constant* region data are still somewhat limited, but the sequences that are available suggest that a value of approximately 60% interspecies homology is a reasonable estimate (Kehoe and Capra, 1972; Kehoe et al., 1973). In contrast, that section of the heavy chain variable region just up to the first hypervariable region (Capra, 1971) shows a 90% intrasubgroup homology among species, no matter how the comparisons are made. This latter point is illustrated by the series of myeloma protein sequences that is displayed in Fig. 3.

Thus, a sampling of V_H III myeloma proteins from all the species in which they are currently available suggests that a striking interspecies conservation of variable region sequence is characteristic of some, if not all, of the proteins of the humoral immune response in these animals.

2. Pools of Immunoglobulins

The approach used in the analysis of the distribution of the V_H III subgroup (*vide supra*) showed, as a corollary, that it was possible to obtain meaningful sequence data on *pooled* IgG from a number of species (Capra et al., 1973b). In fact, there is a precedent for such an approach in the success of Porter and his colleagues (Mole et al., 1971; Wilkinson, 1969) in obtaining primary structure data from pooled rabbit IgG (which is principally a blocked, non-V_H III sequence). Also, Cebra (see, for example, Cebra et al., 1971) has been able to sequence the heavy chain variable region of IgG pools from inbred strains of guinea pigs. Nonetheless, the findings that such data were obtainable, outside hypervariable regions, from a considerable variety of species came as a consider-

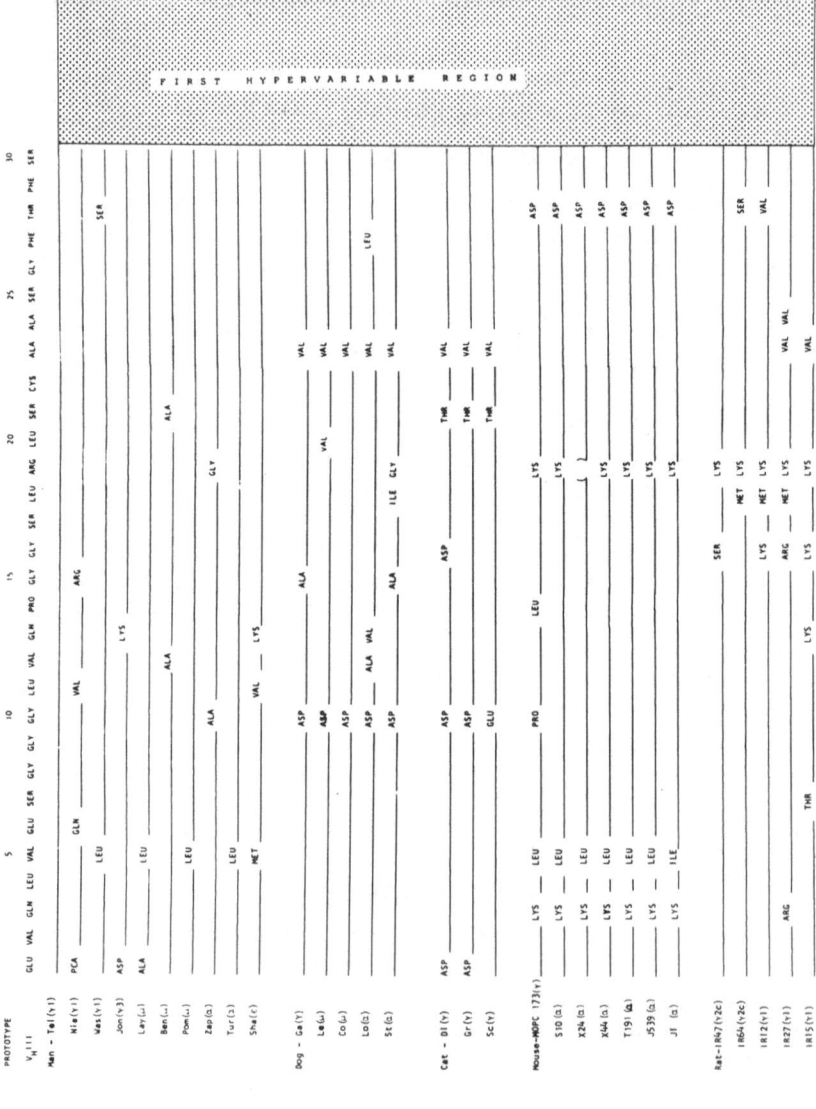

Figure 3. Amino terminal sequences of V_HIII heavy chains from myeloma proteins isolated from various mammalian species. The mouse MOPC 173 γ chain is from Bourgois and Fougereau (1970). The mouse α chain is from Rudikoff *et al.* (1973). The human Nie protein is from Ponstingl *et al.* (1970). All other determinations were made in this laboratory.

V_HIII PROTOTYPE (Human)

5 10 15 20

GLU VAL GLN LEU VAL GLU SER GLY GLY GLY LEU VAL GLN PRO GLY GLY SER LEU ARG LEU SER CYS ALA ALA

Man ——— 1 ——— 2 ——— 3 ———

Mouse ——— LYS ——— ——— LYS ———

Rat ——— 4 ———

Guinea Pig

Dog ——— ASP ——— 5 ——— VAL ———

Cat ASP ——— ASP ——— THR ——— VAL ———

Mink ——— ASP ——— VAL ———

Pig ——— GLU ——— ——— ( ) ——— VAL ———

Seal ——— LYS ——— ASP ———

Sea lion ——— ASP ———

Opossum ——— ILE ——— ASP ———

1. 10% Aspartic Acid   4. 15% Aspartic Acid

2. 15% Leucine   5. 10% Alanine

3. 10% Alanine

Figure 4. Results of amino acid sequence analysis of pooled IgG heavy chains from various mammalian species. The guinea pig data are from Cebra et al. (1971). All other sequences determined in this laboratory.

able surprise and has been interpreted to mean that a marked conservation of structure is characteristic of "normal" antibodies from a number of animal species. Sequences so obtained on pooled material are displayed in Fig. 4, together with the results obtained by Cebra *et al.* for guinea pig pools.

Two additional aspects are noteworthy on the basis of these findings. First, there is a striking homology between these pool sequences and the data obtained for the various myeloma proteins (Fig. 3) and, second, the various interspecies comparisons here show homologies of the same order of magnitude (90%) as did the myeloma proteins. Taken together, these two kinds of data imply that a remarkable restriction of primary structure is characteristic of major segments of certain heavy chains of immunoglobulin molecules from a wide variety of mammalian species.

3. Sequence Studies of Pooled Immunoglobulins from Submammalian Species

To date, sequence data on submammalian immunoglobulins is very sparse, especially for heavy chains. Kubo *et al.* (1971) have reported sequence data for chicken antidinitrophenyl antibodies, whose amino terminal sequence bore a close resemblance to the mammalian $V_H III$ proteins discussed previously. Recently, this laboratory has been investigating heavy chains prepared from pooled IgG isolated from various avian species (Wasserman *et al.*, 1974). The results of sequence studies on pooled IgG heavy chains from five avian species is shown in Fig. 5. For the avian species, all but six positions of the sequence stretch shown contained a single amino acid, which was obtained in greater than 95% yield. The marked similarity to the mammalian prototype sequence is readily apparent.

The combined avian sequences can be used to generate an avian prototype sequence as shown at the bottom of Fig. 5. For that section of the variable region represented here, the avian prototype shows seven differences from the mammalian prototype (positions 1, 5, 13, 16, 17, 21, and 23), indicating a 71% sequence homology. Sequence comparisons of immunoglobulin *constant* regions (Pink *et al.*, 1970) have suggested that immunoglobulin molecules have diverged at the rate of 1 residue/100 residues/$4-5 \times 10^6$ years. If this rate is applied to the avian–mammalian variable region prototype sequences, it would suggest that avian and mammalian divergence occurred approximately 130 million years ago. Since a considerable body of ancillary evolutionary evidence has placed the actual avian–mammalian divergence point at 250–300 million years ago, it appears that the stated constant region rate is not applicable to at least certain sections of the $V_H III$ variable region, which seem to be diverging at a relatively slower rate.

With regard to the shark heavy chain data obtained by Sledge *et al.* (1974), an unquestioned similarity is apparent between this sequence and both the mammalian and avian prototype $V_H III$ sequences (Fig. 6). For the 24 amino

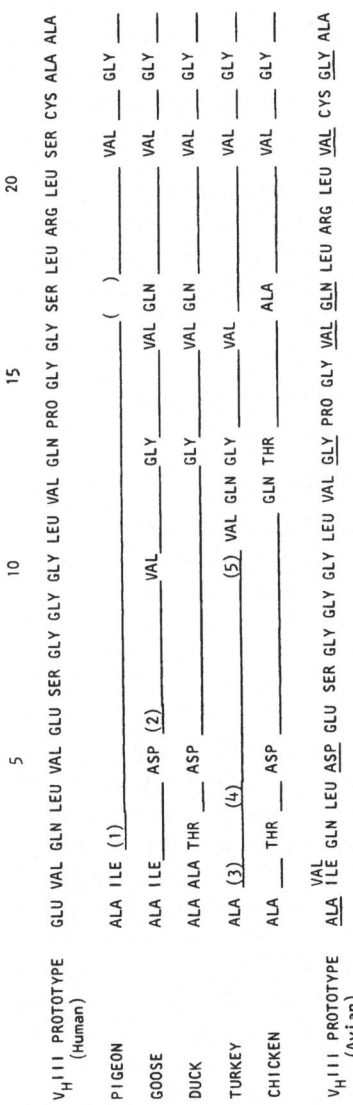

Figure 5. Sequence results obtained on pooled avian heavy chains from various species. The distinct residues of the avian prototype as compared with the human prototype are underlined.

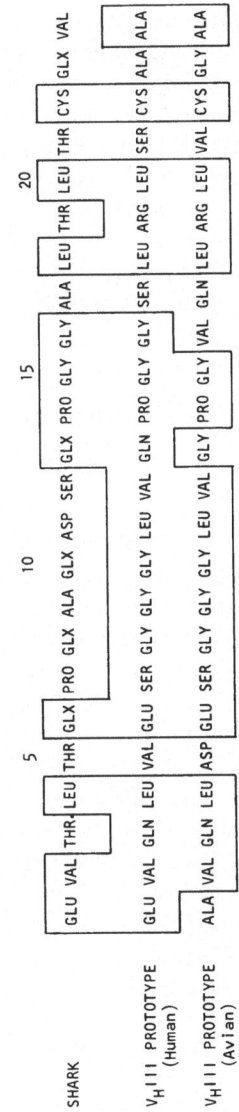

Figure 6. Comparison of a shark heavy chain sequence (Sledge et al., 1974) with the human and avian prototypes. The various sequence identities are blocked in for emphasis.

terminal residues for which a comparison can be made, the avian prototype shows 8 and the human prototype 11 identities with the available shark sequence. It would be premature, however, to assert that these shark proteins are *bona fide* members of the V_H III subgroup.

The conservation of certain heavy chain variable region amino acids across a wide phylogenetic spectrum is nonetheless very clear here because of the following pattern: in all eight positions in which the avian and shark sequences are identical, the mammalian prototype has the same amino acid as well (positions 2, 4, 6, 14, 15, 18, 20, and 22). Of these positions, 14, 15, 18, 20, and 22 are invariant in all mammalian and avian pools studied and, with few exceptions, are also invariant in all V_HIII human, mouse, cat, and dog myeloma proteins sequenced to date. In addition, the proline at position 14 and the cysteine at position 22 are also invariant in *all* of the known human V_H subgroups.

D. Phylogenetically Associated (Species-Specific) Residues within Immunoglobulin Polypeptide Chains

1. Occurrence of Such Residues

As previously discussed, analyses of a series of heavy chains prepared from both myeloma proteins and pooled immunoglobulins showed 90% similarity of sequence up to the first hypervariable region among various species. A corollary to this observation was the finding that at least the first heavy chain hypervariable region occurs at exactly the same position within the chain in all of the species studied. However, a most important question could be asked regarding the area up to that first hypervariable region. Are there any unique features about the approximately 10% differences that were observed among the various species? As pointed out previously (Kehoe and Capra, 1972; Capra *et al.*, 1973b), certain of these differences showed the characteristics of "species-specific" or "phylogenetically associated" residues. That is, some of the 10% differences are amino acids which are characteristic of a certain phylogenetic group and are found in a majority of instances at a given position *within a given variable region subgroup* (Kehoe and Capra, 1972). The principle involved can be illustrated by reference to Fig. 3 and 4. As an example, at position 21 most of the human myeloma proteins and the human V_H III pool show a serine residue. The same residue is present in all the dog myeloma proteins and the dog pool. The cat however, shows a threonine in position 21 in the three available myeloma proteins and in the pool. Comparable assignments can be made for the other species cited. As another example, position 23 can be considered. Here the human myeloma proteins and the pool shows alanine, while the dog and the cat have exclusively valine here, and the other species the residues shown in the figures. Positions 21 and 23 thus qualify as "phylogenetically associated" since

Table II. Phylogenetically Associated Residues for
Various Positions of V_H III Heavy Chains from Various Species[a]

Species	Position							
	1	2	3	10	19	21	23	37
Man	Glu	Val	Gln	Gly	Arg	Ser	Ala	Val
Dog	Glu	Val	Gln	Asp	Arg	Ser	Val	Val
Cat	Asp	Val	Gln	Asp	Arg	Thr	Val	Val
Guinea Pig	Glu	Val	Gln	Gly	Arg	Ser	Val	Ile
Pig	Glu	Glu	Gln	Gly		Ser	Val	
Mouse	Glu	Val	Lys	Gly	Lys	Ser	Ala	Val
Rat	Glu	Val	Gln	Gly	Lys	Ser		
Opossum	Glu	Ile	Gly	Asp				
Mink	Glu	Val	Gln	Asp	Arg	Ser	Ala	
Pigeon	Ala	Ile	Gln	Gly	Arg	Val	Gly	
Goose	Ala	Ile	Gln	Val	Arg	Val	Gly	
Duck	Ala	Ala	Thr	Gly	Arg	Val	Gly	
Turkey	Ala	Val	Gln	Gly	Arg	Val	Gly	
Chicken	Ala	Val	Thr	Gly	Arg	Val	Gly	

[a] Guinea pig data are from Cebra et al., 1971. The other determinations were made in this laboratory.

they show variation that is correlated with the species of origin. As emphasized previously, however, the term "species-specific" is not entirely appropriate since the residues in question are not unique to a given species (e.g., position 23 in Figure 3) and must be defined in relation to a particular variable region subgroup (*vide infra*).

Additional sequence studies on a variety of immunoglobulin preparations from various species has enlarged the catalog of phylogenetically associated residues that are identifiable for V_H III proteins. Table II illustrates assignments of such residues for a number of species, as determined either from myeloma proteins or heavy chain pools. For example, the sequence studies described above for the pools of avian heavy chains have revealed the existence of such residues in birds (Fig. 5, Table II). Positions that are so "avian-associated" include 1 (Ala), 21 (Val), and 23 (Gly). It would seem of particular interest that positions 21 and 23 are also prominent phylogenetically associated residues in the mammalian species studied (Table II).

Also, examination of these available avian heavy chain sequences disclosed another interesting correlation. The goose and the duck are known to be more closely related to each other than either is to any of the other avian species studied. The goose and the duck showed four positions (5, 13, 16, and 17) where they share an amino acid that is not universally present among the other avian species (Fig. 5). Similarly, the turkey and chicken are more closely related to each other than to the other species, and they share a residue at position 12 that is not possessed by the others. These relationships reinforce the inferences that can be drawn from the phylogenetically associated residues presented in Table II.

An important point to appreciate about phylogenetically associated residues is that these residues are *multiple* within the heavy chain variable region of any given species. In consequence, if multiple germ-line immunoglobulin genes are assumed, an *ad hoc* explanation of the existence of such residues in immuno-globulin pools must assume either a number of different mutational events spaced in time, or a number of simultaneous events occurring on a given gene from which additional multigene families are ultimately derived ("gene expansion" of Hood and Talmage, 1970). The findings can be more readily accounted for on a paucigene basis by simply assuming that mutational events occurred on single genes at various points in evolutionary time to generate those residues identifiable today as phylogenetically associated. According to this view, a given mutation in one of these genes (e.g., serine to threonine at position 21 during the phylogenetic development of the cat) would then appear in all of the V_H III polypeptides produced by this zoologic line, until the same codon mutated again. A back mutation at one of the positions involved is most assuredly a realistic possibility which must be taken into account in any analysis of the distribution of the phylogenetically associated residues. As we have previously pointed out (Capra *et al.*, 1973b), nothing in this conception precludes some limited variable region gene duplication *after speciation,* as has presumably occurred with some heavy chain constant region genes to give rise to the immunoglobulin subclasses (Pink *et al.,* 1970). The available sequence data imply that such variable region gene duplications are not numerous and are not incompatible with a paucigene basis for the generation of diversity.

2. Relationship of Phylogenetically Associated Residues to Different Subgroups

Because of the paucity of data for different heavy chain variable region subgroups, such a relationship is difficult to study. In fact, the only species for which such an analysis is approachable at all at this time is man, where some V_H I and V_H II myeloma proteins have been sequenced (Fig. 1). Inspection of positions 3, 10, 21 and 23 in V_H I and V_H II proteins, which positions have been established as phylogenetically associated residues in V_H III heavy chains, shows that no commonality of amino acid is assured for these positions across subgroups *within* the species. Position 23 of the human proteins shows the most extensive deviation, even with the limited data, in having a different amino acid present in each subgroup. Such a pattern reinforces the previously stated conclusion that phylogenetically associated amino acids must be considered on a subgroup-specific basis. It suggests further that the genes coding for the various V_H subgroups diverged well before mammalian speciation. The variable region *subgroups* thus evidently preceded the constant region *subclasses* which, as noted previously, are believed to have followed speciation (Pink *et al.*, 1970).

E. Summary and Conclusions

Sequence studies of immunoglobulin heavy chains from a variety of species have shown that a striking, and unanticipated, structural unity is characteristic of the variable regions of such proteins, particularly among mammals. This unity of primary structure can be seen by the analysis of myeloma proteins from various species, but is even more clearly evidenced by the observation that certain large segments of proteins prepared from *pools* of immunoglobulins are also sequenceable, and can be compared among species. Such a result would, of course, be unobtainable were not the individual proteins within the pool closely similar in sequence, and thus implies a marked restriction in primary structure for at least certain segments of these variable regions. Comparisons of the sequences obtained from the pools of various species fully support the close *interspecies* sequence homologies that are apparent in available myeloma proteins.

Additional features of interest appear when the sequence differences that *do* exist in the variable region segments are considered. Such differences very often show a correlation with the phylogenetic status of the species in question and can be referred to as "phylogenetically associated" residues. Unless certain *ad hoc* assumptions are made, the presence of such residues would seem to place constraints on the number of germ-line genes that are initially present in the genomes of the various species. In contrast, their presence can be rationalized rather easily under a paucigene conception as the basis for explaining the origin of antibody variability.

Studies of heavy chains from various species have also shown that, at least for the V_H III subgroup, the proportion of a given subgroup used in the humoral immune response compared with others differs from species to species. Moreover, the similarity in the extent of utilization of the V_H III subgroup by different species correlated with the closeness of their phylogenetic relationship, as determined by classical zoological criteria.

Additional relevant information bearing on these aspects of the humoral immune response will have to await additional research. Among the immediate questions that remain open are the following:

1. What is the distribution pattern of the V_H I and V_H II subgroups among various species? Do the patterns parallel in any manner the patterns seen for the V_H III subgroup?

2. Are there any additional, presently unappreciated heavy chain subgroups present in some lower species?

3. Exactly how far down the phylogenetic scale is the V_H III subgroup represented?

4. Are all the hypervariable regions located at precisely the same locations within the variable regions of immunoglobulins in the different species?

These, and other questions, will very likely be posed often by immunologists in the immediate years ahead. Among other approaches, additional amino acid sequence data on a wide variety of proteins will aid in obtaining the requisite answers.

ACKNOWLEDGMENTS

The authors acknowledge the assistance of Ms. Bonnie Gerber, Ms. Ellen Bogner, and Ms. Donna Atherton in various phases of this work. A significant portion of the data used here has formed a part of the thesis research of Mr. Richard Wasserman, and the authors gratefully acknowledge his contributions.

REFERENCES

Bazin, H., Deckers, C., Beckers, A., and Heremans, J. F., 1972, *Int. J. Cancer* **10**:568.
Bourgois, A., and Fougereau, M., 1970, *FEBS Letters* **8**:265.
Capra, J. D., 1971, *Nature New Biology* **230**:61.
Capra, J. D., and Kehoe, J. M., 1973, *Proc. Natl. Acad. Sci. U.S.*, **71**:845.
Capra, J. D., Chuang, C., Kaplan, R. D., and Kehoe, J. M., 1973a, IgA Symposium, Birmingham, Alabama.
Capra, J. D., Wasserman, R. L., and Kehoe, J. M., 1973b, *J. Exp. Med.* **138**:410.
Cebra, J. J., Ray, A., Benjamin, D., and Birshstein, B., 1971, in Amos, B. (ed.) *Progress in Immunology*, Academic Press, New York, pp. 269–284.
Cunningham, B. A., Pflumm, M. N., Rutishauser, U., and Edelman, G. M., 1969, *Proc. Natl. Acad. Sci. U.S.* **64**:997.
Hilschmann, N., and Craig, L. C., 1965, *Proc. Natl. Acad. Sci. U.S.* **53**:1403.
Hood, L., and Talmage, D. W., 1970, *Science* **168**:325.
Kabat, E. A., and Wu, T. T., 1971, *Ann. N.Y. Acad. Sci.* **190**:382.
Kehoe, J. M., and Capra, J. D., 1971, *Proc. Natl. Acad. Sci. U.S.* **68**:2019.
Kehoe, J. M., and Capra, J. D., 1972, *Proc. Natl. Acad. Sci. U.S.* **69**:2052.
Kehoe, J. M., Bourgois, A., Capra, J. D., and Fougereau, M., 1973, *Biochemistry*, in press.
Kohler, H., Shimizu, A., Paul, C., Moore, V., and Putnam, F. W., 1970, *Nature* **227**:1318.
Kubo, R. T., Rosenblum, I. Y., and Benedict, A. A., 1971, *J. Immunol.* **107**:1781.
Milstein, C., 1967, *Nature (Lond.)* **216**:330.
Mole, L. E., Jackson, S. A., Porter, R. R., and Wilkinson, J. M., 1971, *Biochem. J.* **124**:301.
Pink, J. R. L., Buttery, S. H., De Vries, G. M., and Milstein, C., 1970, *Biochem. J.* **177**:33.
Ponstingl, H., Schwarz, J., Reichel, W., and Hilschmann, N., 1970. *Hoppe-Seyler's Z. Physiol. Chem.* **351**:1591.
Potter, M., 1972, *Physiol. Rev.* **52**:631.
Potter, M., and Boyce, C., 1962, *Nature* **193**:1086.
Querinjean, P. J., Bazin, H., Beckers, A., Kehoe, J. M., Schulman, J., and Capra, J. D., 1974, *Fed. Proc.* (abs.) **33**:809.
Rudikoff, S., Mushinski, E. B., Potter, M., Glaudemans, C. P., and Jolley, M. E., 1973, *J. Exp. Med.* **138**:1095.

Sledge, C., Clem, L. W., and Hood, L., 1974, *J. Immunol.*, **112**:941.

Wang, A. C., Fudenberg, H. H., and Pink, J. R. L., 1971, *Proc. Natl. Acad. Sci. U.S.* **68**:1143.

Wasserman, R. L., Kehoe, J. M., and Capra, J. D., 1974, *Fed. Proc.* (abs.) **33**:809.

Wilkinson, J. M., 1969, *Biochem. J.* **112**:173.

Wu, T. T., and Kabat, E. A., 1970, *J. Exp. Med.* **132**:211.

Separation Methods for Lymphocyte Populations[1]

Ken Shortman[2]

The Walter and Eliza Hall Institute of Medical Research
Melbourne, Australia

I. INTRODUCTION

The immune system consists of a complex array of specialized and inter-acting cells, a fact that challenges, delights, and confuses the immunologist. A direct experimental approach to this situation would be to separate out and classify individual types of cells so that their immunological responses and the nature of their interactions could be studied under controlled experimental conditions. The technology for sorting out cells from the dauntingly complex mixtures in lymphoid organs is a recent development, and "biological" separa-tion of cells, or the use of cell-specific antisera, has been responsible for the major advances so far. For example, the use of bursectomized or thymectomized animals, and the use of antilymphocyte antisera has led to the functional distinction between B and T lymphocytes.[3] However, the complexity of lym-phocyte populations extends beyond this primary division, and it is evident that in future, separation procedures will be of major importance.

Cell separation procedures may be used with a number of different objec-tives. They may be used simply to separate two types of cells, in order to study their relative role or interaction, without necessarily purifying them, for exam-ple, separating macrophages from lymphocytes. They may be used to purify a

---

[1] This is Publication No. 1934 from the Walter and Eliza Hall Institute.
[2] Mailing Address: The Royal Melbourne Hospital P.O., Victoria, 3050, Australia.
[3] Abbreviations: B cell, bone marrow/bursa-derived lymphocyte; T cell, thymus-derived lymphocyte; AFC, antibody-forming cell; CL, cytotoxic lymphocyte or killer cell; EDTA, ethylenediamine tetraacetate; HEPES, N-(2-hydroxyethyl)piperazine-N-(2-ethane)sulfonic acid.

given type of cell or a cell bearing a given function, for example, cytotoxic lymphocytes. They may be used to separate out different stages in the development of a given type of cell, for example, separating B lymphocyte AFC progenitors from mature AFC. Finally, they may be used analytically to define and characterize new developmental and functional subclasses in an objective manner.

This review will emphasize methods which are of general application, which are well controlled and established experimentally, which give good recovery of viable cells, and which are sufficiently precise and reproducible to be used analytically. Since no one separation procedure is likely to solve all experimental problems, several techniques may have to be used sequentially; this will only be effective if the methods chosen depend on different properties of the cells. Therefore, the procedures reviewed have been classified according to the theoretical basis of the separation, and an attempt has been made to select procedures which are the most efficient applications of this separation principle. The review is not exhaustive and represents a personal assessment of the techniques currently most useful for an experimental immunologist.

II. PRELIMINARY STEPS: PREPARATION OF CLEAN CELL SUSPENSIONS

A. Preparation of Single Cell Suspensions from Solid Tissue

Separation procedures should ideally commence with a clean, debris-free, nonaggregating viable cell suspension containing in good yield a fully representative sample of the cells originally present in the lymphoid tissue or circulating fluid. Just to arrive at this starting point can be the major problem with many cells from solid tissue. Fortunately, lymphocytes are very easily released from lymphoid organs by simple mechanical breakdown of the tissue. Procedures in use range from slow and tedious teasing with needles to more rapid and violent grinding procedures. As long as shearing forces which will break open cells are avoided, both extremes can give about the same total yield of viable lymphocytes with the same spectrum of cells present, the main difference being the greater speed and the greater associated damaged cells and debris with the more violent procedures. A good compromise procedure that is fast and efficient, and still minimizes cell damage, is to cut the tissue into small pieces with sharp scissors, then to extrude the cells by gently pushing the fragments against a stainless steel sieve immersed in suspension medium, using the flat end of the plunger of a glass syringe. Fibrous material is left on the sieve and rejected. Suspension is then completed by mixing the extruded cells in medium with a pasteur pipette.

A wide variety of suspension media can be employed, but some general points should be noted. The very common use of tissue culture media designed for CO_2 incubators is poor technique, since in the absence of high CO_2 pressure the bicarbonate buffer becomes extremely alkaline, and this can inactivate cells. Buffering at $pH \sim 7.2$ is best accomplished by a nontoxic organic buffer such as HEPES. A balanced salt solution best preserves cell integrity, and no advantage in terms of minimizing cell aggregation seems to be gained by omitting divalent metals. Likewise, addition of heparin usually has no effect on reducing cell clumping. Cell viability is generally improved in media containing serum, for example, 20% fetal calf serum. To maintain cells close to their normal state the medium should be isoosmotic with the serum of the species used, and this can vary markedly from most laboratory media, which are normally designed to be isoosmotic with human serum (Williams et al., 1972). For most procedures it is advisable to arrest cell metabolism immediately by working in ice-cold medium; under these conditions additional nutrients are not required in the medium. An example of a useful suspension medium is given by Shortman et al. (1972d).

Freshly prepared cell suspensions contain a high proportion of fine cell debris and large aggregated clumps which would interfere with separation procedures and which are generally reduced by first settling out the large clumps, then "washing" the cells by low-speed (400g, 7 min) centrifugation to leave fine debris in suspension. The efficiency of these steps can easily be improved by a simple "zonal" procedure, i.e., by settling the suspension over a layer of fetal calf serum, then spinning the cells through the layer (Shortman et al., 1972d). Speed of handling and cell viability are improved by reducing the number of times cells are centrifuged to a pellet, and this procedure gives a clean preparation with one spin.

B. Removal of Damaged Cells

Mechanical disintegration of lymphoid tissue inevitably produces a proportion of damaged cells (typically 30% in spleen, 10% in thymus), which are usually visualized by their uptake of stains such as eosin or trypan blue. Being similar in size to intact cells, they are not normally eliminated by settling or washing procedures. Such damaged cells may interfere with many immunological studies, and they often cause severe problems with cell separation techniques because (i) they add to the cell separation load and so limit the number of viable cells that can be separated; (ii) their tendency to adhere nonspecifically to a solid matrix interferes with adherence and affinity chromatography; (iii) they are the cause of severe clumping and aggregation effects.

Several procedures have been devised to eliminate damaged cells. Filtration of suspensions through a column of cotton wool or grass wool or glass beads (Kovařík, 1963; Shortman, 1966) has been used, but such columns will also selectively eliminate certain classes of viable lymphocytes (see later discussion of adherence columns) and for this reason should be avoided.

Damaged cells are normally much denser than viable cells, presumably because of leakage of light cytoplasm, and this has served as the basis of a simple, one-step separation procedure (Shortman *et al.*, 1972d). In this procedure a cell pellet of up to 10^9 cells is dispersed directly into 5 ml of dense ($\sim$1.094 g/cm^3 for mouse cells) isoosmotic, pH 5.1 albumin medium. Further dense medium is layered underneath, light medium is layered above, and the interfaces are deliberately mixed to eliminate sharp density discontinuities. Centrifugation at 3500g for 10 min sediments all damaged cells, leaving viable and fully functional cells in the supernatant, with nearly complete recovery. Low pH albumin is used to reduce cell aggregation; if lower cell loads can be accepted, neutral pH albumin may be employed. Cells damaged by enzyme treatment differ from those damaged mechanically, since they swell and become less dense at low pH; in this case separation can only be effected with neutral pH medium.

The density procedure, although simple, demands the careful preparation of isoosmotic albumin media. An equally effective and simpler alternative has been presented by von Boehmer and Shortman (1973). Damaged cells show a marked tendency to aggregate, and partial separation can be achieved simply by standing suspensions for long periods, allowing aggregated damaged elements to settle out. However, this aggregation and stickiness of damaged cells is greatly enhanced in medium of low ionic strength. Accordingly, cells are dispersed in cold buffered medium of ionic strength 10 to 20% of normal, the osmotic balance being maintained by glucose and sorbitol. Damaged cells preferentially clump and become exceptionally adherent, and are completely eliminated by rapid filtration at 0°C through a thin layer of cotton wool. No selective loss of viable lymphocytes or phagocytes is seen under these conditions, and functional cells are recovered in high yield. The maximum load is 5 $\times$ 10^7 cells per ml, and 10^9 cells can readily be handled with large volumes and several filtering tubes.

C. Elimination of Erythrocytes

With tissues such as spleen or bone marrow, erythrocytes are a major component and may complicate immunological tests and contribute to overloading separation procedures. Although many of the separation techniques described later will effectively separate lymphocytes from erythrocytes, a simple preliminary removal step is often advisable. At neutral pH, red cells are denser than most lymphocytes, and the same density cut procedure used to eliminate damaged cells, but operated at pH 7.2, can be used to remove erythrocytes and damaged cells simultaneously (Shortman *et al.*, 1972d). However, a definite and possibly selective loss of lymphocytes is associated with this neutral pH procedure.

An alternative method is the selective lysis of red cells by suspension in ammonium chloride solution. This depends on the fact that red cells are effectively permeable to NH_4Cl, whereas lymphocytes are not, so that red cells are lysed by the unbalanced osmotic pressure of their colloid and cation contents. With mouse cells, 10 min suspension in 0.17 M NH_4Cl at 0–4°C will eliminate red cells without affecting either the physical properties or the biological activity of lymphocytes (Shortman *et al.,* 1972d). Longer exposure, or incubation at 37°C, will cause some loss of immunological function. With other types of erythrocytes (for example, human), lysis of red cells requires 10 min at approximately room temperature, and possible selective loss of activity should be checked before using this procedure.

D. Elimination of Erythrocytes and Isolation of Lymphocytes from Blood

The preliminary steps in blood fractionation involve separating lymphocytes from the vast excess of erythrocytes and also, if necessary, from platelets and phagocytes. Most of the separation procedures to be considered are capable of sorting out these elements, but the vast overload of erythrocytes would render the separation inefficient. A very extensive literature on separation of blood cells exists, and has been reviewed by Cutts (1970). Several successful commercial machines have been developed to sort out the basic categories of blood cells [the IBM-NCI closed continuous-flow centrifuge (Judson *et al.,* 1968); the Technicon Lymphocyte Separator (Lichtenstein *et al.,* 1971)]. These will not be considered in detail. While many of the techniques developed are fast and effective for many applications, the majority have definite limitations for the experimental immunologist. Lymphocyte purity is often low, and typically recovery from whole blood is poor (~30%), making the selective loss of particular types of lymphocytes a likely event. The following procedures combine high recovery with high lymphocyte purity.

Erythrocytes in blood tend to associate in the form of rouleaux large enough to sediment faster than blood leukocytes, although an individual erythrocyte normally sediments more slowly than a white cell. Under appropriate conditions, merely standing the blood to allow red cells to selectively sediment is an effective, mild, and simple procedure. Fresh blood with a suitable anticoagulant (20 units preservative-free heparin/ml) is used, since defibrination may cause selective loss of certain lymphocytes. When using mice, the animals should be injected with heparin (20 units/animal) before bleeding. Sedimentation is faster if the blood is diluted twofold with a suitable suspension medium, and if the procedure is carried out at room temperature. Red cells from the blood of certain species (e.g., mouse) sediment poorly. In these cases, fibrinogen (human fibrinogen, outdated blood bank material will suffice) is added in the dilution medium to a final level of 5–10 mg/ml to induce rapid sedimentation (R Miller, personal communication). In all cases, the minimum time to complete sedimentation (20–45 min standing) should be used to minimize white cell loss. The efficiency of separation can be increased by a simple procedure introduced by Hulliger and Blazkovec (1967). The fresh, heparinized, diluted, and, if necessary, fibrinogenated blood is layered over a dense, isotonic solution containing a high-density radioopaque material such as Isopaque or Urographin, as well as a red cell agglutinin such as methyl cellulose. Only red cells are sufficiently dense to penetrate this layer. As the sedimentation rouleaux enter this phase, they agglutinate and rapidly sediment to the bottom. The result is an upper layer of plasma and white cells readily removed from the red cells, and recovery of leukocytes is around 95%. The red cell: white cell ratio is reduced typically to around 5:1. If necessary, the ammonium chloride treatment procedure can be used to remove these residual red cells.

To separate lymphocytes from other white cells, the active-adherence column procedure described in detail later may be directly applied to the supernatant from the red cell sedimentation. The purity of the resultant lymphocytes is then 96–100%, with 85–90% overall recovery from the original blood. A special class of adherent lymphocytes would be lost on the column, but these are in very low concentration in blood, if present at all. Any terminal removal of residual red cells with NH_4Cl is best applied after column separation.

III. SEPARATION BASED ON PHYSICAL PARAMETERS OF CELLS

Cells may differ in size, in overall chemical composition, and in the chemical nature of their surface, and a variety of methods have been developed to exploit these differences (Shortman, 1972). Such procedures are potentially capable not only of separating certain types of cells from each other, but also of providing a precise and objective characterization based on the physical parameters of the cell. However, to be capable of this analytical aspect the methods need to be rigorously controlled and standardized, and numerous engineering problems intervene before even a fairly simple separation principle can be made effective. One of the main problems is that cells are not fixed entities, but change their properties with the environment, i.e., with factors such as osmotic pressure, pH, or temperature. While small changes may not be severe enough to kill a cell, they may cause marked effects on the very property being used for separation.

A. Sedimentation-Velocity Separation

1. Theoretical Aspects

A spherical cell moving through a uniform stable medium under the influence of a constant gravitational field rapidly reaches a constant velocity that represents a balance between the applied field and the resistance to movement in the fluid. This constant velocity is given by

$$v = 2(\rho_c - \rho_m)gr^2/9\eta$$

where ρ_c is the density of the cell, ρ_m the density of the medium, g the gravitational field, and r the radius of the cell.

The sedimentation velocity of a cell is therefore determined by *both* the cell diameter and cell density. In practice, if the density of the medium is kept low and the cells do not differ too widely in density, size difference becomes the predominant factor in separation. Separations based purely on cell size can be obtained by preselecting a restricted density range of cells for fractionation by using a preliminary "density cut" procedure, which will be considered later.

When sedimentation separation is carried out in a centrifuge using steep density gradients to avoid turbulence, the centrifugal field and the viscosity and density of the medium vary with the position in the tube. The equation of motion then becomes more complex, and solution for a given set of conditions requires extensive calculation. Computer programs have been used to predict and interpret results, and solutions are available for some conditions (Boone *et al.*, 1968; Pretlow *et al.*, 1969; and Pretlow, 1971).

2. Systems Available

Zonal centrifugation, in a direct adaptation of techniques used for subcellular particles, has been used for cell separation. Many modifications of the usual procedures are needed because of the very rapid sedimentation rate of cells and their relatively narrow size distribution, and because stabilizing gradient media such as sucrose cause osmotic effects. Boone *et al.* (1968) and Pretlow (1971) have used low-speed centrifugation in viscous gradients of Ficoll to produce cell separation. This approach holds promise for rapid, large-scale separation of cells in zonal rotors, and the hardware is available in most laboratories. However, many engineering problems have not as yet been examined, such as (i) the streaming limit for cell loading, (ii) the wall effects when using centrifuge tubes, and (iii) the effects of Ficoll on cell aggregation and medium osmolarity.

Other approaches include centrifugal elutriation in the counterstreaming centrifuge of Lindahl (Lindahl, 1948, 1956; McEwen *et al.*, 1968) currently under commercial development but so far limited to a two-fraction separation; continuous-flow separation at unit gravity in the STAFLO apparatus devised by Mel (Mel, 1964a,b,c; Mel *et al.*, 1965), not commercially available and probably not of adequate resolution for most lymphocyte studies; multiple sedimentation at unit gravity in a thin-layer countercurrent distribution apparatus, an interesting approach developed by Albertsson and Walter (Albertsson, 1972; Walter and Albertsson, 1971) and useful if the commercially available apparatus is at hand.

However, the simplest, the mildest, the most precise and effective, and so far the most rewarding technique has been zonal sedimentation at unit gravity in the STAYPUT device, as introduced by Peterson and Evans (1967) and Miller and Phillips (1969).

3. Unit-Gravity STAYPUT Separation

The basic apparatus is a wide cylindrical chamber with a conical base leading to an entry port with a baffle. A cell suspension is run into the chamber, and suspension medium containing a shallow stabilizing density gradient is pumped in underneath, lifting the cell suspension through the widening cone and into the cylindrical chamber until it forms a thin band at the top of the cylindrical region. The cells are then allowed to settle through the static stabilizing gradient for several hours. At the end of this period the contents are flowed out of the chamber, and fractions containing cells that have sedimented various distances are collected. Because of the width of the chamber and the stability of the system, a small sedimentation difference between cells becomes a large volume difference which may be separated into many fractions.

The conditions for high and optimum resolution, the limits of the system, and the basis of the separation have been thoroughly established in the original studies of Miller and Phillips (1969) and have recently been described in full detail by Miller (1973). The basic apparatus is simple to construct and may be purchased commercially (Johns Scientific, Toronto, Canada). The cell suspension should be as free as possible of debris, damaged cells, and cell aggregates. The cell load on the system must not exceed a certain critical limit above which "streamers" of the cell suspension flow into the gradient instead of the cells sedimenting as individual units. This streaming limit can be increased by making a gradient that is steep just under the cell layer and shallow thereafter. The streaming limit for lymphoid cells will then be around 4×10^6 total cells/ml. This restricts the maximum load on a small (say, 15-cm-diameter) chamber to 10^8 cells in an input cell band of 2.5 ml. The load will increase with the square of the chamber diameter. The stabilizing gradient is best prepared with 5–30% fetal calf serum, but shallow gradients of other marcromolecules such as Ficoll or albumin may be effective. An overlay of salt solution above the cell zone helps provide a flat starting band. A baffle of critical shape and positioning at the streamlined entry port is essential to reduce turbulence during filling of the apparatus. After sedimentation of 1–4 hr at 0–4°C cell fractions are collected either by reversed flow out the entry port, or by upward flow out a separate baffle-free exit cone as suggested by Peterson and Evans (1967) and Mage et al. (1968, 1969) but with some streamlining of the exit port to avoid turbulence (Kraft and Shortman, 1972). Different chambers have been designed for use with larger, rapidly sedimenting cells (Miller, 1973). For analytical work it may be necessary to allow for sedimentation during the filling and emptying of the chamber, as well as during the statis phase, and to allow also for small changes in viscosity and density of the gradient medium (Miller, 1973; Kraft and Shortman, 1972).

4. Some Applications

Cells in Cycle. During the mitotic cycle a cell gradually increases in size, then halves its volume at cell division. During this period there is normally little change in cell buoyant density. Sedimentation-velocity separation should therefore separate different stages of the cell cycle and spread them over a range of sedimentation rates which can vary by a factor of 1.59. A study of L cells in tissue culture by Macdonald and Miller (1970) showed this to be the case, with cells in individual fractions being synchronized for the phase of the cell cycle. In mice, antierythrocyte IgM-producing AFCs near the peak of response were shown by Phillips and Miller (1970) to sediment as expected of a cycling cell population. Unit-gravity sedimentation has been used by Williams and Moore (1973) to characterize and separate cycle stages of granulocytic progenitor cells in monkey hemopoietic tissue. The technique is particularly valuable for studying dividing lymphoid cells, since all stages of the cycle can be simultaneously isolated from a nonsynchronized population.

Blood Cells. Good separation of various human blood elements has been obtained by Brubaker and Evans (1969), the order of sedimentation rate being platelets, erythrocytes, lymphocytes, monocytes, and granulocytes. This separation was as would be predicted from the order of cell size, with the added effect that high cell density caused erythrocytes to sediment close to lymphocytes and increased the sedimentation of granulocytes relative to monocytes.

B Cells and T Cells. The small lymphocytes of B or T lineage are known from morphological evidence to be of roughly similar size, and it would not be expected that large differences in sedimentation rate exist. Sedimentation rate

Figure 1. The unit-gravity sedimentation characteristics of C3H/C57BL6 F1 mouse spleen T (θ+ve) and B (θ−ve) lymphocytes. The T cells were assayed by an anti-θ cytotoxic assay. θ-ve cells were predominantly B cells, but would include lymphocytes lacking defined markers, as well as some nonlymphoid nucleated cells. The curves reflect the absolute B and T cell distribution, not the percentage per fraction. The curves are normalized so that the area under each curve is proportional to the relative concentration of each class. The S values are for separations in media isoosmotic with human (not mouse) serum, performed at 4°C. In the regions through which the cells sediment, the mean density of the medium was 1.010 g/cm³ and the viscosity was close to that of water. The figure was kindly provided by Dr. R. Miller.

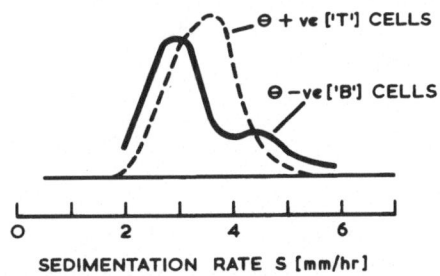

separation of T and B cells from mouse spleen, as shown in Fig. 1, gives marked overlap between the populations and little useful net separation. However, analytically the two lymphocyte classes are clearly different, and there is heterogeneity in the B cell population and possibly also in the T cell population. This may be related to the differentiation states considered below.

B Lymphocyte Differentiation. During the antigen-independent development of B cells from pluripotent stem cells, and during the antigen-dependent development of AFC from B cells, there are several marked overall changes in cell size, additional to cell cycle-dependent variations. Thus sedimentation-rate separation can select out and characterize discrete steps in this developmental pathway. Figure 2 is a summary by Dr. R. Miller of the changes in sedimentation rate of cells at defined stages of this B cell pathway, as demonstrated in the studies of Lafleur, Miller, Phillips, and associates (Phillips and Miller, 1970; Miller and Phillips, 1970; Edwards *et al.*, 1970; Lafleur *et al.*, 1972a, 1972b, 1973). These represent basically the noncycling stages, and the predicted additional changes in sedimentation rate are observed when the cells are in the division cycle. Further intermediates in the pathway can also be demonstrated. For example, shortly after antigen-activation, B cells enlarge and show increased sedimentation, as shown by Diener *et al.* (1973), and very marked cell size and sedimentation rate changes occur in toad spleen AFC during the development of the immune response (Kraft and Shortman, 1972). Marked enrichment (20- to 140-fold) of AFC is obtained by unit-gravity sedimentation (Phillips and Miller, 1970; Kraft and Shortman, 1972; Mage *et al.*, 1968, 1969).

T Lymphocyte Differentiation. T cell differentiation is also characterized by pronounced changes in the sedimentation rate of the cells, as demonstrated by Macdonald *et al.* (1973a,b) and summarized in Fig. 3. Typical slow-sedimenting (and therefore small) T cells initiate a cytotoxic response to alloantigen. The earliest, least mature cytotoxic lymphocytes have a high sedimentation rate, indicating they are large T cells. However, the sedimentation rate of active cells gradually returns toward that of the smaller T cell progenitors as the response develops.

B. Density Separation

1. General Comments

The density of a cell reflects its average chemical composition, i.e., its relative protein, nucleic acid, carbohydrate, lipid, and water content. Most cells have similar proportions of these components, and the density range of cells is therefore relatively narrow. However, sensitive methods relying on these small density differences are now extensively used for lympocyte separation. In operation, density separation is independent of cell size, although the two

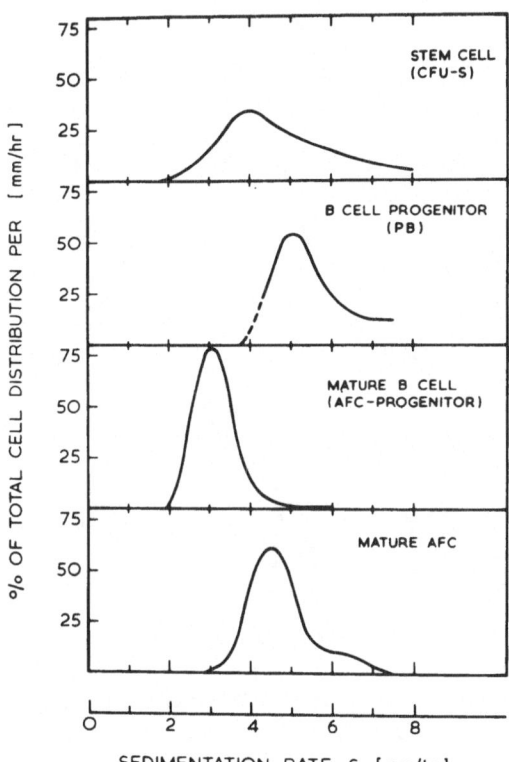

SEDIMENTATION RATE S [mm/hr]

Figure 2. Unit-gravity sedimentation-rate separation
of cells in various stages of the B cell developmental
pathway. Conditions are as for Fig. 1. In all cases
functional assays were used to establish the distribution curves. Stem cells from bone marrow were assayed as colony-formed units (CFU) in spleen after
transfer to irradiated recipients. Both the B cell and
the pre-B cell assays were based on an adoptive
immune response to sheep erythrocytes in irradiated
recipients. AFCs were direct plaque-forming cells in
an antisheep erythrocyte hemolysis assay. In all cases
a major portion of the cells studied were in a noncycling state. Intermediates between these various
categories, probably involving cell division cycles,
have also been demonstrated. The figure was kindly
provided by Dr. R. Miller, and is based on results of
Lafleur, Miller, Phillips, and associates, as detailed in
the text.

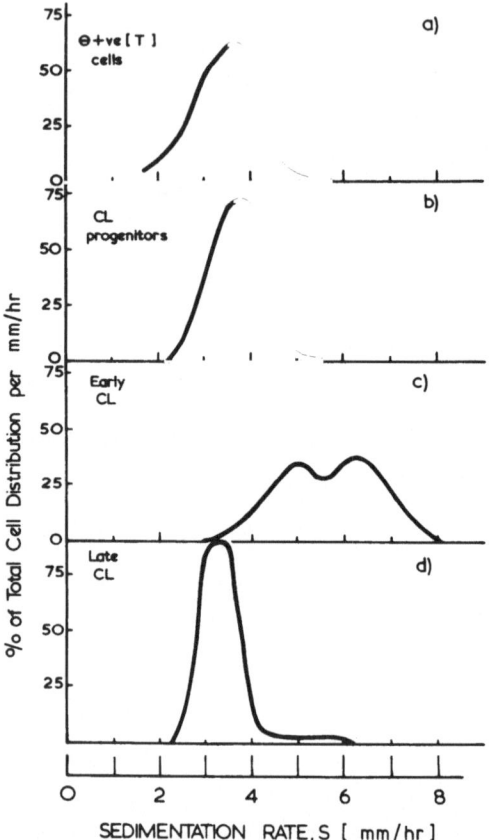

Figure 3. Unit-gravity sedimentation-rate separation
of T cells at various stages of a cytotoxic response to
allogenic cells. Conditions were as for Fig. 1. The
assay for all T cells in mouse spleen involved anti-θ
antiserum. Other profiles were based on functional
assays. The sedimentation profile for cytotoxic
lymphocyte (CL) progenitors was identical for
spleen and thymus, and was measured as the ability
to produce CL in culture. CLs developed from spleen
cells and were measured by a chromium release assay
using labeled allogenic mastocytes. The less mature
CLs were obtained either after transfer to irradiated
allogenic recipients, or by four days of culture with
allogenic cells. Mature or late CLs were obtained 23
days after a tumor allograft into intact animals. The
figure was provided by Dr. R. Miller, and is based on
results of Macdonald, Phillips, Miller, and associates,
as detailed in text.

parameters sometimes vary in parallel. For example, large cells tend to be lighter, in part due to an increased ratio of light cytoplasm to dense nucleus. However, this is only a general rule, and there are now many examples of dense large and light small cells. In many cases, density and sedimentation-rate separation complement each other and can provide a useful two-dimensional approach to cell separation.

2. Systems Available

Many different centrifugation systems have been proposed for separation of cells on the basis of their buoyant density, and these fall into three general categories: (i) neutral density separation, or density cut procedures, where cells are suspended in a medium of given density and centrifuged to give two fractions, the denser sedimented pellet cells and the lighter supernatant cells; (ii) discontinuous-gradient separation, where cells are centrifuged in a medium consisting of a series of layers of increasing density, and cells collect at the interfaces marking regions above and below their own buoyant density; (iii) centrifugation to equilibrium in continuous-density gradients, where cells reach equilibrium in the region corresponding exactly to their buoyant density. These will be discussed in order, with particular emphasis on the analytical, continuous-gradient approach. Some technical problems common to all procedures are considered in the detailed discussion of continuous gradients. Only procedures shown to be effective for lymphocytes are considered. More extensive reviews of density separation have been provided by Shortman (1969b, 1970, 1972) and Leif (1970).

3. Density Cut Procedure

A fast and simple, but nevertheless precise and efficient neutral density separation procedure using albumin media of defined density was introduced by Shortman et al. (1972d). Although originally used for damaged cell and red cell removal as detailed earlier, the same approach with an appropriate choice of albumin concentration can be used to produce a "cut" into cells above and below any given density. A cell pellet is dispersed directly into the density medium in a centrifuge tube, and the same dense medium is layered below and lighter medium is layered above this cell zone. The sharp interfaces are then deliberately mixed to provide a more gradual density change; this minimizes cell aggregation and concentration at the interface and thereby increases the loading capacity and improves separation. Centrifugation for 10–15 min at 4000g in the swing-out head of a refrigerated centrifuge then separates the population into cells lighter and denser than the albumin medium. Two such steps in succession can isolate cells of any given density range.

The procedure is most useful when the choice of the density cut value is made by reference to a cell or activity-density distribution profile established by prior continuous-gradient cell distribution analysis. For example, from Fig. 6, a cut at density 1.075 g/cm³ will produce nonsedimenting cells from CBA mouse thymus enriched ~20 times in PHA-responsive lymphocytes. The procedure is especially useful as a preliminary step to select constant-density cells for sedimentation-rate analysis, since the latter procedure will then give a pure size-based separation. The simple cut procedure has been used by Moore *et al.* (1971, 1973) to produce on a routine basis almost complete separation of normal from leukemic macrophage-granulocyte progenitor cells in human blood and bone marrow, and to extensively purify monkey bone marrow "stem" cells.

4. Discontinuous Density Gradients

Discontinuous, or step, density gradients have been extensively used to separate lymphocyte populations into a number of predetermined density fractions. They offer the advantages of simplicity in generating the "gradient" and simplicity in collecting the cells after centrifugation, since the cells concentrate at the region of the interface between the density steps. Two widely used protocols are those of Dicke *et al.* (1968), Dicke (1970), and Raidt *et al.* (1968). However, this approach has some fundamental limitations and additional restrictions due to the way it is often employed. The operative part of the gradient is in fact the zone at the interface, the true "gradient," and in contrast to a continuous gradient this is only a small proportion of the total tube volume. The maximum cell load for good resolution on a discontinuous gradient is therefore low. This maximum load is often exceeded, giving rise to aggregation and trapping of cells in the "wrong" interface band. In addition the normal practice of layering cells on the top of the gradient produces marked wall effects as radially sedimenting cells encounter the parallel tube walls, and this reduces the efficiency of separation. The technique is often used in such a way that factors such as medium osmolarity and pH are not controlled, resulting in variation in results from one batch of medium to another. For many purposes the previously mentioned density cut procedure is both simpler and more efficient, and the continuous-gradient procedures have greater precision, resolution, and loading capacity. Discontinuous gradients may be the choice in intermediate situations, when a cut into 3–6 separate density fractions is all that is required, and when the cells to be separated are widely different in density.

5. Continuous Gradient Separation

The first precise and effective isopycnic, continuous-density gradient separation of cells was the procedure developed by Leif and Vinograd (1964) for the study of human erythrocytes. Modifications of this procedure have since been extensively used by Shortman (1968, 1969b, 1970, 1972; Williams *et al.*, 1972) and others to produce efficient separation and analysis of lymphocyte populations. The discussion will for convenience center on the basic procedure of the author, with the different approaches used by other workers presented in a comparative manner in the discussion of technical aspects.

The density medium used in the Shortman procedure is bovine serum albumin, usually 16–29% w/w, in a balanced salt solution of precisely controlled osmolarity and *p*H. Normally the *p*H is 5.1, and the medium isoosmotic with the serum of the species studied. The whole procedure is carried out in the cold. A maximum of 10^9 lymphoid cells are dispersed directly into 7.5 ml of the dense medium, and a continuous linear gradient of 15 ml volume prepared using a single-chamber, peristaltic-pump-driven mixing apparatus described elsewhere (Shortman, 1972). The sealed tube is then centrifuged at 4000*g* for 30 min in the swing-out head of a refrigerated centrifuge; these conditions bring the cells to equilibrium. About 20–30 fractions of precise volume are collected by upward displacement out a conical exit, using a time-based peristaltic-pump-driven apparatus described elsewhere (Shortman, 1972). The precise density (± 0.00005 g/cm^3) of each fraction is measured on microdroplet samples, using a nonaqueous, bromobenzene–petroleum spirit gradient in a calibrated burette tube (Shortman, 1968). Cells are then recovered by dilution and centrifugation of each fraction. The method gives high cell and activity recoveries (75–100%) in a very wide range of immunological applications. It is capable of high resolution, especially if narrow-range gradients are used (Shortman, 1968; 1971). Buoyant density values are reproducible to ± 0.0003 g/cm^3, about one quarter of a fraction, so that cells can be characterized on the basis of their density under defined conditions.

6. Technical Aspects

Osmolarity Control: Choice of Medium. Cells act as osmometers and undergo marked density shifts due to water exchange in media of different osmolarity. This parameter must be rigidly controlled if reproducible buoyant density values are to be maintained; if possible it should be checked with a vapor-pressure osmometer. The osmolarity of sera varies substantially from one species to another (Williams *et al.*, 1972) and this factor must be considered, preferably by making the separation gradient isoosmotic with the species studied. The problem of maintaining a constant osmolarity in the face of a varying concentration of density-gradient material is solved in principle by using a substance of high molecular weight, which then contributes little to total osmolarity, rather than using a substance such as sucrose. Albumin has been used in the above procedures of Shortman and of Leif and Vinograd. Others have used Ficoll (Gorczynski *et al.,* 1970; Bach and Brashler, 1970. Noble and Cutts, 1968) or colloidal silica (Pertoft, 1969, 1970; Pertoft and Laurent, 1969; Pertoft *et al.,* 1968). Any small osmotic contribution of the macromolecule itself may be compensated for by adding a small calculated amount of water to the balanced salt solution used as the basic medium. Even consideration of these factors does not ensure constant osmolarity, for in practice "contaminants," such as salt or water in commercial preparations of macromolecules, can have an overwhelming effect on the final osmotic pressure of the medium; such components must be eliminated, for example, by extensive dialysis followed by complete drying of albumin powder. Another complication is that macromolecules may change the effective osmotic pressure by binding significant quantities of either salts or water; thus high Ficoll concentrations appear to "bind" water and cause the dense regions of Ficoll gradients to be markedly hypertonic (Williams *et al.,* 1972; Bach and Brashler, 1970). Under some conditions albumin may induce small osmotic changes by binding salts (Gorczynski *et al.,* 1970), but direct testing of the media prepared by Shortman's procedure showed they were precisely isoosmotic (Williams *et al.,* 1972).

Aggregation Effects: Choice of Medium. Most macromolecules used as gradient media appear to enhance cell association, resulting in either overt clumping or simply an increased proportion of doublets and small aggregates. This is a major factor limiting the resolution of density separation, since cells then band at the mean density of the aggregate, rather than reaching equilibrium at their own buoyant density. Ficoll causes more extensive aggregation than albumin, but both induce aggregation at neutral pH (Shortman, 1972), both in the cold and at room temperature. Lowering the pH of albumin media to around 5.1 eliminates visible signs of aggregation and improves resolution; this is readily achieved by using nonneutralized albumin, which then acts as an excellent buffer near its low isoelectric point (Shortman, 1968, 1972). To reduce aggregation in Ficoll, both low pH and the addition of a dispersing agent have been employed (Gorczynski *et al.,* 1970; Hilal *et al.,* 1964; Shortman, 1968, 1972). Other steps taken to reduce cell association and improve resolution are (a) reducing the total cell load on the gradient, (b) dispersing cells into the gradient before separation, and (c) using relatively high centrifugal forces to pull apart interacting cells that differ in density (Shortman, 1968, 1969b, 1970, 1972).

Wall Effects and Streaming. If cells are applied as a band at the top of a density gradient, two hydrodynamic effects causing lack of resolution may occur. Since the load is usually well above the streaming limit discussed earlier for sedimentation separation, the upper layer streams into the gradient as blobs of medium and cells (Hilal *et al.,* 1964) rather than the cells moving as individual units. This can be overcome by dispersing cells directly into the gradient medium itself (Shortman, 1968, 1972; Leif and Vinograd, 1964) or by increasing the viscosity of the medium used in the initial cell band (Leif *et al.,* 1972). A second effect occurs as some of the radially sedimenting cells meet the cylindrical tube walls and adhere, rather than move to the region of their buoyant density. This can be overcome by using zonal rotors or sector-shaped tubes or by applying a washer to restrict cells to the central gradient regions (Leif *et al.*, 1972). Alternatively wall effects and streaming can both be overcome by mixing cells into the lower regions of the gradient initially, so that sedimentation is away from the tube walls (Shortman, 1968, 1972; Leif and Vinograd, 1964).

Linearity of Density Gradients. If the shape of a density gradient departs from linear, the distribution of cells in fractions collected on a volume basis will be altered. This is no more than an inconvenience when separation alone is the objective. However, when cell populations are being characterized analytically the problem becomes crucial, since false peaks can readily be generated and the apparent distribution profile will vary. It is technically difficult to generate strictly linear gradients with viscous solutions of macromolecules, and conventional gradient-generation systems are inadequate. Leif (1968a,b) has developed a special pump-and-gradient system making strictly linear gradients, but unfortunately the rather complex apparatus is not yet available commercially. The gradient-generation-and-collection system employed by Shortman (1972) based on the earlier system of Leif and Vinograd (1964) produces very nearly linear gradients if a relatively stiff (e.g., Tygon) rather than soft (e.g., Silastic) tubing is used in the peristaltic pump. One way to avoid the effects of gradient shape on the apparent cell density distribution is to plot all results as cells per density increment *vs.* density (which is the mathematically correct form) rather than as cells per fraction or as cells per unit volume. This approach demands very accurate density determinations on each fraction, which can be accomplished by the microdroplet procedure used by Shortman (1968, 1969b, 1970).

Rebanding Experiments. A basic control for the validity of density separation experiments is the ability to reband cells from one fraction as a single peak with identical density on a second gradient. Leif and Vinograd (1964) and Leif *et al.* (1972) have demonstrated excellent rebanding of erythrocytes with albumin gradients at neutral *p*H, and Gorczynski *et al.* (1970) obtained exact rebanding of mouse spleen cells using Ficoll gradients. AFC fractions were successfully rebanded in isoosmotic *p*H 5.1 albumin gradients by Williams *et al.* (1972). However, a disturbing observation is that thymus lymphocytes usually fail to reband and show an increase in density on the second spin (Shortman, 1968; Williams *et al.*, 1972; Williams and Shortman, 1972). There is evidence that no density shift occurs in the course of one single run. This effect is possibly due to the stress induced by a second centrifugation, which affects the permeability properties of only particular types of cells, such as the more labile thymocytes. The effect is reduced by working under isoosmotic conditions (Williams *et al.*, 1972), by reducing the centrifugal force used (Shortman, 1968), and, surprisingly, by working at acid rather than neutral *p*H (Williams and

Shortman, 1972). The results do serve as a warning that the separation procedure may affect the propeties of cells, despite the excellent biological recoveries usually obtained.

Effect of pH on Cell Buoyant Density. Changing the pH of the medium to avoid aggregation effects can result in changes in the apparent buoyant density of various cells. The most obvious case is erythrocytes, which show a reversible increase in volume and decrease in density at acid pH (from 1.11 g/cm^3 at pH 7.4 to 1.087 g/cm^3 at pH 5.1, for mouse erythrocytes at mouse osmolarity) (Legge and Shortman, 1968; Williams and Shortman, 1972). This has served on the basis of a procedure for separating erythroid from lymphoid cells (Shortman and Seligman, 1969). The reason for the volume and density change is the specialized anion permeability—cation impermeability properties of the erythrocyte membrane. As the pH decreases, the charge on the red cell hemoglobin becomes more positive, and anions enter the cell across the membrane in accordance with the Donnan equilibrium. The resultant increase in anions, predominantly Cl$^-$, causes the cell to swell osmotically. This interpretation was challenged by Kneece and Leif (1971), but has been substantiated by control experiments of Williams and Shortman (1972).

Lymphocytes do not normally display these selective permeability properties. They do not change volume with pH under normal conditions (Legge and Shortman, 1968; Shortman and Seligman, 1969; Williams and Shortman, 1972), and do not change density with pH when tested in a simple, nonaqueous neutral density separation procedure (Williams and Shortman, 1972). However, they do display definite pH-induced density shifts in continuous aqueous gradients of Ficoll (Gorczynski *et al.*, 1970) or albumin (Williams and Shortman, 1972). The density change of lymphocytes with pH is about half that observed with erythrocytes, and is reversible. Surprisingly, the buoyant density of lymphocytes at acid pH in isoosmotic albumin media is close to the apparent "true" density in serum, and it is the banding density at pH 7.2 which is anomalous (Williams and Shortman, 1972). The results suggest that some stress on the cell membrane during centrifugation can cause unusual permeability changes, giving pH-induced effects similar to red cell characteristics.

Fine Structure and Heterogeneity in Lymphocyte Density Distribution Profiles. A characteristic of the density distribution of lymphoid cell populations, as seen with the low pH albumin procedure of Shortman, is the density heterogeneity, with a series of closely spaced density peaks in the cell distribution profile (Shortman, 1968, 1971), such as obtained in Figs. 4, 5, and 6. These density "peaks" can only be fully resolved with high-resolution, narrow-range gradients, and the failure of some investigators to detect such heterogeneity has been due to the use of very-wide-range gradients with few fractions. A range of control experiments has suggested that these peaks represent valid physical entities (Shortman, 1968, 1971; Williams *et al.*, 1972), and immunological studies are revealing functional differences between the density peaks. It is possible that the density subpopulations represent discrete stages in the differentiation of lymphocytes. Nevertheless, there is no positive evidence that all peaks represent valid biological entities, and the anomalous rebanding and pH effects leave room for some degree of complexity induced by the method itself. Gorczynski *et al.* (1970) suggested that the generation of osmotic gradients by salt binding in albumin media could explain the density heterogeneity of AFC. In a test of this possibility, Williams *et al.* (1972) demonstrated the absence of osmotic gradients in the albumin media, and attributed differences in apparent AFC heterogeneity to biological differences in the source of AFC used for study (see, for example, Fig. 5). However, the possibility remains that some more subtle effect, such as differential salt binding or differential cell permeability, could cause some part of the buoyant density heterogeneity.

Effect of Temperature. Most separation procedures are carried out at low temperature to prevent metabolic activity and to conserve cell viability. However, at temperatures below 20°C there may be phase changes in the lipids of the lymphocyte surface, and this could affect properties such as cell permeability. A series of comparisons in which AFC and thymus lymphocytes were separated at 22°C or 4–7°C showed that the resulting density distribution characteristics were very similar. Heterogeneity and fine structure in the distribution profile of lymphocyte populations were unchanged, cell recoveries were the same, and similar pH effects were observed. The only difference appeared to be the predictable small shift to lighter buoyant density with increasing temperature (Shortman, unpublished data).

7. Some Applications

Blood Cells. Continuous-density gradients of many types, employing albumin, Ficoll, and colloidal silica density media, have been applied to human blood cells to test the effectiveness of separation. Basically similar results have been reported in all cases (Pertoft and Laurent, 1969; Pertoft *et al.*, 1968; Zucker and Cassen, 1969; Oberjat, 1970; Williams *et al.*, 1974; Noble and Cutts, 1968). Erythrocytes give a single peak, but with a wide density dispersion due to the continuous age distribution of the population (Leif and Vinograd, 1964; Shortman, 1968). As discussed previously, erythrocytes are the densest blood elements above pH 7.0, but swell to lower densities as the pH is reduced. The next densest elements are granulocytes, with some separation between basophils, neutrophils, and eosinophils (Pertoft and Laurent, 1969; Pertoft *et al.*, 1968; Oberjat, 1970; Zucker and Cassen, 1969; Williams *et al.*, 1974). Although there is a clear distinction between dense granulocytes and lighter mononuclear cells, there is only partial separation between human blood lymphocytes and monocytes. Most workers have found blood monocytes to be generally lighter than lymphocytes (Pertoft and Laurent, 1969; Pertoft *et al.*, 1968; Zucker and Cassen, 1969; Oberjat, 1970), in line with the light density of tissue macrophages as compared to small lymphocytes (Shortman *et al.*, 1970), but Noble and Cutts (1968) reported they were denser, a result that may have been due to incomplete density equilibrium. However, recent results of Williams *et al.* (1974) indicate that monocytes are heterogeneous, with components denser and less dense than lymphocytes. Most workers have reported that lymphocytes form a single homogeneous density peak, but the wide range of the gradients used would preclude detection of any fine structure. Recent studies of Williams *et al.* (1974) using narrow-range, higher-resolution conditions confirmed the relatively narrow density range of lymphocytes, but showed substantial density heterogeneity with distinct peaks within this range. Part of this was due to B cells distributing differently from T cells.

B and T Lymphocytes. Both B and T lymphocytes are heterogeneous in density and show a wide density dispersion with substantial overlap between the two populations (Shortman *et al.*, 1972c), as shown in Fig. 4. Similar results are obtained with human blood lymphocytes (Williams *et al.*, 1974). Thus the method is not useful as a general procedure for separating all B cells from all T cells, although particular subpopulations can be isolated and characterized. The density subpopulations may differ in biological function. Thus recirculating B and T cells are denser than most of those in the spleen (Fig. 4), and of the T cells in the spleen only the denser appear to be able to respond to the mitogen phytohemagglutinin (Fig. 6) (Shortman *et al.*, 1973). The denser spleen T cells also are more effective "helper" cells in a humoral response to sheep erythro-

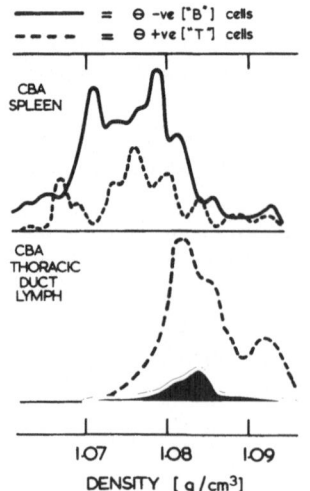

Figure 4. The density distribution of T (θ+ve) and B (θ−ve) lymphocytes in CBA mouse spleen and thoracic duct lymph. The T cells were assayed by an anti-θ antiserum cytotoxic assay. The θ-ve cells were predominantly B cells but included lymphocytes lacking defined markers and some nonlymphoid nucleated cells. The curves represent the absolute T and B cell distribution, not the percentage per fraction. The ordinate is cells per density increment, with the values normalized so that the area under the curve is proportional to the relative numbers of cells of that class. The separation was at pH 5.1, in mouse osmolarity albumin media, under conditions similar to the detailed results of Shortman, Cerottini, and Brunner (1972c). Each curve represents the mean of three separate gradients.

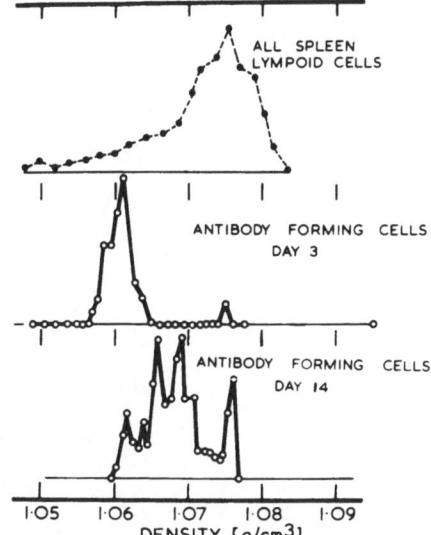

Figure 5. The density distribution of mature and immature AFC in toad spleen. The animals (*Bufo marinus*) were injected with polymerized bacterial flagellin and spleen cells separated at the times stated. AFC were enumerated with a cytoadherence assay. The separation was in albumin at pH 5.1, isoosmotic with toad serum. The figure is derived from data of Kraft and Shortman (1972) and Kraft, Shortman, and Marchalonia (1971).

cytes, and this allows effective density separation of collaborating B and T cells from mouse spleen (Gorczynski *et al.*, 1971).

Antibody-Forming Cell Development. An example of the use of continuous-density gradients to isolate and characterize steps in lymphocyte differentiation is the study of AFC development in toad spleen by Kraft *et al.* (1971) and Kraft and Shortman (1972), illustrated in Fig. 5. The earliest AFCs detected after antigenic stimulation are relatively homogeneous, light density cells, significantly enriched by the separation procedure. They were shown to be very large dividing cells. As the response develops progressively denser AFCs appear, apparently in a sequential, stepwise manner. The end-product AFCs late in the response are predominantly dense, nondividing, small, lymphocyte-like elements. This clearcut progression for AFC development has not as yet been demonstrated for mammalian systems; this may reflect the relative lack of synchrony of AFC differentiation in higher animals.

T Cell Differentiation. Density separation is proving a valuable tool in the study of the maturation pathway of immunologically functional T cells (Shortman *et al.*, 1973; Shortman *et al.*, 1972a; Shortman *et al.*, 1972c). In the thymus an immunologically active subpopulation can be isolated and substantially purified in the light density regions of continuous albumin gradients, as illustrated in Fig. 6. These light density cells represent mostly the minor subpopulation of thymocytes with the surface antigenic constitution of peripheral T cells, namely TL⁻, low θ, high H2. The major population of dense and antigenically distinct thymocytes is immunologically inactive. However, in peripheral lymphoid tissues

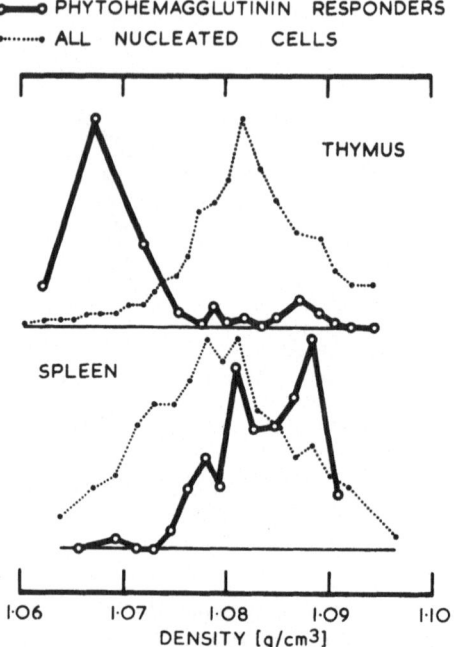

○━━○ PHYTOHEMAGGLUTININ RESPONDERS
●········● ALL NUCLEATED CELLS

THYMUS

SPLEEN

1·06   1·07   1·08   1·09   1·10
DENSITY [g/cm³]

Figure 6. The density distribution of T cells responding to phytohemagglutinin (PHA) mitogen in thymus and in spleen. The results are on CBA mice, with the separations performed in pH 5.1 albumin media of mouse serum osmolarity. The total distributions of PHA-responsive elements were obtained by (a) culturing a fixed number of cells from each fraction with or without PHA; (b) determining the mitogenic response by the incorporation of tritiated thymidine into cellular DNA; (c) subtracting the background values to give a per-culture PHA response; (d) multiplying the per-culture response by the total cells per fraction to give an absolute PHA response per fraction; (e) expressing this as PHA response per density increment, normalized to a peak value of 100%. The figure was drawn from data of Shortman, Byrd, Cerottini, and Brunner (1973).

the functionally active T cells are generally dense, differing in this property from their counterparts in thymus, suggesting further maturation steps are involved after migration from the thymus (Fig. 6).

C. Electrophoretic Separation

1. Theoretical Aspects

The surface charge on a lymphoid cell is a biologically important param-eter, and separation on the basis of this property should reflect quite different aspects of the cell than the sedimentation or buoyant density procedures. All animal cells carry a net negative charge at physiological pH, but this charge can vary with cell type, with stage of cell differentiation, and with the species studied. Electrophoretic separation can be employed to separate on the basis of rate of migration toward the anode. The movement of cells in an electric field is determined by the properties of both the cell and the medium. In a medium containing ions, the effective charge and mobility of a cell are greatly reduced by a layer of opposite charge which forms around the cell. The electrophoretic mobility of the cell then becomes directly dependent on the electrokinetic potential, the ζ potential at the outer part of this double layer, according to the formula

$$v = \zeta \epsilon E / 6 \pi \eta$$

where v is the velocity of migration, ϵ the dielectric constant, E the field strength, and η the medium viscosity. It should be noted that v becomes independent of cell size and, under constant conditions of medium and field strength, will directly reflect cell surface charge.

The effects of changing medium ionic strength on electrophoretic mobility are given by the general relationship $v_1/v_2 \simeq (I_2/I_1)^{1/2}$, where I is the ionic strength.

A major engineering problem in cell electrophoresis systems has been to stabilize the conducting medium against turbulence, without resorting to a porous solid phase which would interfere with cell migration. This bears on the problem of obtaining a sufficient degree of cell migration. To maximize cell migration, one can increase field strength or lower ionic strength. High field strength generates heat which must be removed from the system to avoid thermal turbulence, and this can be the limiting problem under practical condi-tions. Most cell separations must therefore be carried out at ionic strengths well below normal physiological levels, and addition of nonionic sugars must be made to conserve osmotic balance.

2. Free Continuous-Flow Electrophoresis

Only recently have electrophoretic systems suitable for preparative and analytical separation of lymphoid cells become available commercially, and the only well established system is that developed by Hannig (1964, 1969, 1971, 1972) (VAP$_4$ manufactured by DESAGA, Heidelberg, Germany, marketed as Elphor VAP$_4$ by Bender and Hobein, Munich, Germany, and FF4 by Brinkmann Instruments, Westbury, New York). The electrophoresis chamber consists of two closely spaced vertical glass plates. A homogeneous electric field is applied across the chamber by platinum electrodes separated from the chamber by ion-exchange membranes. Efficient cooling is accomplished electronically by Peltier batteries attached to a cooling plate at the back of the chamber. A film of buffered medium flows in continuously from the top and is collected in 96 fractions via a pump at the bottom. Cooling produces a slight decreasing temperature gradient from top to bottom, contributing to stability by the formation of a slight density gradient. A lymphoid cell suspension (maximum of 12×10^6 cells/ml) is introduced as a continuous stream at a single inlet point. Cells migrate toward the anode to distribute into about 20 fractions. The short residence time (less than 5 min) and the low operating temperature ($\sim 5°C$) allows good recovery of viable cells.

The medium for cell separation must have a low conductivity (about 0.0014 $\Omega^{-1} \cdot cm^{-1}$), must be well buffered at neutral pH, must conserve full viability, and must be isoosmotic for the cells studied. Hannig (1971) has suggested a number of media, and one very suitable for lymphoid cells, based on HEPES buffer and glucose and sorbitol to maintain osmotic balance, has been employed by von Boehmer et al. (1974). The use of such low ionic strength medium markedly heightens cell association and aggregation problems. This becomes a limiting problem with material such as spleen suspensions, where much of the aggregation is due to the presence of damaged cells. Prior elimination of damaged cells, without selective loss of viable cells, may be accomplished by the procedure of von Boehmer and Shortman (1973) discussed earlier, and this then allows effective separation (von Boehmer et al., 1974).

The Hannig procedure allows high recovery of fully viable cells, and can handle around 10^8 lymphoid cells per hour. The validity of the separation achieved and the degree of resolution was checked by experiments showing exact rebanding of separated cells (Hannig and Zeiller, 1969; von Boehmer et al., 1974). There may be some fluctuation (± one fraction) in the position of a given cell type from one experiment to another due to slight variations in temperature, voltage, or flow rate. For analytical work the separation profiles can be normalized from one run to another by reference to the migration of a small number of red cells, a suitable standard and a normal contaminant of many lymphoid suspensions (von Boehmer et al., 1974).

3. Some Applications

Blood Cells. Red cells are the fastest migrating blood elements, although the degree of migration and separation from leukocytes varies with the species

(Ganser *et al.,* 1968; Hannig and Krüsmann, 1968; von Boehmer *et al.,* 1974). Hannig and Krüsmann (1968) and Ganser *et al.* (1968) found that granulocytes, monocytes, and lymphocytes all displayed different electrophoretic character- istics, with partial separation between the different elements. Granulocytes were electrophoretically heterogeneous, showing two peaks of mobility.

T and B Cells. The electrophoretic properties of T and B lymphocytes differ, with less overlap between these populations than is obtained with density or sedimentation-rate separation (Fig. 7). Some reports suggested complete

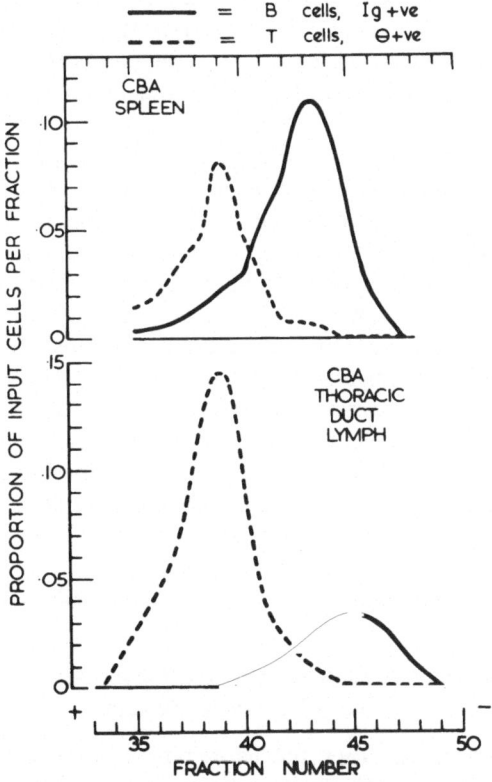

Figure 7. The electrophoretic distribution of T and B lymphocytes from mouse spleen and tho- racic duct lymph. T cells were assayed by anti-θ antiserum cytotoxic assay. B cells were assayed directly by autoradiographic determination of cells with a high density of immunoglobulin receptors. The small proportion of lymphocytes in spleen lacking either marker was found between the B and T cell peaks. The figure is derived from data of von Boehmer, Shortman and Nossal (1974).

separation of mouse spleen T and B cells could be obtained (Nordling *et al.,* 1972; Wioland *et al.,* 1972), but this appears only to be true if a nonrepresentative fraction of spleen cells, obtained by adherence or sedimentation preselection, is used for analysis. In spleen, von Boehmer *et al.* (1974) found that T cells are predominantly of fast mobility, while B cells are mainly of low mobility but with a significant high-mobility component (see Fig. 7). The fast-moving B cells overlapping the T cell peak are large adherent cells and include AFC. This conclusion agrees with earlier studies of Zeiller *et al.* (1972), who used functional rather than direct antigenic markers for the subpopulations. Zeiller *et al.* (1970) demonstrated marked changes in electrophoretic mobility during the differentiation of B cells to AFC. However, despite this partial overlap of T and B cells in spleen, the separation is still extensive, and with thoracic duct lymph cells completely pure T and B cells are readily obtained (Fig. 7) (von Boehmer *et al.,* 1974).

Cells Involved in Mixed Lymphocyte Reactions. Clear examples of the application of electrophoretic separation of T and B cells from mouse spleen are the recent studies of von Boehmer (1974a,b), who has used the technique to separate the lymphocyte classes and so to clarify the nature of the cells responding and the cells stimulating in mixed lymphocyte reactions (MLR). Of the electrophoretically separated elements, only T cells are capable of recognizing an allogenic stimulus, but even mitomycin-treated T cells can do this, despite their inability to divide. As a consequence of this recognition event, some nonspecific factor appears to cause all types of untreated lymphocytes, both T and B, both allogenic and syngenic, to proliferate. In contrast to the recognition process, both T and B cells can serve as the foreign stimulus in an allogenic mixed lymphocyte reaction. A different result is obtained for the newly discovered syngenic mixed lymphocyte reaction, in which a small population of thymus T cells respond to spleen lymphocytes. In this case the stimulating peripheral cell is a B lymphocyte, and peripheral T cells are ineffective.

D. Counter-Current Distribution in Aqueous
Polymer Two-Phase Systems

A second physical separation procedure reflecting differences in cell surface characteristics, and particularly surface charge, is based on the relative distribution of cells between two immiscible aqueous polymer solutions. This procedure will only be outlined briefly, since it has as yet had little application to lymphocyte separations. A more complete review has been given elsewhere (Shortman, 1972) and excellent accounts have been provided by Albertsson (1971), who developed the procedure, and by Walter (1969), who has extensively applied it to the separation and characterization of cells.

Basically the procedure involves solutions of certain polymers, such as dextran and polyethylene glycol, which separate into two distinct phases above a certain concentration. Cells introduced in the system may distribute between the two phases according to the Brönsted formula

$$K = e^{s\lambda}/RT$$

where K is the partition coefficient, S the cell surface area, R the Boltzmann constant, and λ a constant characteristic of the system depending on the cell surface and the nature of the polymers.

If conditions for a useful K value are obtained, cells may then be separated by repetitive distribution in the thin-layer counter-current apparatus devised by Albertsson (1965) and available commercially (Incentive Research and Development, Bromma, Sweden; Buchler Instruments Division, Nuclear-Chicago Corp., Fort Lee, New Jersey). Cell viability is conserved during this process.

Cell surface charge appears to be the major factor determining cell partition between the phases (Walter, 1969; Walter *et al.*, 1967, 1968; Brooks *et al.*, 1971) despite the unchanged nature of the polymers used, probably because of a small but definite unequal partition of ions between the two phases (Seaman and Walter, 1971). Although this means the results will be generally similar to those obtained by electrophoresis, the charge properties of the cell seem to be reflected in a somewhat different way (Walter *et al.*, 1972), and the potential exists for developing separations reflecting other membrane properties.

The potentialities of the procedure, particularly as a tool to follow cell surface changes during differentiation, have been clearly demonstrated by the detailed study of red cell differentiation and development by Walter and colleagues (Walter *et al.*, 1969a; Walter, 1969; Albertson, 1971). Blood lymphocytes and polymorphs have been successfully partitioned (Walter *et al.*, 1969b), and both cell types were found to be heterogeneous, each forming two main peaks, a result that agrees with electrophoretic separation. Partial separation between the cells was obtained, the effectiveness varying with the species studied. The application most relevant to immunological investigation was the partial separation, after relatively few transfers, of AFC, hemopoietic colony-forming cells, and granulocytes from mouse spleen by Brunette *et al.* (1968). Good recovery of activity was obtained. It is unfortunate that this promising approach to lymphocyte separation has not been pursued further.

IV. ADHERENCE SEPARATION OF LYMPHOCYTES AND PHAGOCYTES

The passage of cells, generally blood leukocytes, through columns is now a routine technique for separating lymphocytes from phagocytes. The column materials used are beads of glass or various plastics, or fibrous material such as glass wool, nylon wool, or cotton wool. Most of the standard procedures are relatively inefficient, and interpretation of the results is often complicated by the variety of factors that may cause cell adherence, especially when cell suspensions from lymphoid organs are studied. One attempt to sort out these factors (Shortman et al., 1971) led to a description of four different separation effects, namely: (a) an active, metabolism-dependent adherence of phagocytic elements; (b) a passive, "physical," metabolism-independent adherence of certain distinct subclasses of lymphoid cells; (c) a passive adherence or retention of damaged cells, regardless of type or column conditions; (d) a "filtration" effect, selecting out larger cells on a size basis, and only operative with small channel size, e.g., with beads below 100μ diameter.

Attempts to use columns to remove damaged cells or to select out small lymphocytes achieved some success (Shortman, 1968; 1969a), but other procedures discussed previously now accomplish these ends much more effectively. Two useful column procedures will be considered: the separation of phagocytes from lymphocytes by active-adherence columns (where effects (a), (b), and (c) are *all* operative) and the passive-adherence separation of different lymphocyte subpopulations (where effects (b) and (c) are operative).

A. Active-Adherence Separation of Phagocytes from Lymphocytes

The active attachment of cells to surfaces seems to be correlated with phagocytic function, since macrophages, monocytes, and granulocytic cells all display this effect. The conditions for effective attachment have been studied in detail by Garvin (1961) and Rabinowitz (1964), and the following factors seem essential:

(a) A period of incubation (10–30 min at 37°C) in a tissue culture medium under conditions allowing active metabolism. Adhesion is insignificant below 15°C. Nor is it obtained above 45°C, when the cells are killed, or when metabolic inhibitors are present.

(b) A heat-labile factor in fresh serum or plasma. Generally, isologous serum is required. Heat-inactivated serum is ineffective.

(c) The presence of both calcium and magnesium ions. Chelating agents used as anticoagulants (e.g. EDTA) must be avoided during the adherence phase. EDTA may be used to help remove adherent phagocytes from the solid substrate.

Rabinowitz (1964) separated human blood leukocytes on columns of siliconized glass beads or glass wool. The cells suspended in fresh plasma were run onto a dry column, then incubated for 30 min at 37°C. Washing out the column with plasma–salt solution produced first pure lymphocytes, then platelets. Phagocytic cells were eluted with medium containing EDTA and free of Ca^{++} and

Mg^{++}, which produced a peak of polymorphs followed by a peak of monocytes. Recovery of phagocytes, especially monocytes, was sometimes poor with this procedure. In addition, when this procedure was applied to cells from lymphoid organs, a high proportion of the input lymphocytes were trapped in the column.

The Rabinowitz column procedure was modified by Shortman et al. (1971) to increase the efficiency of separation and to minimize lymphocyte trapping. Larger siliconized glass beads, around 450 μ in diameter, were used. Both the column and the cell suspension were preequilibrated at 37°C, with pH 7.0 tissue culture medium containing 50% homologous serum. The cells were passed through the column in 10 min as a continuously moving band to give a phagocyte-free filtrate. Adherent cells were recovered by first eluting with medium containing EDTA, then gently disrupting the bed of beads. Damaged cells mechanically released from the beads were again trapped by reforming the column and washing released viable cells through with EDTA medium. This procedure gives good recoveries of viable cells, including the adherent cells, free of damaged elements. Up to 10^9 lymphoid cells can be handled on large (2.5 cm diameter $\times$ 15 cm) columns. The method is applicable to blood, peritoneal exudate, spleen, and lymph node cells. Applied to mouse spleen preparations the active, filtrate lymphocytes are over 500-fold depleted of active macrophages, and over 50-fold depleted of active polymorphs (Shortman et al., 1970; 1971).

This column procedure has now been used extensively to study the role of adherent or A cells, presumed to be macrophages or a macrophage subclass, in the immune response to antigens in cell culture. The results obtained are summarized in Table I, drawn from the studies of Shortman et al. (1970), Shortman and Palmer (1971), Palmer (1973), Feldmann and Palmer (1971), and Feldmann (1972). Macrophage-depleted lymphocytes fail to respond to certain A-cell- and T-cell-requiring antigens, such as foreign erythrocytes, but respond normally to certain polymeric antigens that appear to prime B cells directly. The effectiveness of separation may be judged by the fact that the secondary response to sheep erythrocytes, which has a definite but quantitatively small macrophage requirement, was also absent in the nonadherent lymphocytes (Table I) (Feldmann and Palmer, 1971). The procedure has also been effective in removing phagocytic cells from mouse bone marrow, producing a filtrate fraction which contains small- to medium-sized lymphoid and erythroid cells and is enriched for stem cells (Metcalf et al., 1971).

This procedure has one substantial disadvantage shared with all active-adherence methods, namely that certain subclasses of lymphocytes also adhere to the columns. These then contaminate the adherent, phagocyte fraction. This also complicates the interpretation of results, since any loss of activity in the filtrate could be due to the loss of a special lymphocyte subclass, as well as to the loss of phagocytes. For example, separate checks were required to establish that the results of Table I were due primarily to removal of macrophage-like

Table I. The Effect of Active-Adherence Column Separation
on Immune Responses in Culture

| Antigen | Nature of response | Activity (mean AFC generated per 10^6 cells cultured) | | "Macrophage" requirement |
		Unfractionated cells	Column filtrate cells	
Donkey erythrocytes	primary, IgM	68	1	+
Sheep erythrocytes	primary, IgM	150	5	+
	secondary, IgM	397	34	+
	secondary, IgG	286	32	+
Sheep erythrocyte, membrane fragments	primary, IgM	20	17	−
Polymerized flagellin	primary, IgM	86	83	−
DNP'hapten (conjugated, to polymerized flagellin)	primary, IgM	49	40	−

The results demonstrate the effects of active-adherence column macrophage depletion by the procedure of Shortman et al. (1971) on humoral immune responses in cell culture. The values given are simply the means of all available published data, from the work cited in text. Within individual experiments, culture-to-culture variation in response was 10–15%, while the reported absolute values from one series of experiments to another varied over a three-fold range. However, the effect of column fractionation was consistent and independent of the absolute response of the culture system. Primary indicates the response of unprimed cells; secondary, the response of cells from animals previously exposed to antigen. The results demonstrate that the response to certain antigens requires macrophage-like cells, while the response to other antigens does not. Separate experiments using specific anti-macrophage antisera established that the results were not due to loss of active adherent lymphocytes.

cells, and not just to lymphocyte redistribution. This adherent lymphocyte problem is much less bothersome with blood, or peritoneal exudate (where 80–100% of the lymphocytes pass through the column), than with spleen (where 40–60% of the lymphocytes are trapped).

Other procedures have been used for separating phagocytes from lymphocytes. Differential adherence to plastic petri dishes is extensively used in a number of variations of the method introduced by Mosier (1967) in the first demonstration of an adherent-cell requirement in the immune response. Although simple in operation, most versions of the procedure are relatively inefficient and fail to reduce adherent cells to the low levels obtained by column procedures. Efficiency of separation may be increased by repetitive separation, but the final yield of nonadherent cells is then no more than 50%, giving the same opportunities for selection within lymphocyte subpopulations as with column separation.

Another approach to eliminate phagocytes from lymphocytes was designed to directly reflect the actual phagocytic activity of the cells. The cell suspension is mixed with some form of heavy or magnetic particles (often coated with some material enhancing phagocytosis). Phagocytes ingesting the material may then be eliminated by their enhanced sedimentation or by an applied magnetic field (Levine, 1956; Lichtenstein et al., 1971). This is the basis of one commercial lymphocyte separator (Technicon) and produces blood lymphocytes around 96% pure with 80–90% recovery, a result comparable with column separation. It is not clear, however, that separation depends on the actual ingestion of the magnetic particles. The basis of separation may still be adherence of cells to particles, and if so the method would still cause selection of adherent from nonadherent lymphocytes.

B. Physical Adherence Column Separation between Lymphocyte Subpopulations

Although the trapping of lymphocytes in active-adherence columns is a disadvantage when attempting separation between macrophages and lymphocytes, the phenomenon can be exploited to give separation of different subclasses of lymphocytes. Plotz and Talal (1967) first noted that certain types of AFC from immunized spleens adhered to glass-bead columns along with macrophages and granulocytes, and this was confirmed by others (Salerno and Pontieri, 1969). The basis for the adherence of lymphoid cells was studied in more detail by Shortman et al. (1971, 1972b). Adherence to glass-bead columns is a basic property of certain lymphocytes and is not just the result of nonspecific trapping. Lymphocyte adherence is effective at 4–7°C, as well as at 37°C, and is therefore a metabolism-independent passive process, in contrast to phagocyte adherence. Adherent lymphocytes tend to be larger in size, although their size as such does not cause the trapping in the columns. Also, they are generally lighter in density than the nonadherent elements. Although adherent cells are slightly enriched for B cells, there is no striking B cell–T cell separation with mouse spleen, both major lymphocyte classes containing adherent and nonadherent elements. Basically, adherent lymphocytes include "activated" forms, such as AFC and most cytotoxic T lymphocytes, as well as the larger dividing blast cells. Nonadherent lymphocytes include the typical, small, nondividing lymphocyte, the type considered capable of recirculation.

Marked separation of functionally different lymphocytes has been obtained on glass-bead adherence columns designed to divide splenic lymphocytes into two fractions: the 60% least adherent and the 40% most adherent (Shortman *et al.* 1971). The columns have been run at 37°C or 6–7°C with identical results. As mentioned before, AFCs may be separated from many non-AFCs although the degree of separation depends on the antigenic system used (Shortman *et al.* 1972b). Cells responding to the mitogen phytohemagglutinin are primarily nonadherent, whereas cells responding to pokeweed mitogen are concentrated in the adherent fraction (Shortman *et al.,* 1972b; 1973). Recently Schlegel and Shortman (1974) have found differences in the adherence properties of AFC progenitors, depending at least in part on their past history of antigenic contact or prestimulation.

The adherence separation approach has been extended by Adams (1973a,b), who has developed a two-stage, cold-column procedure for selecting out the 15% most adherent and the 15% least adherent cells. Under these conditions B cell–T cell separation becomes more striking. The least adherent fraction contains both B and T cells, but the filtrate is at least 90% pure T cells. Adherent and nonadherent T cells seem to be functionally different. The 15% least adherent elements are a very effective and enriched source of collaborating or helper T cells, restoring the response to sheep erythrocytes of T-cell-depleted populations.

V. METHODS BASED ON SPECIFIC CELL SURFACE RECEPTORS AND ANTIGENS

The separation techniques considered so far demand quite extensive differences in the basic adherence properties or the physical parameters of cells. These techniques alone are inherently incapable of separating lymphocytes on the basis of the property that most fascinates an immunologist, namely, the biological specificity provided by receptors at the cell surface. There is a need for techniques to select, from among a group of physically and biologically similar lymphocytes, just those cells with receptors specific for a given antigen, or with receptors specifically binding immunoglobulins, antigen–antibody complexes, or lectins. A related requirement occurs when two biologically distinct cells (such as T or B lymphocytes) have by chance very similar overall physical characteristics, but differ markedly in the antigenic makeup of their cell surface. It would be an advantage to make direct use of the selectivity of antisera in the isolation of cells.

Such methods are relatively recent, but are being reported with increasing frequency and increasing success. No universally applicable procedure has yet emerged, so the following is a comparative survey of the various methods that have been fruitful to date, with some indication of their limitations.

A. Affinity-Column and Fiber Fractionation

1. Affinity-Column Separation

One general approach is to fix antigens or antibodies, or lectins to a solid matrix and then to pass the cell suspension through a column of this coated material; only cells with the specific receptor or surface antigen should be bound. Attempts to achieve such separation with lymphocytes have been reviewed by Wigzell (1970; 1971), Wigzell and Andersson (1971), and Wofsy (1972). The initial attachment of antigens or antibodies to the bead surface in sufficient concentration to bind cells has not been a major problem. This has been achieved in several ways, namely: (a) simple adsorption onto glass or acrylic beads (Wigzell and Andersson, 1969), or polyurethane foam (Evans et al., 1969); (b) adsorption of antibody followed by a second layer of excess antigen to create a double layer (Wigzell et al., 1972; Mage et al., 1969); (c) covalent coupling of antigens, antibodies, or lectins to polyacrylamide or polysaccharide beads (Truffa-Bachi and Wofsy, 1970; Edelman et al., 1971). Covalent coupling to a derivatized matrix should produce a stabler and more defined product and would now be the preferred procedure.

A major problem with the first attempts using coated glass or acrylic beads was the high degree of nonspecific retention of cells by the columns. Thus Wigzell and Andersson (1969) found that 25% of input cells were trapped by columns coated with syngenic mouse serum only, and this 25% included some AFCs and memory cells. This phenomenon is clearly the same as the "physical" or passive lymphocyte adherence described in more detail earlier, and would be strongly selective for certain subpopulations of lymphocytes. Because of this, very little purification of the specifically adherent cells could be expected. In addition, the cells passing through the column would be depleted not only of the specific binding population, but also of special subclasses of adherent lymphocytes.

These problems have been markedly reduced by the use of polyacrylamide or polysaccharide beads, where nonspecific binding of cells is reduced (Wofsy, 1972; Schlossman and Hudson, 1973; Kishimoto and Ishizaka, 1972). Under careful conditions nonspecific binding can be less than 1% of the input (Truffa-Bachi and Wofsy, 1970). The use of large beads ($> 600 \mu$ diameter) and rapid flow rates is also important in reducing nonspecific binding. In an alternative system using a reticulated polyurethane foam as a matrix, nonspecific adsorption was reduced to 8% or less by slow rotation of a horizontal column, which allowed unbound cells to fall away from the matrix when the relative direction of the gravitational field changed (Evans et al., 1969).

The second major problem, and the one currently limiting the general application of affinity chromatography, is the recovery of the enriched, specifically bound cells from the column. The binding of cells to the solid matrix is a complex process which may involve, after the specific interaction, shape changes in the cell surface and secondary nonspecific binding forces. The thermodynamics of specific binding would also be markedly dependent on the distribution and frequency of ligands on the matrix, which would determine the number of receptors or antigenic sites on the cell surface involved in the attachment. The ideal chromatographic method for releasing antigen-bound cells would be elution with a specific hapten. Unfortunately, the existence of multiple specific bonds and of secondary nonspecific adherence effects may make hapten elution an impossible or at least inefficient approach for thermodynamic reasons. Although free hapten effectively prevents binding of cells if added before passage through the column, the general experience has been that cells once bound cannot readily be eluted, even with high hapten concentrations. However, cells specific for β-lactoside determinants have recently been bound to polyacrylamide columns, then recovered with reasonable yield and extraordinary purification by elution with free hapten (Henry et al., 1972). This may have been due to the reversal of specific binding, or alternatively to the release of cells by receptor turnover, with the hapten serving to block further interaction. As yet no comparable results have been reported with other antigenic determinants.

As an alternative approach, mechanical disruption of the column or a fast flow rate of medium can generate sufficient shearing forces to release bound cells. However, this may involve damage to the cells by tearing the cell membranes. Recoveries of active cells by such methods have generally been poor. However, in one report disruption of antigen-coated glass-bead columns released immunologically active and specific cells (Abdou and Richter, 1969), and specifically bound cells have been released from polyurethane columns by squeezing the foam matrix (Evans et al., 1969).

Introduction of some form of labile or reversible bond in the matrix–ligand–cell linkage may in future provide the means of releasing bound cells without damage. A new but somewhat unwieldy approach of this type has been to release bound cells with good recovery by totally digesting the Sephadex bead matrix with dextranase (Schlossman and Hudson, 1973). Another novel approach currently being developed by Haas (1974) is the use of low-melting-point gelatin as a matrix; temperatures of 25–37°C are sufficient to melt the matrix and release viable and enriched specific lymphocytes.

2. Derivatized Fiber Separation

An alternative to column-based affinity chromatography has been developed by Edelman et al. (1971) and Rutishauser et al. (1972), who covalently coupled antigens, antibodies, or lectins to nylon fibers, and then used fibers strung in parallel onto a supporting collar, or used a fiber mesh, to bind specific cells. Despite the basic similarity to column procedures, the system displays some different properties and offers some particular advantages in analytical studies of the properties of antigen-binding cells. The degree of coupling of ligand to the fibers may be closely controlled, and may be manipulated to provide various geometric arrays of binding surfaces. The actual adhesion of cells can be observed microscopically and quantitated, an enormous advantage when establishing new separation conditions (see Fig. 8). Many studies can be performed with bound cells still on the fiber, thus bypassing the need to elute viable cells from the matrix. Nonspecific binding of cells to the fibers appears to be extremely low, at least 50% of the attached cells being specifically bound. Damaged cells do not adhere to the fibers. Although column procedures are inherently more efficient in maximizing contact between the cells and the matrix surface, complete depletion of binding cells from a suspension can still be achieved by a 1 hr incubation with fiber mesh.

Release of specifically bound cells from the fibers has presented the same problems as release from columns. Although some release was obtained by the competitive inhibitors of binding, high concentrations were required and release was slow. Mechanical procedures, in particular plucking the taut fiber, are more effective, causing immediate quantitative release of bound cells (Edelman *et al.*, 1971). Although the freshly released cells have membrane damage, as assessed by vital stains, the cells apparently retain a capacity to repair this damage on incubation in serum-containing medium. No data have as yet been presented on the immunological competence of the released cells.

A different and promising approach to the release of bound cells has recently been presented by Kiefer (1973). He observed that cells bound to fiber mesh at 4°C spontaneously release on incubation at 22°C, presumably by a normal process of receptor turnover. The released cells were of high viability. It remains to be determined if the cells are immunologically active, and if the binding-and-release process has triggered the cells into an immune response.

3. Some Applications and Results of Column and Fiber Affinity Separation

Purification and Study of Antigen-Reactive Lymphocytes. A primary aim has been to isolate from cell suspensions lymphocytes with receptors specific for a given antigen. These may be B or T cells, and may represent either the antigen-responsive progenitor cell or the activated, effector product. Surprisingly, fibers and columns appear to differ in the class and type of specific cell bound. Columns appear to bind B cells, both AFC progenitors and AFC, but there is no evidence for T cell binding (Wigzell, 1971; Wofsy, 1972). In contrast, fibers appear to effectively bind both B and T cells (Rutishauser and Edelman,

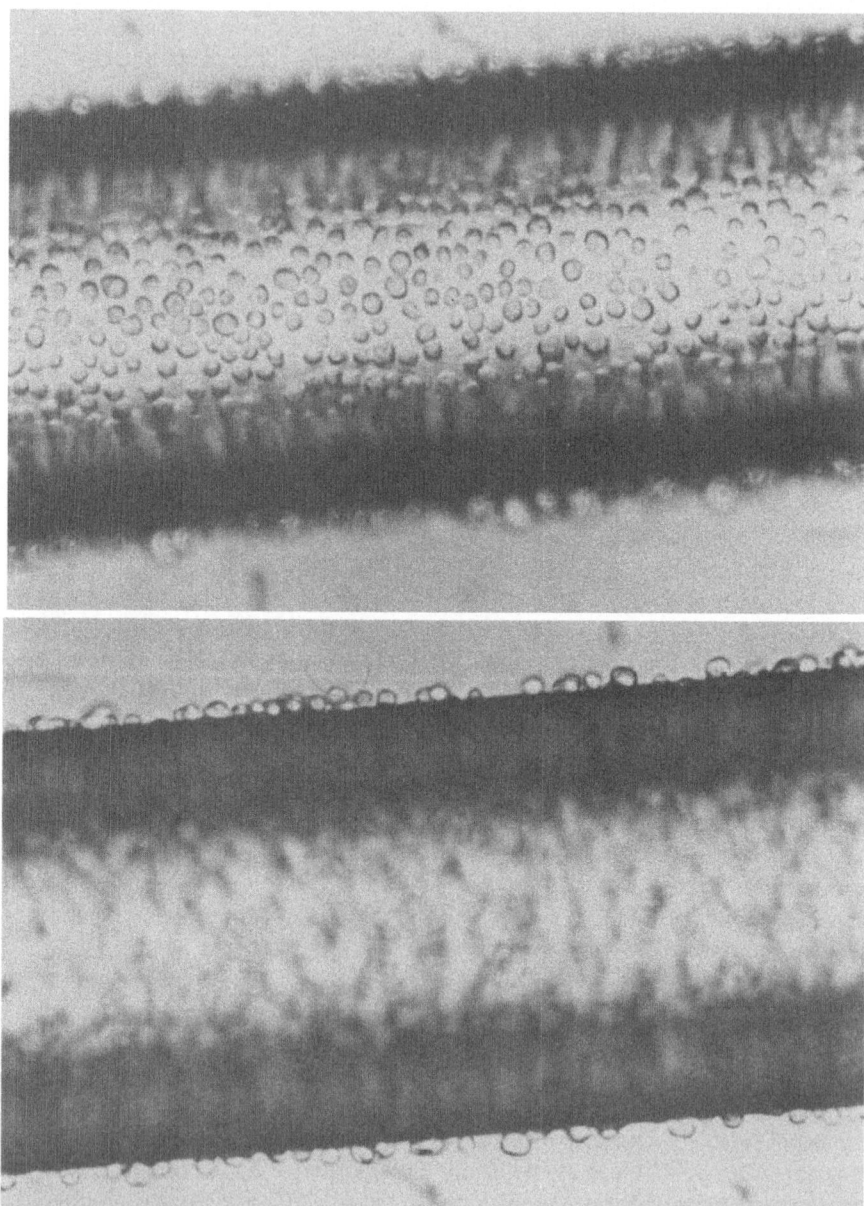

Figure 8. Mouse thymus lymphocytes bound to a nylon fiber derived from concanavalin A. The field was focused on the face of the fiber in the upper portion and on the edge of the fiber in the lower portion; in both cases at ×150 magnitification using bright-field microscopy. The photograph is from Edelman, Rutishauser, and Millette (1971) reproduced with the kind permission of Dr. Edelman and his publishers.

1972), but do not bind AFC (Rutishauser *et al.*, 1972). This presumably reflects differences in the nature, frequency, and turnover rate of receptors on the various cell types.

The complete or nearly complete purification and recovery of immunologically active, specific AFC progenitor cells has been the elusive goal of all the studies in this field, and the only convincing realization of this goal to date is the work of Henry *et al.* (1972). They obtained about 3000-fold enrichment of B-cell progenitors for an antibody response to azophenyl–β-lactoside, using hapten elution from a derivatized or polyacrylamide-bead column.

Affinity columns have been extensively used to study the properties of antigen-reactive cells and their surface receptors, without the need to actually purify or recover the active cells. Wigzell and colleagues (1970, 1971) in particular have used well designed depletion experiments to establish that cells initiating humoral immune responses have a restricted range of specific receptors on the cell surface, and to demonstrate that these receptors are similar to the final immunoglobulin product. The exact nature of the surface immunoglobulin receptors on progenitor cells is being studied by using columns coupled to the appropriate antiimmunoglobulin antiserum (Wigzell *et al.*, 1972; Kishimoto and Ishizaka, 1972). A much more detailed study of the properties of the binding cells should now be possible by direct observation of cells bound on fibers (Rutishauser and Edelman, 1972) (Fig. 8).

B Cell–T Cell Separation. Column procedures have been used for a simple B cell–T cell separation without reference to the antigenic specificity of the cells. The use of a broad-specificity antiimmunoglobulin antiserum attached to a bead matrix has been used to bind B cells on the basis of the high density of surface immunoglobulin receptors, while T cells pass into the effluent (Wigzell *et al.*, 1972; Schlossman and Hudson, 1973). An alternative approach not requiring the specific antiimmunoglobulin antiserum has made use of a receptor for antigen–antibody complexes present on all B cells (Basten *et al.*, 1972). Spleen cells were incubated with antiserum, then incubated on a column containing antigen-coated beads. B cells were retained via the formation of antigen–antibody complexes bound to cells, and T cells (91% pure) were recovered in the effluent. In both approaches the recovery and efficiency will depend on the choice of appropriate matrix and selection of conditions which give effective specific and minimum nonspecific binding.

B. Specific Modification of Physical Properties

1. Rosette Separation

Although separation procedures based on gross physical properties of cells cannot themselves detect differences in the binding specificity of lymphocyte receptors, it is often possible to cause a marked specific change in some physical parameter as an indirect result of the specific binding of reactive cells to antigenic material. The best known example is the separation of cells which specifically bind and form "rosettes" with foreign erythrocytes. These rosettes may be separated on the basis of an effective increase in size and thus of sedimentation rate (Edwards *et al.*, 1970; Osoba, 1970; Haskill and Marbrook, 1972). Since a variety of materials can be bound to the erythrocyte surface, the method can be made applicable to a wide range of antigens and haptens, in fact to all those used in modified hemolytic plaque assays. Although the rosettes may be used as such for some immunological assays, the problem of eliminating erythrocytes bound to the specific lymphocytes limits some applications of the method. Natural receptor turnover at metabolizing temperatures can be employed to shed the red cells, or they can be reduced to membrane fragments by selective destruction with NH_4Cl.

The actual sedimentation-rate separation of rosettes from nonreactive cells is best accomplished in a flat, shallow "pancake" modification of the unit-gravity separation procedure, as described by Edwards *et al.* (1970) and Miller (1973). If the specific lymphocyte-depleted, nonrosette fraction is also to be recovered, the stability of the displacement step after sedimentation should be improved by using a further shallow-stabilizing density gradient for the displacement solution. This procedure can give around 50% pure rosettes, the chief contaminants being aggregated cells, especially aggregated polymorphs.

As an alternative to sedimentation separation, the density increase due to the binding of dense red cells may be used to effect specific separation of rosettes (Moav and Harris, 1970). Since erythrocytes have an exceptionally high density only at neutral *p*H (see earlier discussion), neutralized albumin or other media around *p*H 7 should be used. The simplified density cut procedure previously described could make this a simple and rapid separation.

2. Electrophoretic Deflection

A different specific separation approach is now possible with the development of continuous cell electrophoresis. The binding of antigens, lectins, or antibodies of appropriate charge should induce a specific deflection in the electrophoretic mobility of reactive lymphocytes. Because of the high mobility of erythrocytes, rosettes should be separable by this approach. However, it has a wider potential application, especially for the isolation of hapten-specific lymphocytes.

C. Cytotoxic Antisera and Damaged Cell Removal

The specificity of cytotoxic antisera is frequently used to eliminate a particular lymphocyte class by incubation of cells with antiserum and a source of complement. This procedure leaves the damaged cells in the suspension, a disadvantage in many applications. The damaged cell removal procedures described earlier may be coupled with an efficient and specific cytotoxic procedure to produce a clear, viable, and purified cell suspension. Antiimmunoglobulin antisera may be used to selectively eliminate B cells, anti-θ-antiserum to eliminate T cells. To be effective, the antiserum used should be specific and of high titer, and a nontoxic, absorbed complement (preferably rabbit complement) should be employed. Optimum conditions can be established with a small-volume cytotoxic assay, then scaled up in cell number and volume, with allowance for the extra time taken to reach temperature equilibrium on incubation. Either the low-ionic-strength filtration technique (von Boehmer and Shortman, 1973) or a density cut at neutral pH (Shortman *et al.*, 1972d) may be used to completely eliminate the damaged cells. An example of this procedure is given by Shortman *et al.* (1973) for the preparation of B cells in mouse spleen by elimination of θ-bearing T cells. The same procedure may be modified for selective elimination of high-θ cells from mouse thymus, leaving a pure preparation of the low-θ subpopulation (Shortman and Jackson, 1974).

VI. ELECTRONIC CELL SORTING

An entirely different approach to the bulk handling of cell suspensions considered so far is to classify and separate cells one at a time, using a high-speed electronic cell-sorting apparatus. Selection may be on the basis of either the physical parameters of the cell, or the specific receptors or antigens on the cell surface. The effective instruments to date have used a sensing unit coupled with a device for first breaking a liquid stream into droplets and for then separating those droplets containing particular cells. The drop deflection methods were developed by Sweet (1965) and employ a low-power ultrasonic vibrator to reduce a liquid stream into droplets of precise size and uniform spacing, a charging pulse to impart selected droplets with a given electrostatic charge, and a transverse electrostatic field to deflect charged droplets.

The first such separation device was developed by Fulwyler (1970; Fulwyler *et al.*, 1969) and separates on the basis of cell volume, using the Coulter principle for the electronic measurement of the size of individual cells passing through an aperture. The instrument thus can simultaneously produce precise data on the size distribution on cell populations, as well as samples of size categories for biological testing. The expense and complexity of the apparatus, the low cell load that can be handled, and the small number of fractions separated (generally two) make sedimentation-velocity separation a simpler and more practical alternative for most investigators.

The Fulwyler approach has been extended by the group at Stanford (Bonner *et al.*, 1972 and Hulett *et al.*, 1969), who have produced a machine of wider application capable of selecting viable, biologically specific cells by using cell fluorescence as the separation parameter. Living cells are rendered differentially fluorescent by direct staining or by binding of fluroescent labeled antibodies or antigens. The cylindrical liquid stream of cells is illuminated with a laser beam, and fluorescent light from the activated dye on labeled cells is used to generate a signal pulse for the deflection of droplets containing labeled cells. The instrument has been well calibrated in terms of reproducibility and sensitivity, and is sufficiently quantitative in response to differentially separate cells with high or low levels of associated fluorescence.

An impressive demonstration of the potential of the instrument has been the separation of antigen-binding cells using fluorescent labeled antigen. These were shown to be active as precursors of specific AFC (Julius *et al.*, 1972), About 50% of the purified cells were antigen binders, and activity enrichment factors of about 500 could be obtained. This compares well with the best recent results from affinity chromatography, and has the advantage that adaptation to different antigens would be relatively simple. However, to date only antigen-binding B cells appear to be separated. The lower binding capacity of T cells under these conditions may be below the current sensitivity of the device (Julius *et al.*, 1972).

Although the machine is in commercial development, its expense and electronic complexity will probably limit it to a small number of research groups. Its application is also restricted by the relatively small cell load (about 5×10^7 cells) that can be handled in a reasonable time. The presence of fluroescent labeled antigen or antibody on the surface of the separated cells may also be a problem for some applications. However, because of its versatility, the machine should prove a major advance in the study of the immunological specificity of lymphocytes.

REFERENCES

Abdou, N. I., and Richter, M., 1969, *J. Exp. Med.* **130**:141.
Adams, P. B., 1973a, *Cell Immunol.*, **8**:356.
Adams, P. B., 1973b, *Cell Immunol.*, **8**:372.
Albertsson, P.-Å., 1965, *Anal. Biochem.* **11**:121.
Albertsson, P.-Å., 1971, *Partition of Cell Particles and Macromolecules*, 2nd ed., John Wiley and Sons, New York.
Albertsson, P.-Å., 1972, *Exp. Cell Res.* **73**:161.
Bach, M. K., and Brashler, J. R., 1970, *Exp. Cell Res.* **61**:387.
Basten, A., Sprent, J., and Miller, J. F. A. P., 1972, *Nature New Biol.* **235**:178.
Bonner, W. A., Hulett, H. R., Sweet, R. G., and Herzenberg, L. A., 1972, *Rev. Sci. Instr.* **43**:404.
Boone, C. W., Harell, G. S., and Bond, H. E., 1968, *J. Cell. Biol.* **36**:369.
Brooks, D. E., Seaman, G. V. F., and Walter, H., 1971, *Nature New Biol.* **234**:61.
Brubaker, L. H., and Evans, W. H., 1969, *J. Lab. Clin. Med.* **73**:1036.
Brunette, D. M., McCulloch, E. A., and Till, J. E., 1968, *Cell Tissue Kinet.* **1**:319.
Cutts, J. H., 1970, *Cell Separation: Methods in Hematology*, Academic Press, New York.

Dicke, K. A., 1970, *The Separation of Hemopoietic Cell Suspensions,* van Bekkum, D. W., and Dicke, K. A. (eds.), Radiobiological Institute TNO, Rijswijk ZH, The Netherlands, p. 64.

Dicke, K. A., van Hooft, J. I. M., and van Bekkum, D. W., 1968, *Transplantation* 6, 562.

Diener, E., Kraft, N., and Armstrong, W. D., 1973, *Cell. Immunol.* 6:80.

Edelman, G. M., Rutishauser, U., and Millette, C. F., 1971, *Proc. Nat. Acad. Sci. U.S.* 68:2153.

Edwards, G. E., Miller, R. G., and Phillips, R. A., 1970, *J. Immunol.* 105:719.

Evans, W. H., Mage, M. G., and Peterson, E. A., 1969, *J. Immunol.* 102:899.

Feldmann, M., 1972, *Eur. J. Immunol.* 2:130.

Feldmann, M., and Palmer, J., 1971, *J. Immunol.* 21:685.

Fulwyler, M. J., 1970, *Automated Cell Identification and Cell Sorting,* Wied, G. L., and Bahr, G. F. (eds.), Academic Press, New York, p. 97.

Fulwyler, M. J., Glascock, R. B., Hiebert, R. D., and Johnson, N. M., 1969, *Rev. Sci. Instr.* 40:42.

Ganser, M., Hannig, K., Krüsmann, W. F., Pascher, G., and Ruthenstroth-Bauer, G., 1968, *Klin. Wochschr.,* 46:809.

Garvin, J. E., 1961, *J. Exp. Med.,* 114:51.

Gorczynski, R. M., Miller, R. G., and Phillips, R. A., 1970, *Immunology* 19:817.

Gorczynski, R. M., Miller, R. G., and Phillips, R. A., 1971, *Immunology* 20:693.

Haas, W., 1974, in preparation.

Hannig, K., 1964, *Hoppe Seylers Z. Physiol. Chem.* 338:211.

Hannig, K., 1969, *Progress in Separation and Purification, Vol. 2, Modern Separation Methods of Macromolecules and Particles,* Gerritsen, Theo (ed.), John Wiley and Sons, New York, p. 45.

Hannig, K., 1971, *Methods in Microbiology,* Norris, J. R., and Ribbons, D. W. (eds.), Vol. 5B, Academic Press, London, p. 513.

Hannig, K., 1972, *Techniques of Biochemical and Biophysical Morphology,* Glick, D., and Rosenbaum, R. (eds.), John Wiley and Sons, New York, p. 191.

Hannig, K., and Krüsmann, W. F., 1968, *Hoppe Seylers Z. Physiol. Chem.* 349:161.

Hannig, K., and Zeiller, K., 1969, *Hoppe Seylers Z. Physiol. Chem.* 350:467.

Haskill, J. S., and Marbrook, J., 1972, *Cell Immunol.* 3:448.

Henry, C., Kimura, J., and Wofsy, L., 1972, *Proc. Nat. Acad. Sci. U.S.* 69:34.

Hilal, S. K., Mosser, D. G., Loken, M. K., and Johnson, R. W., 1964, *Ann. N.Y. Acad. Sci.* 114:661.

Hulett, H. R., Bonner, W. A., Barrett, J., and Herzenberg, L. A., 1969, *Science* 166:747.

Hulliger, L., and Blazkovec, A. A., 1967, *Lancet* 1:1304.

Judson, G., Jones, A., and Kellogg, R., 1968, *Nature* 217:816.

Julius, M. H., Masuda, T., and Herzenberg, L. A., 1972, *Proc. Nat. Acad. Sci. U.S.* 69:1934.

Kiefer, H., 1973, *Eur. J. Immunol.* 3:181.

Kishimoto, T., and Ishizaka, K., 1972, *J. Immunol.* 109:1163.

Kneece, W. C., and Leif, R. C., 1971, *J. Cell. Physiol.* 78:185.

Kovařík, S., 1963, *Folia Biol. (Prague)* 9:388.

Kraft, N., and Shortman, K., 1972, *J. Cell. Biol.* 52:438.

Kraft, N., Shortman, K., and Marchalonis, J., 1971, *Immunology* 20:919.

Lafleur, L., Miller, R. G., and Phillips, R. A., 1972a, *J. Exp. Med.* 135:1363.

Lafleur, L., Underdown, B. J., Miller, R. G., and Phillips, R. A., 1972b, *Ser. Haematol.* 5:50.

Lafleur, L., Miller, R. G., and Phillips, R. A. 1973, in press.

Legge, D. G., and Shortman, K., 1968, *Brit. J. Haematol.* 44:323.

Leif, R. C., 1968a, *Anal. Biochem.* 25:271.

Leif, R. C., 1968b, *Anal. Biochem.* 25:283.

Leif, R. C., 1970, *Automated Cell Identification and Cell Sorting,* Wied, G. L., and Bahr, G. F. (eds.), Academic Press, New York, p. 21.

Leif, R. C., and Vinograd, J., 1964, *Proc. Nat. Acad. Sci. U.S.* 51:520.

Leif, R. C., Kneece, W. C., Warters, R. L., Grinvalsky, H., and Thomas, R. A., 1972, *Anal. Biochem.* 45:357.

Levine, S., 1956, *Science* 123:185.
Lichtenstein, B., Paseltiner, L., Wiengard, R., and Widmark, R., 1971, Technical bulletin from Technicon Instrument Corporation, Tarrytown, N.Y. U.S.A.
Lindahl, P. E., 1948, *Nature* 161:648.
Lindahl, P. E., 1956, *Biochim. Biophys. Acta* 21:411.
Macdonald, H. R., and Miller, R. G., 1970, *Biophys. J.* 10:834.
Macdonald, H. R., Phillips, R. A., and Miller, R. G., 1973a, *J. Immunol.* 111:565.
Macdonald, H. R., Phillips. R. A., and Miller, R. G., 1973b, *J. Immunol.* 111:575.
Mage, M. G., Evans, W. H., and Peterson, E. A., 1968, *Proc. Soc. Exp. Biol. Med.* 127:478.
Mage, M. G., Evans, W. H., and Peterson, E. A., 1969, *J. Immunol.* 102:908.
McEwen, C. R., Stallard, R. W., and Juhos, E. T., 1968, *Anal. Biochem.* 23:369.
Mel, H. C., 1964a, *J. Theoret. Biol.* 6:159.
Mel, H. C., 1964b, *J. Theoret. Biol.* 6:181.
Mel, H. C., 1964c, *J. Theoret. Biol.* 6:307.
Mel, H. C., Mitchell, L. T., and Thorell, B., 1965, *Blood* 25:63.
Metcalf, D., Moore, M. A. S., and Shortman, K., 1971, *J. Cell. Physiol.* 78:441.
Miller, R. G., 1973, *New Techniques in Biophysics and Cell Biology*, Vol. 1, Pain, R., and Smith, B. (eds.), John Wiley and Sons. London.
Miller, R. G., and Phillips, R. A., 1969, *J. Cell. Physiol.* 73:191.
Miller, R. G., and Phillips, R. A., 1970, *Proc. Soc. Exp. Biol. Med.* 135:63.
Moav, N., and Harris, T. N., 1970, *J. Immunol.* 105:1522.
Moore, M. A. S., Williams, N., and Metcalf, D., 1971, *J. Cell. Physiol.* 79:283.
Moore, M. A. S., Williams, N., and Metcalf, D., 1973, *J. Nat. Cancer Inst.* 50:603.
Mosier, D. E., 1967, *Science* 158:1573.
Noble, P. B., and Cutts, J. H., 1968, *J. Lab. Clin. Med.* 72:533.
Nordling, S., Andersson, L. C., and Hayry, P., 1972, *Eur. J. Immunol.* 2:405.
Oberjat, T. E., 1970, Personal communication.
Osoba, D., 1970, *J. Exp. Med.* 132:368.
Palmer, J., 1973, submitted for publication.
Pertoft, H., 1969, *Exp. Cell Res.* 57:338.
Pertoft, H., 1970, Dissertation. University of Uppsala, Uppsala, Sweden.
Pertoft, H., and Laurent, T. C., 1969, *Progress in Separation & Purification, Vol. 2, Modern Separation Methods of Macromolecules and Particles*, Gerritsen, Theo (ed.), John Wiley and Sons, New York, p. 71.
Pertoft, H., Bäck, O., and Lindahl-Kiessling, K., 1968, *Exp. Cell Res.* 50:355.
Peterson, E. A., and Evans, W. H., 1967, *Nature* 214:824.
Phillips, R. A., and Miller, R. G., 1970, *Cell Tissue Kinet.* 3:263.
Plotz, P. H., and Talal, N., 1967, *J. Immunol.* 99:1236.
Pretlow, T. G., 1971, *Anal. Biochem.* 41:248.
Pretlow, T. G., Boone, C. W., Shrager, R. I., and Weiss, G. H., 1969, *Anal. Biochem.* 29:230.
Rabinowitz, Y., 1964, *Blood* 23:811.
Raidt, D. J., Mishell, R. I., and Dutton, R. W., 1968, *J. Exp. Med.* 128:681.
Rutishauser, U., and Edelman, G. M., 1972, *Proc. Nat. Acad. Sci. U.S.* 69:3774.
Rutishauser, U., Millette, C. F., and Edelman, G. M., 1972, *Proc. Nat. Acad. Sci. U.S.* 69:1596.
Salerno, A., and Pontieri, G. M., 1969, *Clin. Exp. Immunol.* 5:209.
Schlegel, R., and Shortman, K., 1974, in preparation.
Schlossman, S. F., and Hudson, L., 1973, *J. Immunol.* 110:313.
Seaman, G. V. F., and Walter, H., 1971, *Federation Proc.* 30:1182A.
Shortman, K., 1966, *Australian J. Exp. Biol. Med. Sci.* 44:271.
Shortman, K., 1968, *Australian J. Exp. Biol. Med. Sci.* 46:375.
Shortman, K., 1969a, *Progress in Separation and Purification, Vol. 2, Modern Separation Methods of Macromolecules and Particles*, Gerritsen, Theo (ed.), John Wiley and Sons, New York, p. 91.
Shortman, K., 1969b, *Progress in Separation and Purification, Vol. 2, Modern Separation Methods of Macromolecules and Particles*, Gerritsen, Theo (ed.), John Wiley and Sons, New York, p. 167.

Shortman, K., 1970, *The Separation of Haemopoietic Cell Suspensions,* van Bekkum, D. W., and Dicke, K. A. (eds.), Radiobiological Institute TNO, Rijswijk ZH, The Netherlands, p. 43.

Shortman, K., 1971, *J. Cell. Physiol.* 77:319.

Shortman, K., 1972, *Ann. Rev. Biophys. Bioeng.* 1:93.

Shortman, K., and Jackson, H., 1974, *Cellular Immunology,* in press.

Shortman, K., and Palmer, J., 1971, *Cell. Immunol.* 2:399.

Shortman, K., and Seligman, K., 1969, *J. Cell. Biol.* 42:783.

Shortman, K., Diener, E., Russell, P., and Armstrong, W. D., 1970, *J. Exp. Med.* 131:461.

Shortman, K., Williams, N., Jackson, H., Russell, P., Byrt, P., and Diener, E., 1971, *J. Cell Biol.* 48:566.

Shortman, K., Brunner, K. T., and Cerottini, J.-C., 1972a, *J. Exp. Med.* 135:1375.

Shortman, K., Byrd, W. J., Williams, N., Brunner, K. T., and Cerottini, J.-C., 1972b, *Australian J. Exp. Biol. Med. Sci.* 50:323.

Shortman, K., Cerottini, J.-C., and Brunner, K. T., 1972c, *Eur. J. Immunol.* 2:313.

Shortman, K., Williams, N., and Adams, P., 1972d, *J. Immun. Methods* 1:273.

Shortman, K., Byrd, W., Cerottini, J.-C., and Brunner, K. T., 1973, *Cell. Immun.* 6, 25.

Sweet, R. G., 1965, *Rev. Sci. Instru.* 36:131.

Truffa-Bachi, P., and Wofsy, L., 1970, *Proc. Nat. Acad. Sci. U.S.* 66:685.

von Boehmer, H., 1974a, *J. Immunol.* 112:70.

von Boehmer, H., 1974b, submitted for publication.

von Boehmer, H., and Shortman, K., 1973, *J. Immun. Meth.* 2:293.

von Boehmer, H., Shortman, K., and Nossal, G. J. V., 1974, *J. Cell Physiol.,* in press.

Walter, H., 1969, *Progress in Separation & Purification, Vol. 2, Modern Separation Methods of Macromolecules and Particles,* Gerritsen, Theo (ed.), John Wiley and Sons, New York, p. 121.

Walter, H., and Albertsson, P.-A., 1971, *Exp. Cell Res.* 67:218.

Walter, H., Selby, F. W., and Garza, R., 1967, *Biochim. Biophys. Acta* 136:148.

Walter, H., Krob, E. J., and Garza, R., 1968, *Biochim. Biophys. Acta* 165:507.

Walter, H., Krob, E. J., Garza, R., and Ascher, G. S., 1969a, *Exp. Cell Res.* 55:57.

Walter, H., Krob, E. J., and Ascher, G. S., 1969b, *Exp. Cell Res.* 55:279.

Walter, H., Tung, R., Jackson, L. J., and Seaman, G. V. F., 1972, *Biochem. Biophys. Res. Commun.* 48:565.

Wigzell, H., 1970, *Transplant. Rev.* 5:76.

Wigzell, H., 1971, *Progress in Immunology, Vol. 1,* (B. Amos, ed.), p. 1105, Academic Press, New York.

Wigzell, H., and Andersson, B., 1969, *J. Exp. Med.* 129:23.

Wigzell, H., and Andersson, B., 1971, *Ann. Rev. Microbiol.* 25:291.

Wigzell, H., Sundqvist, K. G., and Yoshida, T. O., 1972, *Scand. J. Immunol.* 1:75.

Williams, N., and Shortman, K., 1972, *Australian J. Exp. Biol. Med. Sci.* 50:133.

Williams, N., and Moore, M. A. S., 1973, *J. Cell Physiol.* 82:81.

Williams, N., Kraft, N., and Shortman, K., 1972, *Immunology* 22:885.

Williams, N., Moore, M. A. S., Shortman, K., Condon, L., Pike, B., and Nossal, G. J. V., 1974, *Aust. J. Exp. Biol. Med. Sci.,* in press.

Wioland, M., Sabolovic, D., and Burg, C., 1972, *Nature New Biol.* 237:276.

Wofsy, L., 1972, Third International Convocation on Immunology: Specific Receptors of Antibodies, Antigens and Cells, Buffalo, New York, in press.

Zeiller, K., Pascher, G., and Hannig, K., 1970, *Hoppe Seylers Z. Physiol. Chem.* 351:435.

Zeiller, K., Holzberg, E., Pascher, G., and Hannig, K., 1972, *Hoppe Seylers Z. Physiol. Chem.* 353:105.

Zucker, R. M., and Cassen, B., 1969, *Blood* 34:591.

Radioelectrocomplexing:
A General Radioimmunoassay Procedure for the Detection of Primary Binding of Antigen by Antibody

Malcolm J. Simons

WHO Immunology Research and Training Centre
University of Singapore
Singapore, Singapore

and

Albert A. Benedict

Department of Microbiology
University of Hawaii
Honolulu, Hawaii

I. INTRODUCTION

Of the numerous *in vitro* methods available for estimating the concentration of antigen or antibody in biological fluids those based on the determination of the primary interaction between antigen and antibody have certain advantages over methods in which secondary interactions are measured. The chief advantages are that (1) meaningful thermodynamic and stoichiometric characterization of the reaction can be obtained when antibody and hapten are employed, and (2) nanogram amounts of antigen or antibody can be measured relatively simply and rapidly if the antigen is radioactively labeled.

Among the first to employ radioimmunoassay (RIA) procedures were Berson *et al.* (1956) and Farr (1958). Since these early studies there has been an increasing use of RIA for the detection of antibodies and a variety of antigens. In a recent volume entitled "Radioimmunoassay Methods" (Kirkham and Hunter, 1971) the view was expressed that "no single method of measurement [in endocrinology] has been adopted so rapidly and applied so widely as the RIA. Because of its general simplicity, sensitivity potential, and wide applicability, it is rapidly becoming the method of choice for the measurement of most protein and polypeptide hormones."

RIA is also finding increasing use in the fields of immunology, enzymology, microbiology, and oncology. As an indication of the range of application, RIA methods have been described for the detection of chlamydial and rickettsial agents (Gerloff and Watson, 1967; Tabert and Lachman, 1965), Hepatitis B viral antigen (HBAg) (Walsh et al., 1970) and antibody (HBAb) (Lander et al., 1971), carcinoembryonic antigens (Thomson et al., 1969), alpha-fetoprotein (AFP) (Ruoslahti and Seppala, 1971; Purves and Geddes, 1972), and prostaglandins (Levine and van Vunakis, 1970; Caldwell et al., 1971).

A requirement common to all RIA methods is the availability of purified antigens which can be radiolabeled. In the procedure itself, two stages are involved: (1) an incubation period for the reaction between the test sample and the reagents to approach equilibrium and (2) separation of free radiolabeled reagent from that bound in immune complexes. In different RIA procedures the incubation period varies from less than 1 hr to more than 72 hr. Separation of free from bound radiolabeled molecules in the second stage can be achieved by numerous methods (Hunter, 1967) including (1) electrophoresis (paper, cellulose acetate, polyacrylamide), (2) gel filtration, (3) ion-exchange resins, (4) adsorption (to dextran-coated charcoal, powdered silica or talc, cellulose powder, starch grains), (5) salt precipitation, (6) solvent fractionation, (7) double antibody precipitation, and (8) antibody bound to solid phase. Each of these procedures has its advantages and its adherents. All have limitations due to the time taken in the separation process or to the need for centrifugation, washing, or other steps which cannot easily be automated.

An ideal RIA would be one which is (1) sensitive, (2) specific (yet able to reveal nonspecific effects, such as radiation damage), (3) simple to perform, (4) simple to interpret, (5) rapid, (6) quantitative, (7) capable of showing no labeled antigen in the "bound" antigen fraction in the absence of antibody, (8) capable of showing 100% of the labeled antigen in the "bound" antigen fraction in the presence of excess antibody, (9) conservative of reagents, (10) inexpensive, (11) adaptable to microscale or macroscale, and (12) adaptable to automation.

The RIA described here is a development of the technique of counterimmunoelectrophoresis (CIE). Many antigens have an anodal migration on electrophoresis at high pH values, whereas antibodies migrate toward the cathode. In CIE the reactants move toward each other and form a line of visible precipitation where the antigen and antibody concentrations are at or are near equivalence (Culliford, 1964; Lang, 1955; Watson and Whinfrey, 1958; Bussard, 1959; Feinberg and Hill, 1968).

The RIA adaptation, here called "radioelectrocomplexing" (REC), involves the formation of subvisible complexes of radiolabeled antigen with antibody as a result of counterdirectional movement produced during gel electrophoresis (Simons, 1972). In REC, both immune complex formation and separation of free from bound antigen are achieved by a single electrophoretic process. In most previous RIA methods, electrophoresis has been employed for the separation of free radiolabeled antigen from that bound in immune complexes which had been formed prior to electrophoresis (Yalow and Berson, 1960; Yalow and Berson, 1964; Minden et al., 1969). In the 3 years since the first experiments using REC at least three groups have reported assays employing the principle of radioimmunoassay by counterimmunoelectrophoresis. Tilden and DeLand (1972) described the application of electroosmophoretic RIA to the detection of HBAg and HBAb. In 1972, Capalbo reported on a radioelectroimmunodiffusion assay for the detection of nanogram amounts of bovine serum albumin. In the same year Coller et al. disclosed a radioimmunoelectrophoretic binding assay for the detection of carcinoembryonic antigen, which was subsequently described in more detail (Coller et al., 1973).

Of importance to any discussion on antigen—antibody interaction are the concepts of "affinity" and "avidity." Distinction between the two is especially important when considering multideterminant antigens, such as those which are usually involved in RIA. "Affinity" is a thermodynamic value which describes the binding strength between an antibody binding site and an antigenic determinant or univalent hapten, and which is expressed by the average intrinsic association constant (K_o). "Avidity" is a relative measure of binding which is based on the multivalency of antigens and immunoglobulins. Thus, an IgM antibody with more than two binding sites would be expected to form less dissociable complexes with a multivalent antigen than an IgG antibody which is bivalent, even though the two antibodies had the same affinity constants. In this connection, Hornick and Karush (1969; 1972) have distinguished the "intrinsic affinity" from the "functional affinity" of IgG antibody; that is, the binding ability of IgG antibody to the polyvalent ligand is several orders of magnitude greater than that for the binding to the monovalent ligand.

The interaction between antibody and antigen, whether a single determinant on a multideterminant antigen or a univalent hapten, can be represented by the reversible equation

$$H + Ab \underset{k_d}{\overset{k_a}{\rightleftharpoons}} AbH$$

where k_a and k_d are the association and dissociation constants, respectively. According to the law of mass action, the intrinsic association constant (affinity) is

$$K_a = \frac{(AbH)}{(Ab)(H)}$$

In studying the rates of complex formation several investigators have noted a rather limited range of constants, whereas dissociation rates seem to vary more extensively (Day et al., 1963; Hornick and Karush, 1972). It has been suggested that the strength of antibody–hapten association is governed by the rate of dissociation (Froese, 1968) and, as pointed out by Hornick and Karush (1972), the rate of dissociation of bivalent antidinitrophenyl (anti-DNP) antibody from a multivalent DNP–protein antigen is considerably less than the rate of dissociation from a monovalent DNP hapten.

Since avidity or functional affinity of an antigen–antibody system is an important variable influencing the rate of dissociation of immune complexes, the question of the effect of electrophoresis on dissociation arises. Kleczowski (1959) demonstrated that the degree of dissociation occurring during electrophoresis depended on the quality of the antibody; dissociation was greater when antibody formed during the early phase of a primary response was used and was less using hyperimmune serum. In their use of electrophoresis for the separation of free radiolabeled insulin from that bound in immune complexes, Yalow and Berson (1960) observed some trailing of free radiolabeled insulin, which they attributed to immune complex dissociation during the 16-hour period of electrophoresis. They noted that the dissociation was less likely to occur using antisera characterized as "high avidity." Similarly, Weigle and Deichmuller (1960) regarded dissociation of soluble antigen–antibody complexes as partly responsible for the diversified electrophoretic distribution of bovine serum albumin-I^{125} (BSA-I^{125}) activity in sera containing BSA-I^{125} / anti-BSA complexes. Other workers employing free boundary electrophoresis found only a small amount of dissociation of soluble complexes when the complexes were prepared in vitro with hyperimmune sera and excess antigen (Singer and Campbell, 1955; Ishizaka et al., 1959). Minden et al. (1969) also observed that the strength and duration of the electrophoretic force influenced dissociation of antigen–antibody complexes and that such dissociation would effect the sensitivity of primary binding tests, in their case that of radio-gel electrophoresis.

The foregoing theoretical considerations provide a basis on which practical objectives can be defined. For the REC system, the central objective is the determination of the conditions where

1. Association of radiolabeled antigen and antibody is maximized.
2. Separation of bound from free radiolabeled antigen is maximized.
3. Dissociation of bound radiolabeled antigen from immune complexes is minimized.

For each antigen–antibody system it was necessary to investigate a range of variables to determine the optimal REC conditions. In the next section some aspects of antigen–antibody interaction have been investigated by REC using specifically purified anti-DNP and multivalent DNP. This is followed by a detailed description of the determination of optimal REC conditions for human serum albumin (HSA). In the subsequent sections some of the applications of REC are exemplified using AFP and HBAg as radiolabeled antigens.

II. MATERIALS AND METHODS

A. Antigens

2,4-DNP–protein conjugates were prepared by the method of Eisen (1964). Dinitrophenyl–bovine gamma globulin (DNP-BGG) and DNP-HSA had approximately 60 and 40 moles of DNP per mole of protein, respectively. Crystallized HSA (Armour), BSA (Pentax), and egg albumin (EA) were obtained commercially. The dinitrophenyl–protein antigens were provided by Ms. K. Yamaga, Department of Microbiology, University of Hawaii, Honolulu. Radiolabeling of conjugates, HSA, and BSA was performed using either I^{131} or I^{125} by the method of Hunter and Greenwood (1962) or by the method of McConahey and Dixon (1966). Efficiency of iodination was 45–60% as measured by the proportion of radioactivity in the protein peak on Sephadex G-25 gel filtration. The maximum specific activity of the labeled HSA was 4.5–6.0 μCi/μg. A large percentage of the radiolabel (92–96%) was precipitated by 5% trichloracetic acid. To eliminate material which did not migrate electrophoretically as albumin, DNP-HSA and HSA each were fractionated by starch block electrophoresis and the fastest moving fraction was used as antigen in REC. The concentrations of 2,4-DNP derivatives and 2,4-dinitrophenol (DNP-OH) were determined by their extinction coefficients as given by Little and Donahue (1968).

AFP-I^{125} and AFP standard solutions were obtained commercially (α-feto-125 kit, Dainabot Radioisotope Laboratories, Tokyo, Japan) and I^{125}-labeled preparations of HBAg of *adw, adr,* and *ayw* subtypes were obtained from Dr. R. H. Purcell, National Institute of Allergy and Infectious Diseases, National Institutes of Health, Bethesda, Maryland. Purified preparations of HBAg were provided by Dr. M. F. Warburton, Commonwealth Serum Laboratories, Parkville, Victoria, Australia, and by Professor K. Nishioka, Virology Division, National Cancer Center Research Institute, Tokyo, The Reference Hepatitis B Antigen Panel No. 2, comprising 35 HBAg-positive sera, 10 HBAb-positive sera, and 16 sera nonreactive by current methods was supplied by the Division of Biologics Standards, NIH, Bethesda, Maryland.

B. Antisera

Adult white leghorn chickens were given four intravenous injections of 2 mg DNP-BGG each over a one-year period and were bled seven days following the last injection. From a pool of these sera the anti-DNP antibodies were purified by affinity chromatography (Cuatrecasas *et al.,* 1968) as modified by Wofsy and Burr (1969). Briefly, antisera to which a final concentration of 0.001 M EDTA was added were passed through Sepharose–DNP–lysine columns, and the columns were washed repeatedly with borate buffer (pH 8.2; $\Gamma/2$ = 0.16). The anti-DNP antibodies were eluted first with 0.1 M DNP-OH, followed by elution of the remaining antibodies with 0.1 M DNP-glycine. These antibody preparations will be referred to as "DNP-OH" and "DNP–glycine" antibodies, respectively. The IgG and IgM anti-DNP antibodies in each preparation were separated and recovered by gel filtration on Sephadex G-200.

For some experiments chickens were given either two intravenous injections of 2 mg DNP-BGG 45 days apart, or two intramuscular injections of 2 mg DNP-BGG each in Freund's complete adjuvant 30 days apart. The IgG fractions, referred to as globulin fractions, were isolated by precipitation of the globulins with 18% Na_2SO_4 followed by two cycles of gel filtration on Sephadex G-200 (Benedict, 1967).

Rabbits were given footpad inoculations of 2 mg HSA in Freund's complete adjuvant, bled after 10 days, and the sera pooled (early antiserum). To obtain a late antiserum, the rabbits were given two additional footpad injections of 1 mg HSA in Freund's incomplete adjuvant. The anti-HSA antisera were not fractionated.

Anti-AFP sera were purchased from ULTA, Zaragoza, Spain. A pooled serum from multiply-transfused humans served as the reagent HBAb. The anti-immunoglobulin antiserum was purchased from Hyland Laboratories, California. The antisera to immunoglobulin heavy chains of the gamma, mu, alpha, and epsilon types were provided by Dr. D. S. Rowe, WHO International Reference Centre for Immunoglobulins, Lausanne, Switzerland.

C. Radioelectrocomplexing

Except for minor differences, which will be pointed out later, the methods used for the DNP-HSA/anti-DNP and the HSA/anti-HSA systems were similar. Microscope slides were precoated with agar and covered with 4 ml (10 mm layer) of 1% purified agar (Difco) in veronal buffer (pH 8.6; $\Gamma/2$ = 0.05). For some experiments, agarose (L'Industrie Biologique Française), at the same concentration in veronal buffer, was also tested. Two wells, each 3 mm in diameter and 4 mm apart, were punched in the agar as four parallel pairs; thus, duplicate or triplicate test samples and controls could be run under the same conditions. However, in many experiments duplicate test samples and a single diluent control were run per slide.

Denaturation of chicken antibody preparations was minimized by dilution in a 1:50 dilution of normal chicken serum (NCS), and dilutions of DNP conjugates were made in a 1:100 dilution of BSA. For the DNP-protein studies,

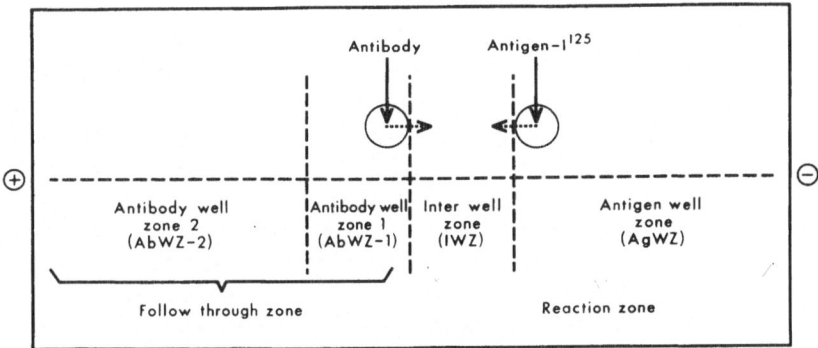

Figure 1. Schematic diagram of radioelectrocomplexing.

borate buffer was used as the diluent. Rabbit anti-HSA antisera were diluted in a
1:64 dilution of normal rabbit serum (NRS). Veronal buffer alone served as the
diluent for HSA. Five-microliter amounts each of antigen and antibody were
placed in their respective wells (Fig. 1), and electrophoresis was carried out at a
constant current of 2.5–10 mA/slide (approximately 200 V) for varying periods
of time using a veronal buffer (pH 8.6; $\Gamma/2$ = 0.05). The concentrations of
DNP-HSA, HSA, and anti-DNP given are those which were actually introduced
into the wells; that is, the concentrations in 5 or 10 μl. After electrophoresis the
agar was cut with a sharp razor blade according to the pattern shown in Fig. 1.
Where antigen was reacted with antibody, radiolabel usually was found in the
antigen well zone (AgWZ) and the interwell zone (IWZ) (Fig. 1). Therefore, the
AgWZ and the IWZ together were considered as the reaction zone (RZ). The
slabs of agar from the RZ and the follow-through zone (FTZ) were placed in
tubes 10 $\times$ 25 mm or 13 $\times$ 100 mm, and the agar was pushed or crushed to the
bottom of the tube with an applicator stick. The radioactivity was determined in
a gamma spectrometer.

After subtraction of background radioactivity from all counts, the percentage of antigen bound in the RZ was calculated for each agar strip by
correcting for the presence of unbound labeled antigen as indicated by controls.
This correction was made according to the formula

$$\text{corr}_{RZ_t} = RZ_t - \left[(RZ_t + FTZ_t) \times \frac{RZ_c}{(RZ_c + FTZ_c)} \right]$$

where t and c represent test and control reactions, and RZ_t, FTZ_t, RZ_c, and
FTZ_c are the observed cpm in the respective zones. Then,

$$\text{corr}_{\%\text{ antigen bound}} = \frac{\text{corr}_{RZ_t}}{\text{corr}_{(RZ_t + FTZ_t)}} \times 100$$

D. Equilibrium Dialysis

The binding constants on the globulin preparations were determined by equilibrium dialysis according to Werblin and Siskind (1972). Duplicate samples of normal and of antibody-containing globulin were dialyzed for 3 days at 4°C against various concentrations of ϵ-DNP-3,5-^{3}H-(N)-L-lysine (New England Nuclear). After dialysis, the protein concentration of each sample was determined by Folin analysis. Samples were counted in Aquasol (New England Nuclear) using a Packard Tricarb scintillation spectrometer until at least 20,000 counts had been registered. The amount of hapten bound at each free hapten concentration was determined for an adjusted globulin concentration of 10 mg/ml. Calculations for total binding sites and affinity constants were performed as described by Werblin and Siskind (1972) with the aid of an APL/360 computer program.

III. QUANTITATIVE STUDIES

A. DNP/anti-DNP

1. Effect of Diluents on Migration of DNP-HSA-I^{125}

It was desirable to use NCS as a diluent to protect nanogram quantities of specifically purified IgG and IgM antibodies from denaturation. For this purpose the lowest concentration of NCS which produced nonspecific retardation of DNP-HSA-I^{125} anodal migration had first to be established. Most NCS diluted 1:8 bound 10–25% of the antigen in the RZ. To give a margin of safety, a 1:50 dilution of NCS was used as the diluent. This dilution did not result in retardation of the antigen in the RZ, but it did retard movement of antigen in the FTZ compared to when borate buffer was used. This is shown in an

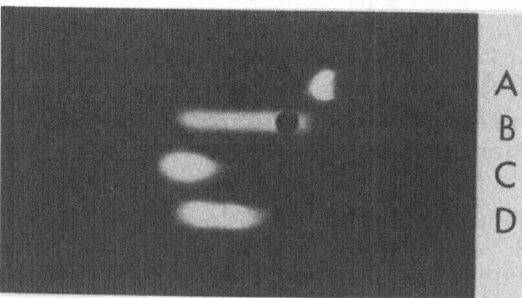

Figure 2. Autoradiograph of DNP-HSA-I^{125} reacted with (A) 600 ng, and (B) 37 ng of specifically purified anti-DNP IgG; (C) borate buffer; (D) 1:50 dilution of normal chicken serum.

autoradiograph (Fig. 2). Nonspecific retardation of radiolabeled antigen by normal sera has been found to vary depending upon the nature of the antigen.

2. Effect of Duration and Electrical Current of Electrophoresis

For each system, variables, such as the length of time of electrophoresis and the electrical current applied, have been studied. In the absence of antibody and employing 2.5 mA/slide, DNP-HSA-I^{125} eventually entered the anodal wick and buffer vessel only after 2.5 hr. With a current of 5.0 mA/slide, the antigen entered the anodal wick after 1.5 hr of electrophoresis. The distribution of bound antigen was studied by autoradiography at various times of electrophoresis at 2.5 mA/slide and 5 mA/slide and with amounts of antibody which would bind 50% (7.0 ng) and 90% (18 ng) of antigen. With 18 ng of antibody, the radioactivity was held in the RZ after 90 min at 2.5 mA; whereas, with a current of 5.0 mA, radioactivity appeared in the RTZ after 50 min. Similarly, with a current of 2.5 mA, radioactivity did not appear in the FTZ until 60 min of electrophoresis with 7 ng of antibody, but at 5.0 mA antigen was detected in the FTZ at 30 min. There was a wide distribution of radioactivity in the FTZ as seen in the autoradiograms, particularly in those of the electrophoretic runs using 5 mA. This was interpreted as representing immune complexes composed of excess antigen, and probably antigen which dissociated from some of the complexes and migrated anodally behind the unbound antigen front. Consistent with this interpretation of complex dissociation was the finding that 18 ng of antibody held antigen in the RZ for 90 min when a current of 2.5 mA was applied, but when the current was increased to 5.0 mA there was a component which migrated with the trailing edge of the antigen. The phenomenon of dissociation is considered more fully in a later section. For the DNP-HSA and anti-DNP system, dissociation of complexes appeared to be minimum when 2.5 mA/slide was applied for 75 min, so these conditions were adopted as the standard.

3. Binding Curves

In Fig. 3a are shown typical binding curves of a preimmune serum, serum obtained 6 days after a single injection of antigen, and serum obtained 8 days after a booster injection of 2 mg of antigen given 30 days following primary immunization. It was mentioned earlier that NCS in dilutions of 1:8 or less bound DNP-HSA to a varying extent. The preimmune serum used in this experiment demonstrated this effect. The binding curve of an anti-DNP globulin fraction, which had a binding constant of approximately 1×10^6 M^{-1}, is shown in Fig. 3b. About 6 ng of antibody globulin bound 50% of the antigen, whereas 40 ng of normal globulin were required to bind a similar amount of antigen.

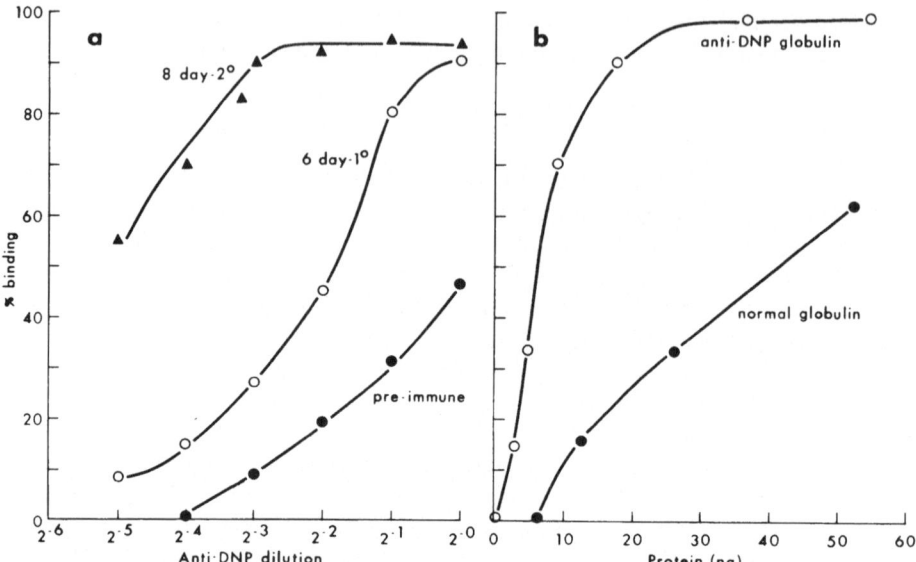

Figure 3. Binding of DNP-HSA-I^{125} by (a) anti-DNP antisera and preimmune serum; and (b) anti-DNP globulin fraction (7 S) and normal 7 S globulin.

To determine the relationship of varying concentrations of antigen and antibody, increasing amounts of antigen were added to varying concentrations of specifically purified anti-DNP IgG antibody. Figure 4a shows the percent binding of antigen at four antibody levels as a function of increasing antigen concentration. If antibody is saturated, then the radioactivity in the RZ should reach a

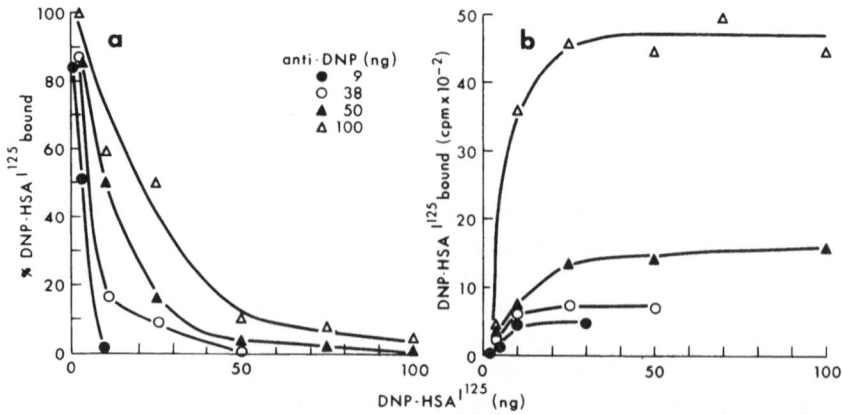

Figure 4. Binding of increasing amounts of DNP-HSA-I^{125} at four different antibody levels. (a) Percent DNP-HSA-I^{125} bound in reaction zone (RZ); (b) radioactivity (cpm) in RZ.

constant level for a fixed amount of antibody. This would be valid if significant dissociation of complexes did not occur under the conditions used. It can be seen in Fig. 4b that at different antibody levels a constant level of radioactivity in the RZ was approached as the antigen concentration was increased.

Based on these relationships, two methods of antibody assay are available. The first involves the determination of concentration of antibody or dilution of antiserum required to give 50% binding of a standard concentration of antigen. For example, the standard concentration of antigen could be established as that amount of antigen required to give 80% binding of a reference serum. A second method of estimating antibody potency is based on reacting a constant amount of antibody with varying amounts of antigen and determining the concentration of antigen which just saturates the antibody (Fig. 4b).

4. Sensitivity for Detection of IgM and IgG Antibody

Approximately 0.31 and 1.25 pmol of specifically purified IgM and IgG anti-DNP antibodies, respectively, gave 50% binding of 3 ng of antigen. Approximately 40 times (12 pmol) and 84 times (105 pmol) more of normal IgM and normal IgG, respectively, were required to bind 50% of the antigen. Thus, as would be expected (Onoue *et al.*, 1968; Ashman and Metzger, 1969) the IgM antibody was more avid than the IgG antibody.

5. Specificity of the Reaction

The specificity of binding was determined by adding a constant amount of DNP-HSA-I^{125} to increasing concentrations of unlabeled DNP–HSA at different antibody levels. As the antibody concentration was increased the amounts of DNP-HSA required to give 50% binding was increased. A plot of the amount of antibody required to bind 50% of labeled antigen *vs* the amount of unlabeled antigen required to give 50% binding yielded a straight line. Thus, REC may be used to determine the concentrations of unlabeled antigens by exploiting the ability of unlabeled antigen to compete with labeled antigen and thereby to inhibit the binding of the labeled antigen. Hapten inhibition studies given below also attest to the specificity of the reaction.

6. Hapten Inhibition of Binding of Antibody with DNP-HSA-I^{125}

The specificites of antibodies and the relative combining constant (K_{rel}) of a hapten with antibody have been studied by the variable ability of different haptens to inhibit the reactions of antibody with conjugated haptens (Landsteiner, 1945; Pauling *et al.*, 1944). Hapten inhibition offers an advantage over other methods for determining K_{rel} in that specifically purified antibody is not

Table I. Comparison of the Relative Binding Constants
of 2,4-DNP Derivatives and Two Antibody Preparations
as Determined by Inhibition of Binding of Anti-DNP
and DNP-HSA-I^{125} in Radioelectrocomplexing

	Antibody preparations			
	DNP-OH[a]		DNP-glycine[b]	
	Concentration of hapten at 50% inhibition of binding		Concentration of hapten at 50% inhibition of binding	
Hapten	$(M \times 10^6)$	K_{rel}[c]	$(M \times 10^6)$	K_{rel}
ε-DNP-lysine	4.5	1.00	9.0	1.0
2,4-Dinitrophenol	110	0.041	1000	0.009
DNP-glycine	20	0.22	40	0.22
ε-DNP-aminocaproate	2.5	1.8	4.5	2.0

[a] Eluted from immunoadsorbent with 2,4-DNP-OH.
[b] Following elution with 2,4-DNP-OH, antibody eluted with DNP-glycine.
[c] Relative binding constant.

required. To determine whether REC was potentially useful for this purpose, the
DNP-OH and DNP-glycine antibody preparations were reacted with various
concentrations of the following DNP derivatives: DNP-OH, DNP-glycine, ε-DNP-
L-lysine, and ε-DNP-aminocaproate. To minimize dissociation of hapten and
antibody during electrophoresis, the inhibiting hapten was added to the agar and
to the buffer in the electrode vessels to the final concentration desired. The
electrode vessels of the electrophoresis apparatus were partitioned with plexi-
glass into five sections so that five different inhibitor concentrations could be
tested under the same conditions of electrophoresis. The amounts of antibody
and DNP-HSA-I^{125} giving 80–85% binding were used. Taking the concentration
of DNP-lysine which gave 50% inhibition as a standard with a K_{rel} = 1.0, the K_{rel}
values for the other ligands at 50% inhibition were calculated. As shown in Table
I, the K_{rel} of the haptens for both antibodies in the order of increasing K_{rel} of
the haptens was DNP-OII, DNP-glycine, DNP-lysine, and DNP-caproate. This
order of increasing affinities was the same as that reported by Eisen and Siskind
(1964), who used fluorescence quenching for measuring affinities.

7. Dissociation of Complexes

To study this problem further, two concentrations of anti-DNP IgG, 70 ng
and 7.0 ng, which formed complexes with 10 ng of antigen in moderate

antibody excess and moderate antigen excess, respectively, were electrophoresed with a current of 5 mA/slide. In previous experiments this amount of current seemed to accelerate apparent dissociation. Slides were removed 20, 30, 50, and 75 min after electrophoresis and one set of each was prepared for autoradiography. The agar of another set of slides was fractionated in a manner as shown in Fig. 5 and the radioactivity of the fractions was determined. A comparison of the radioactivity in the fractions as determined by autoradiography and by actual counts in the fractions is presented in Fig. 5. The complexes formed in antibody excess remained in the RZ (fractions 5, 6, and 7) after 75 min of

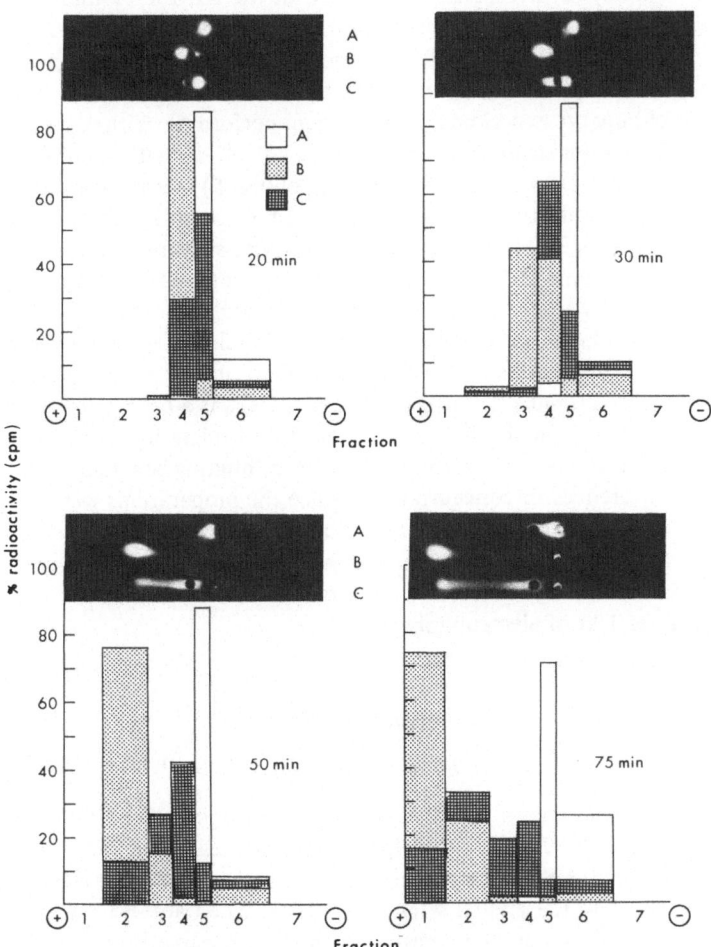

Figure 5. Autoradiographs and radioactivity (percent cpm/fraction) in fractions after various times of electrophoresis at 5 mA/slide.

electrophoresis, whereas, at this time, the complexes formed in antigen excess formed two major zones of radioactivity. One zone had the same rate of migration as the trailing half of the antigen in the buffer control, and the other zone remained in the cathodal end of the FTZ (fractions 3 and 4). Although only 11% of the binding remained in the RZ for the low antibody concentration, antigen was bound as indicated by the activity in fractions 3 and 4. It is reasonable to suggest that complexes of various ratios of antibody to antigen were formed and that they were responsible for the smearing of radioactivity in the FTZ. The complexes formed in antigen excess seemed to be stable under the conditions employed in that they remained in the RZ for 75 min. However, a more rigorous examination of dissociation would be possible if antibody preparations were employed with different known binding constants and the complexes were formed in zones other than that of antibody excess. For this purpose preliminary experiments have been performed with three anti-DNP globulin preparations with binding constants of 1×10^5 M^{-1} (globulin-1), 3×10^6 M^{-1} (globulin-2), and 1×10^8 M^{-1} (globulin-5), respectively. In the first experiments concentrations of globulin-1 and globulin-2, which would bind about 90% of antigen after 1 hr of electrophoresis, were electrophoresed for various periods of time at 2.5 mA/slide. For both preparations, the percentage of bound antigen (RZ) decreased with time; however, the rate of disappearance from the RZ was faster for globulin-1 than for globulin-2. In another experiment these antibody preparations were diluted so that, after 1 hr of electrophoresis, they bound only 30—50% of antigen. Again there was a faster rate of disappearance of globulin-1 from the RZ. The faster rate of migration of globulin-1 from the RZ is best explained on the basis of its lower binding constant rather than as a result of differences in concentrations, since the preparations were equated on the basis of binding of antigen after 1 hr of electrophoresis. Actually more globulin-1 antibody was used than either of the other preparations; 50% of antigen was bound by globulin-1 and only 33% of antigen was bound by globulin-2 after 1 hr of electrophoresis.

B. HSA/anti-HSA

1. Electrophoretic Migration of HSA-I^{125}

In initial experiments the distribution patterns of HSA-I^{125} were investigated by cutting the 76-mm gel strips into narrow zones of 2—3 mm width. In the absence of anti-HSA, labeled HSA migrated anodally under electrophoresis, eventually entering the anodal wick and buffer. When anti-HSA was present in the antibody well, anodally migrating HSA-I^{125} became bound to cathodally moving anti-HSA antibody. With anti-HSA of high antibody titer ("late" immune serum), the anodal direction of migration of HSA-I^{125} was reversed.

Radiolabel was found not only between the wells, but also around the antigen well and even cathodal to it. This was interpreted as indicating the existence of immune complexes formed in relative antibody excess. By contrast, when anti-HSA was tested at dilutions near antibody extinction, radioactivity was present around and immediately anodal to the antibody well. On further dilution of the antiserum, the distribution of radiolabel progressively approached that of antigen which was migrated in the absence of anti-HSA.

Theoretically, the total radioactivity counted in the separate zones (Fig. 1) should be equal to that dispensed into the antigen well. From Table II, for example, it can be seen that the total radioactivity detected in each gel reaction strip was similar. Nonetheless, a variation of ±5–10% in total count occurred between agar strips within an experiment. A small proportion of HSA-I^{125} remained in the RZ even when the solution added to the antibody well did not contain anti-HSA (Table II). The proportion of this "background" radiolabel varied between 5% and 10%. It was less when dilutions of nonantibody-containing sera in buffer were used as controls than when buffer alone was used. No difference was observed when the sera were used at dilutions of 1%, 2%, or 10%. For routine use a 1:64 dilution of NRS in veronal buffer was used both as the diluent for rabbit anti-HSA and as the control.

2. Effect of Gel Composition and Concentration

The proportion of radiolabel in the RZ was less with agarose than with agar when both were tested at concentrations ranging from 1.0% to 2.0%. Agar of less than 1% concentration was too friable for easy transfer to counting rubes. Table II shows the distribution of radiolabel in the four zones when HSA-I^{125} was migrated against dilutions of anti-HSA for varying times using 1% agar and 2% agar as the supporting matrices. The patterns of radiolabel distribution in the 1% and the 2% agar were different by 30 min, but approximately 20% of the radiolabel was still present in the RZ of the control at that time. At 90 min the distribution of the label in the controls was similar in 1% agar and 2% agar; however, more label remained in the RZ when less anti-HSA was tested in 2% agar. The faster anodal migration of label in the reactions in 1% agar between HSA-I^{125} and anti-HSA at 2^{-10} dilution also was seen at 50–70 min. At these times the counts in the RZ of controls in 1% agar were less than in the corresponding zones in 2% agar. Concentrations of agar between 1% and 2% showed intermediary effects. For routine use, 1% agar was chosen since retardation of anodal migration of HSA-I^{125} was least at this concentration.

It should be noted that, although agar was more suitable than agarose for the assay of binding between HSA and anti-HSA, other antigen–antibody systems may require the use of agarose. For example, when antigens which have a relatively low net electronegative charge are to be tested, the electroendosmotic

Table II. Distribution Patterns of HSA-I^{125} when Migrated against Dilutions of Anti-HSA for Varying Electrophoretic Times in 1% Agar and 2% Agar

Anti-HSA dilution	EP time (min)	1% Agar					2% Agar				
		AbWZ-2	AbWZ-1	IWZ	AgWZ	Total cpm	AbWZ-2	AbWZ-1	IWZ	AgWZ	Total cpm
2^0	30	1	2	82	15	2210	2	1	84	13	1926
	50	1	1	82	16	2135	1	0	78	21	1921
	70	1	2	81	16	1981	2	0	81	17	2096
	90	0	2	85	13	1919	1	1	77	21	1981
2^{-5}	30	1	17	84	14	2237	3	1	85	11	1955
	50	1	2	83	14	1846	1	0	84	15	1910
	70	1	1	89	9	1981	1	1	83	15	1887
	90	1	2	89	8	2016	2	0	86	12	1906
2^{-10}	30	6	33	48	13	2085	13	22	54	11	1833
	50	9	27	60	4	2334	11	14	61	14	1956
	70	15	35	44	6	1996	12	15	63	10	1883
	90	13	23	57	7	1900	5	8	77	10	1870
Control	30	55	26	4	15	2193	75	7	8	10	1838
	50	86	3	6	5	1964	79	3	5	13	2069
	70	88	2	3	7	1836	82	3	5	10	2013
	90	90	3	2	5	1846	89	3	3	5	1926

Table III. Distribution Patterns of HSA-I^{125} when Migrated against Dilutions of Anti-HSA under Electrical Currents of 10 mA and 7.5 mA per Slide

Anti-HSA dilution	EP time	10 mA					7.5 mA				
		AbWZ-2	AbWZ-1	IWZ	AgWZ	Total cpm	AbWZ-2	AbWZ-1	IWZ	AgWZ	Total cpm
2^0	40	0	0	92	8	4881	0	1	83	16	4218
	50	0	0	93	7	5002	2	1	89	8	3686
	60	0	0	90	10	4481	1	0	90	9	3638
	90	0	0	93	7	4734	2	0	90	8	3720
2^{-5}	40	4	0	90	6	5096	1	5	83	11	4002
	50	5	0	88	7	5266	1	1	93	5	3808
	60	8	1	87	4	5223	3	2	88	7	3701
	90	3	0	93	4	4746	5	2	89	4	3883
2^{-10}	40	76	16	3	5	4646	7	19	76	8	3777
	50	80	12	3	9	4457	6	14	74	6	356
	60	81	10	4	5	4194	20	19	56	5	4519
	90	85	8	3	4	4784	29	27	39	5	4018
Control	40	89	3	3	5	4658	38	47	6	9	3180
	50	92	2	3	3	4694	72	18	5	5	3614
	60	93	1	2	4	4577	68	20	6	6	3515
	90	94	0	2	4	4075	86	3	5	6	3759

effect of agar may preclude anodal migration. To achieve movement of such antigens counter to that of the corresponding antibody, or at least to obtain differential unidirectional migration, it may be necessary to employ agarose and other buffer conditions, such as that of high pH. These conditions were found to be necessary for the detection of IgE by CIE (Beng et al., 1973).

3. Effect of Electrical Current

In the previous experiment electrophoresis was carried out using a constant current of 10 mA/slide (approximately 200 V). The effects of lesser currents on the migration of antigen are shown in Tables III and IV. Unlike DNP–HSA, using 2.5 mA there was an insufficient anodal migration for differentiation between test reactions and controls to be made. The distribution of antigen achieved using 7.5 mA was similar to that using 10 mA; however, at 50 min and at 70 min approximately 20% of the counts had not passed through the early FTZ in the controls. A current of 5 mA resulted in a distribution of label intermediate to that produced by 7.5 mA and by 2.5 mA. A current of 10 mA/slide was used for subsequent experiments.

4. Effect of Duration of Electrophoresis

Some data relating to the effects of varying electrophoretic times have been shown in Tables II, III, and IV. In Fig. 6 is shown the percentage of radiolabel in the RZ for early and late anti-HSA sera at 60 min at different antibody levels. The proportion of radiolabel in the RZ decreased during the period of electrophoresis. Disappearance of label from the RZ was most marked with the early antiserum. Even the undiluted early anti-HSA showed 20% less counts after 90 min electrophoresis than at 30 min. With the 2^{-3} dilution no counts remained in the RZ after 90 min electrophoresis, although 42% of counts were present in that zone at 30 min.

As pointed out in the discussion of the DNP/anti-DNP system, the disappearance of radioactivity from the RZ with time was due either to migration of immune complexes into the FTZ and/or to dissociation of the complexes with anodal movement of the free HSA-I^{125}. The patterns of radioactivity observed in the four zones using the complete range of dilutions of the late anti-HSA serum favored the latter possibility. The rate of disappearance of antigen from the RZ after 30 min was more pronounced with early antibody than with hyperimmune sera. This effect could be best assessed by comparing those dilutions of the early and the late antiserum which bound equal amounts of HSA-I^{125}. The dilutions of the early and late anti-HSA which bound approximately 80% of the HSA-I^{125} were 2^{-2} and 2^{-8} respectively. Between 30 min and 90 min 66% of the HSA-I^{125} bound to the 2^{-2} dilution of early anti-HSA

Table IV. Distribution Patterns of HSA-I^{125} when Migrated against Dilutions of Anti-HSA under Electrical Currents of 5 mA and 2.5 mA per Slide

Anti-HSA dilution	EP time	5 mA					2.5 mA				
		AbWZ-2	AbWZ-1	IWZ	AgWZ	Total cpm	AbWZ-2	AbWZ-2	IWZ	AgWZ	Total cpm
2^0	40	3	0	84	13	4642	3	2	74	21	3589
	50	1	0	81	18	4067	3	1	78	17	3768
	60	1	0	89	10	4722	2	1	87	10	3644
	90	0	0	88	12	5235	2	2	85	11	3773
2^{-5}	40	3	8	85	4	5341	5	2	80	13	3959
	50	2	3	91	4	5012	1	2	83	14	3516
	60	2	3	88	7	5067	3	2	85	10	3805
	90	4	1	89	6	5165	3	2	88	7	4085
2^{-10}	40	5	75	14	6	4601	5	2	73	20	3955
	50	7	78	9	6	4614	2	55	39	4	3877
	60	28	59	7	6	4408	3	33	47	17	4010
	90	70	20	4	6	4378	2	33	57	8	3620
Control	40	3	70	20	7	4571	8	16	50	26	3674
	50	13	74	6	7	4472	4	24	55	17	3605
	60	43	48	4	5	4525	9	36	35	20	3243
	90	86	4	3	7	4765	3	77	11	9	3970

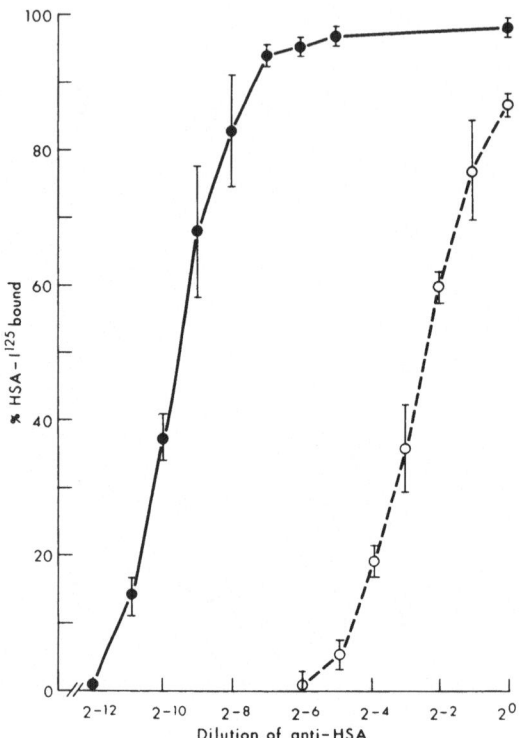

Figure 6. Binding curves of HSA-I^{125} with early and late anti-HSA sera after electrophoresis for 60 min. (Vertical bars represent ± 1 SD of quadruplicate determinations.)

migrated out of the reaction zone, compared to 15% with the higher dilution of the late antiserum. These findings suggested that the difference between the early and the late antisera could be explained on the basis of differing antibody avidity. Thus, in order to minimize dissociation of complexes in REC, it is important to use antibody of high avidity at a dilution which binds the majority of the radiolabeled antigen.

5. Effect of Position of the Wells

Using a current of 10 mA/slide for 60 min, the effects of varying the position of the well pairs were studied. The distribution of radiolabel was very similar in the reactions involving anti-HSA-undiluted and at 2^{-5} dilution. With the 2^{-10} dilution of anti-HSA there was a difference in label distribution between the four positions in that anodal migration of radiolabel was greatest where the well pair was nearest the cathode. A trend was observed in which anodal migration of radiolabel was least when the distance of the well pairs from the cathode was greatest. A standard position was chosen in which the cathodal margin of the antigen well was 3 cm from the cathodal end of the slide. With the well pairs in this position near the center of the slide, a satisfactory rate of HSA-I^{125} anodal movement was achieved. Within the 60 min of electrophoresis the labeled antigen did not migrate beyond the FTZ into the anodal wick and buffer.

6. Binding of HSA-I^{125} by Early and Late Antisera

Some of the characteristics of the binding curves with early and late antisera are depicted in Fig. 6. Undiluted early anti-HSA serum failed to bind all the HSA-I^{125} (86%). A dilution of approximately $2^{-2.5}$ bound 50% of the antigen. With the late anti-HSA, 50 % of the HSA-I^{125} was bound by a dilution of almost 2^{-10}. The slopes of the two binding curves were similar. The relation between the distribution of the radiolabel and the dilution of late anti-HSA is shown in more detail in Table V.

7. Reproducibility of Binding Curves

(a) Within experiments. In Fig. 6 the percentages of bound HSA-I^{125} represent the mean of quadruplicate determinations obtained by testing each

Table V. Distribution Patterns of HSA-I^{125}
when Migrated against Dilutions
of the Late Anti-HSA

Anti-HSA dilution	AbWZ-2	AbWZ-1	IWZ	AgWZ	Total cpm
2^0	0	0	91	9	4721
2^{-2}	0	0	93	7	4970
2^{-4}	0	0	94	6	5032
2^{-6}	0	0	96	4	4714
2^{-7}	0	0	94	6	4818
2^{-8}	11	8	82	6	4614
2^{-9}	60	31	5	4	4883
2^{-10}	83	11	2	4	4556
2^{-11}	91	2	2	5	4387
2^{-12}	92	1	2	5	4589
Control	93	1	2	4	5035

dilution on four different slides. The vertical bars represent ±1 standard deviation (SD) from the mean. Only for the dilutions corresponding to the steepest part of the binding curve were there substantial deviations in individual determinations. Slight differences in partitioning of zones between slides would be expected. The variation between quadruplicate determinations was less when all four replicates were tested on the one slide.

(b) Between experiments. Serial dilutions were made of each of two aliquots of the early and late antisera. Each dilution was further divided into quadruplicate samples. All samples were tested under code. The binding curves for each of the aliquots of the early and late antisera are shown in Fig. 7. The shapes of the curves were very similar, and the 50% binding dilutions were essentially the same for both of the pairs of antisera ($2^{-2.25}$ and $2^{-2.5}$ for the early antiserum and 2^{-9} and $2^{-9.5}$ for the late antiserum).

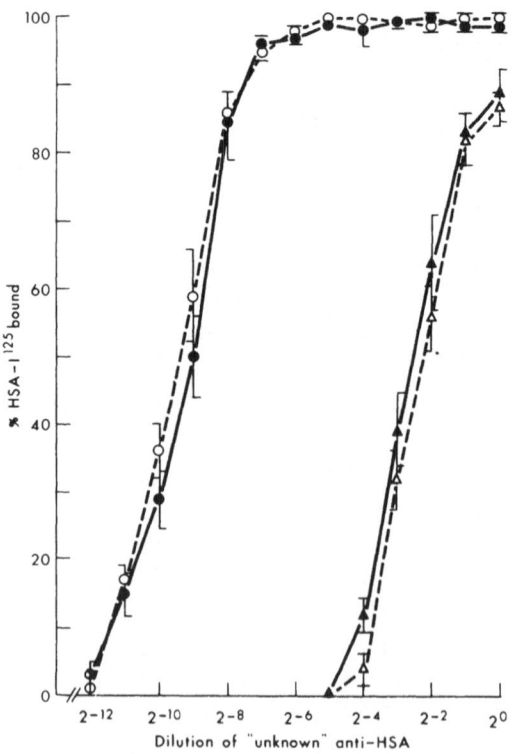

Figure 7. Binding curves of HSA-I^{125} with "unknown" anti-HSA sera.

8. Effect of Amount of HSA-I^{125} on the Binding Curves

Binding curves of serial dilutions of HSA-I^{125} with late anti-HSA showed that there was an inverse relation between the amount of HSA-I^{125} and the antibody dilution binding 50%. As in the DNP–anti-DNP system, the plot of dilutions of antiserum which bound 50% of antigen against HSA-I^{125} dilutions gave a straight line.

9. Immunological Specificity of HSA-I^{125}/anti-HSA Binding

(a) Direct REC of HSA-I^{125} and BSA-I^{131} with anti albumin sera. When HSA-I^{125} was tested against anti-HSA, anti-BSA and anti-EA, binding was greatest with the homologous antiserum. Anti-BSA cross-reacted with HSA-I^{125} but the 50% binding titer (2^{-6}) was lower than that of anti-HSA (2^{-11}). When BSA-I^{131} was used, binding with anti-BSA occurred to a lower titer (2^{-18}). Anti-HSA cross-reacted with BSA-I^{131} to a titer of 2^{10}. Anti-EA did not bind either labeled antigen.

(b) Inhibition of HSA-I^{125} binding with anti-HSA by unlabeled HSA. Known amounts of unlabeled HSA were pipetted into the antigen well. Anti-HSA at dilutions sufficient to bind 97%, 82%, 38%, and 27% of labeled antigen were delivered into the antibody well. Counterdirectional movement was initiated by a short period of electrophoresis (10–15 min). HSA-I^{125} was then pipetted into the antigen well and electrophoresis continued for a further 45 min. The rationale of the initial electrophoresis was to allow time for binding to occur between unlabeled HSA and anti-HSA thereby maximizing the probability of competitive inhibition of binding between the subsequently added HSA-I^{125} and reagent anti-HSA.

Two hundred fifty nanograms of HSA completely inhibited binding. Amounts between 25 ng and 0.025 ng (25 pg) showed partial inhibition. The amount of HSA producing 50% inhibition of binding of HSA-I^{125} for the four dilutions of anti-HSA (2^{-4}, 2^{-5}, 2^{-6}, and $2^{-6.5}$) was 50, 25, 10, and 1 ng respectively. Thus, the sensitivity for antigen detection was dependent upon anti-HSA dilution, being highest nearest to the limiting binding dilution. Amounts of HSA as low as 100 pg could be detected. No inhibition occurred with the same amounts of EA.

10. Quantitation of HSA

Application of REC to the quantitation of HSA follows from the methods employed to establish immunological specificity of the system. Several approaches have been investigated including (1) mixing the HSA solutions with dilutions of anti-HSA prior to delivery into the antibody well, (2) mixing "unknown" HSA solutions with HSA-I^{125} prior to addition to the antigen well, and (3) prefilling the antigen well with the unknown HSA solution. The third method has proved to be the most sensitive, enabling amounts of HSA as low as 100 pg to be detected.

IV. APPLICATIONS OF RADIOELECTROCOMPLEXING

A. Alpha-Fetoprotein

Several proteins have been described which are present in the sera of fetal and newborn animals. One of these is identified by mobility in the alpha region on electrophoresis and is termed alpha-fetoprotein (AFP). In 1963, Abelev and associates first showed that an AFP was synthesized by a transplantable hepato-cellular carcinoma (HCC), and was secreted into the serum of adult mice (Abelev et al., 1963). The presence of AFP in the serum of human patients with HCC was first demonstrated by Tatarinov (1964). In 1966 an international collabora-tive study was initiated involving patients from five African centers, Singapore, and Jamaica (O'Conor et al., 1970). The study established that the presence of AFP detectable by immunodiffusion (ID) in the serum of an adult with liver disease was virtually diagnostic of HCC. Approximately 3 of every 4 biopsy-proven HCC patients had AFP detectable by ID. ID is a relatively insensitive technique, having a lower limit of sensitivity of approximately 3 μg/ml (Purves et al., 1968), so the possibility existed that the 25% of "AFP-negative" HCC patients had levels which were elevated above normal although undetectable by ID.

In the last five years, more sensitive methods for AFP detection have been introduced. Using radiolabeled AFP and autoradiography of ID and electroim-munodiffusion patterns (Abelev et al., 1971; Sizaret et al., 1971), levels of 40-50 ng/ml were detectable. However, the procedures were time-consuming, at least 7 days being required for the autoradiographic component.

Double antibody precipitation radioimmunoassays for AFP quantitation have been described by at least six groups (Ruoslahti and Seppala, 1971; Purves and Purves, 1972; Waldmann and McIntire, 1972; Hirai et al., 1973; Ishii, 1973; Masseyeff et al., 1973). Sensitivity for AFP detection at levels of 0.25 ng/ml has been claimed by one group (Ruoslahti and Seppala, 1971), and of 0.5 ng/ml by another (Masseyeff et al., 1973). The other groups report confidence in detec-tion of AFP in the 5-20 ng/ml range.

There is a great need for standardization in this field, because even the values reported for normal subjects vary by a factor of 5-10 between 2.6 ± 1.6 ng/ml (Masseyeff et al., 1973), 11-13 ng/ml (Purves and Geddes, 1972), and 2-16 ng/ml (Ruoslahti and Seppala, 1971).

AFP testing has been most intensively applied to the study of patients with liver diseases. In many of the countries of Africa and Asia, where HCC occurs most commonly, the relatively sophisticated RIA techniques have not yet been established. In addition to the usual issues of complexity and cost, considerations of radioisotope handling hazards and the lack of radioactivity disposal facilities are also of great relevance to proposals for the introduction of RIA procedures into many countries. The possibility that REC might be suitable as a simple, sensitive, and relatively safe assay for the detection of elevated levels of AFP (>1–10 ng/ml) was investigated.

1. Binding Curves of AFP-I^{125} with Anti-AFP

It was first established that almost all AFP-I^{125} migrated beyond the antibody well under the conditions found to be optimal for HSA. When a current of 10 mA/slide was applied for 60 min, less than 5% of the radiolabel remained in the AgWZ and IWZ when AFP-I^{125} was run against a serum lacking antibody to AFP. Figure 8 shows the binding curve of AFP-I^{125} (1600 cpm/10

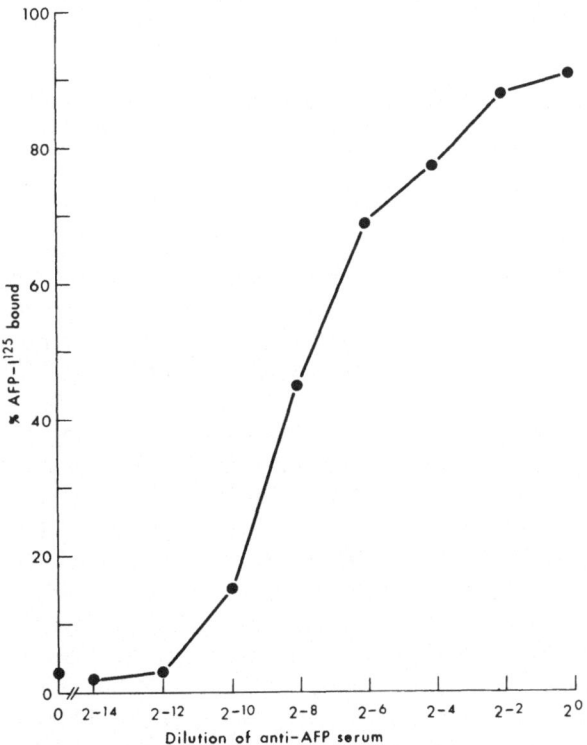

Figure 8. Binding curve of AFP-I^{125} (1600 cpm) with anti-AFP serum.

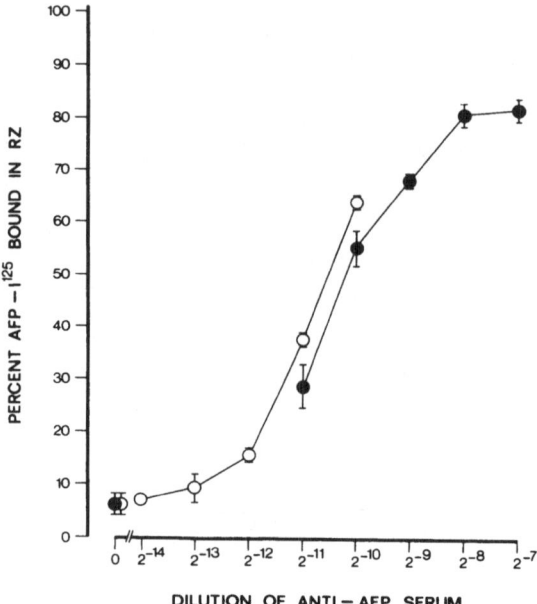

Figure 9. Reproducibility of binding of AFP-I^{125} with
anti-AFP serum using AFP-I^{125} at 400 cpm. (Vertical
bars represent ± 1 SD of duplicate determinations.)

μl) determined by single reactions with fourfold dilutions of anti-AFP serum. In
Fig. 9 the results of two experiments conducted on different days and with
separately prepared dilutions of anti-AFP is shown. The binding curves were
obtained using AFP-I^{125} (400 cpm/10 μl); the vertical bars represent ±1 SD of
duplicate determinations. The "50% binding" dilutions were 2^{-10} and $2^{-10.5}$ in
the two experiments.

Experiments were undertaken to determine the immunological specificity of
the radiolabeled AFP and of the anti-AFP. Table VI shows that the commercial
anti-AFP contained antibody to HSA in that it bound HSA-I^{125}. Binding could
be inhibited by prior electrophoresis of the anti-AFP against HSA. No retardation of the anodal migration of HSA-I^{125} was found when anti-AFP was diluted
to 1:2. Since, for the assay of AFP, anti-AFP was used at a dilution of 1:2048,
the contaminant antibodies would not have influenced reaction specificity.
AFP-I^{125} has been migrated against antiserum to normal serum components
which have an electrophoretic mobility similar to AFP, but no binding has been
observed. Thus, within the limit of sensitivity of REC, the radiolabeled AFP
preparations have been regarded as immunochemically pure.

Quantitation of AFP by Inhibition of AFP-I^{125}
Binding with Anti-AFP

The standard assay for detection of AFP involved the initial filling of the antigen well with dilutions of AFP standard, followed by a short period of electrophoresis (10–15 min) against dilutions of anti-AFP. AFP-I^{125} was then added to the antigen well and electrophoresis continued for 60 min. Figure 10 shows the inhibition curves obtained using anti-AFP at 2^{-7} to 2^{-12} dilutions. It can be seen that sensitivity for detection of low amounts of standard AFP was greater using the higher antibody dilutions. Figure 11 shows the percentage of radiolabel in the AgWZ and IWZ combined after varying periods of electrophoresis using antibody at a dilution binding 30–40% AFP-I^{125} and four amounts of standard AFP for inhibition. One hundred picograms (10 ng/ml) produced an inhibition curve clearly distinguishable from that of the negative control.

For routine screening purposes, 5-μl samples of undiluted serum were tested. Fresh sera invariably emptied from the antigen well within the 15-min initial electrophoresis. However, some sera, usually of small volume which had

Table VI. Detection of Antibody to HSA
in Anti-AFP Serum

EP time (min)	Antiserum	AbWZ-2	AbWZ-1	IWZ	AgWZ	Total cpm
30	anti-HSA2^{-5}	2	3	85	10	3594
	anti-HSA2^{-10}	10	31	48	11	3545
	anti-AFP2^{0}	20	66	3	11	3273
	NRS2^{-6}	58	32	4	6	3245
40	anti-HSA2^{-5}	3	2	84	11	3811
	anti-HSA2^{-10}	12	23	55	10	3369
	anti-AFP2^{0}	75	14	2	9	3449
	NRS2^{-6}	83	5	3	9	3652
50	anti-HSA2^{-5}	3	1	90	6	3604
	anti-HSA2^{-10}	9	23	59	9	3436
	anti-AFP2^{0}	85	9	1	5	3404
	NRS2^{-6}	85	2	3	10	3436
60	anti-HSA2^{-5}	2	1	85	12	3334
	anti-HSA2^{-10}	7	25	58	10	3367
	anti-AFP2^{0}	86	6	1	7	3310
	NRS2^{-6}	88	2	2	8	3502

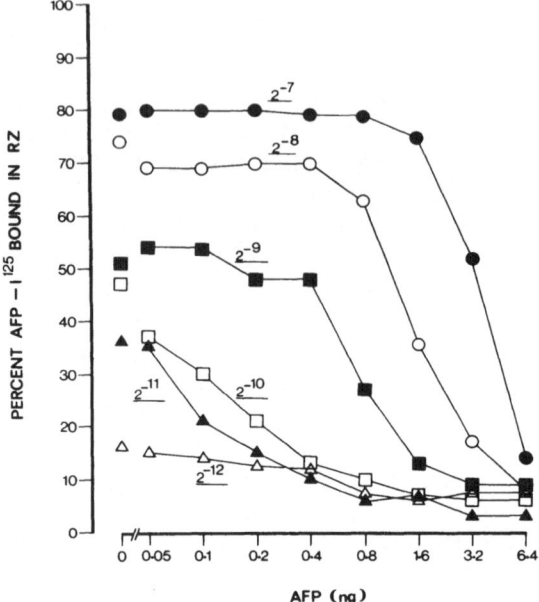

Figure 10. Inhibition of the binding of AFP-I[125] with dilutions of anti-AFP by varying the amounts of an AFP standard solution.

been held for long periods at 4°C, remained in the well. They had to be retested at a dilution of 1:2 or 1:4. Sera producing complete inhibition of AFP-I[125] binding were retested at dilutions of 1:10 and 1:50. This enabled AFP in amounts between 5–10 ng/ml and 16,000 ng/ml to be quantified.

3. Application to Patient Investigation and Population Screening

REC has been applied to the investigation of patients in several disease categories. Evidence has been obtained in support of the findings of Waldmann and McIntire (1972) that children with ataxia–telangiectasia* appear to be unique among those with congenital immune deficiency diseases in that they have raised levels of AFP (Simons and Hosking, 1973). Sera from seven Aus-

*Ataxia–telangiectasia is a rare disorder characterized by cerebellar ataxia, oculocutaneous telangiectasia, recurrent sinopulmonary infections, and a tendency to the development of lymphoid malignancy. An immune deficiency, regularly involving thymic-dependent cell-mediated immunity and frequently also affecting the humoral immune system, underlies the recurrent infections. A range of other abnormalities, including gonadal and hepatic dysfunction, has also been described.

tralian Caucasian patients with ataxia–telangiectasia from three families were tested in Singapore, together with sera from two parents, two normal siblings in one of the families, and twelve other sera, mainly from children with immune deficiency diseases. All seven of the affected children had elevated AFP levels between 40–320 ng/ml. Both parents and both of the normal siblings had levels of <10 ng/ml, a finding which is also in accord with that of Waldmann and McIntire.

In a recent study of 139 Singapore Chinese patients with HCC, AFP was detected at levels of >10 ng/ml in the sera of 128 (92.1%) (Simons *et al.*, 1973). This proportion is similar to that of 93% (99/107) reported by Nishi and Hirai (1973) and of 89% (49/56) reported by Ishii (1973) using double antibody RIA procedures. At the University of Malaya, Kuala Lumpur, Drs. P. Chan and T. K. Ti have adopted REC for studies of AFP and found it to be a simple procedure for quantitation of levels ≥10 ng/ml (Chan and Ti, 1973). They have also found that approximately 90% of HCC patients have detectable levels of AFP.

With the detection of AFP in normal subjects, together with the demonstration of increased levels in patients with diseases other than HCC (hepatitis;

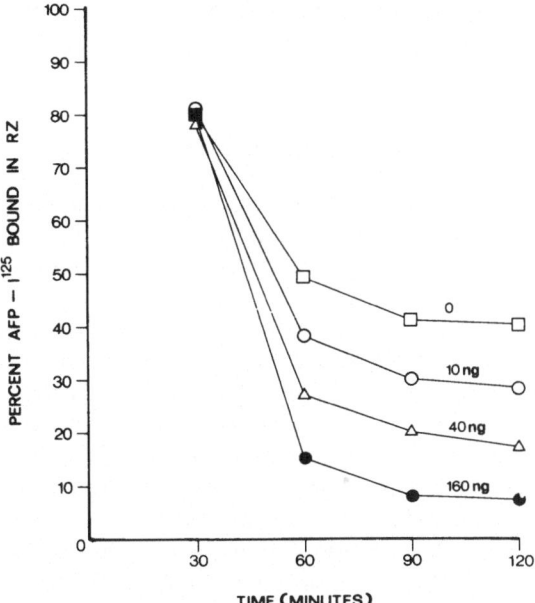

Figure 11. Inhibition of the binding of AFP-I^{125} with a 50% binding dilution of anti-AFP by varying the amounts of AFP/ml of standard solution. Inhibition by 10 ng/ml (0.1 ng/10 μl sample) was detectable after electrophoresis for 60 min.

cirrhosis; gastric, colon and rectal carcinomata), it is apparent that the advantage of increased sensitivity provided by RIA is offset by the loss of specificity for disease diagnosis. ID is therefore still useful as a simple method for routine diagnosis of HCC. RIA is likely to find increasing application to questions such as whether elevated AFP levels, or changes in levels with time, are manifestations of early malignancy and whether decreased levels in HCC patients undergoing therapy have any prognostic significance. Present indications are that RIA will be useful in surveillance of populations for early HCC detection and in monitoring the effects of chemotherapy and surgery in patients with HCC.

Patients with many types of liver diseases, including HCC, have a high frequency of hepatitis B antigenemia (WHO, 1973a). There is some evidence that elevated AFP levels may be associated with the presence of HBAg, particularly in HCC patients. Routine testing of sera from HCC patients for AFP. HBAg, and HBAb is becoming standard practice in many laboratories, and extension to the investigation of patients with acute and chronic liver diseases can be expected. In the next section the application of REC to the detection of HBAb and HBAg will be documented. The availability of an RIA procedure in which the three serum factors can be investigated by testing three 10-μl serum aliquots in adjacent wells of a single slide promises to greatly simplify laboratory testing and thereby to enable a larger number of patients to be more comprehensively investigated.

B. Hepatitis B Antibody

In 1963 Blumberg observed that when the serum of an Australian aborigine was diffused against serum from a multiply transfused hemophiliac patient a band of precipitation developed (Blumberg, 1964). The hemophiliac's serum was shown to contain antibody which precipitated an antigenic substance present in the serum of the aborigine. The name Australia antigen (Au) was given to this antigenic substance. Recently, attempts have been made to standardize the nomenclature of the terms and symbols which have been used to refer to serum factors similar if not identical to Au. Also, there is now very compelling evidence of an association between Au and hepatitis of type B. It has therefore been recommended that the serum antigen be redesignated as HBAg (WHO, 1973a).

Many techniques have been described for the detection and measurement of HBAg and of HBAb. Characteristics of some of these techniques have been tabulated in a recent WHO Technical Report of Viral Hepatitis (Table VII). The footnote to the table states that radioimmunoassay methods are the most sensitive for detecting HBAb, but they are complex to perform and relatively slow. In the last five years there have been numerous reports of radioimmunoassay procedures applied to the HBAg/HBAb system (Walsh et al., 1970; Purcell,

1970; Coller *et al.*, 1971; Lander *et al.*, 1971; Aach *et al.*, 1971; Hollinger *et al.*, 1971; Ginsberg *et al.*, 1972; Tilden and DeLand, 1972; Ling and Overby, 1972). In this section the application of REC to the detection of HBAb is considered.

1. Electrophoretic Migration of HBAg-I^{125}

The migration pattern of HBAg-I^{125} was found to be similar to that of HSA and AFP, but a higher proportion of radiolabel failed to enter the AbWZ-2 despite the application of an electrical current of 10 mA per slide. Table VIII illustrates the distribution pattern of radiolabel when HBAg-I^{125} was migrated against dilutions of reagent HBAb for 90 min and 120 min. In the actual experiment the agar was subdivided into ten zones, but for simplicity the results are presented as the percentage distribution of radiolabel in four zones. The slower migration velocity of HBAg-I^{125} relative to HSA and AFP probably reflects the pleomorphic, particulate nature of the antigenic substance. It has been noticed that the amount of unbound radiolabel which fails to exit from the "bound" zones varies according to the batch and increases with age of the HBAg-I^{125} preparation. To some extent the poorly migrating components can be diminished by centrifugation (15,000–20,000 rpm/30 min) and by utilizing, as HBAg-I^{125}, only those fractions of the total labeled preparation which migrated rapidly on starch block electrophoresis.

2. Evidence for HBAb in Sera of the Reference Hepatitis B Antigen Panel No. 2

In preliminary screening, 3 sera of the Reference Panel (Nos. 221, 231, and 224) were shown by counterimmunoelectrophoresis (CIE) to contain HBAb. These 3 and 8 other sera showed a pattern of reactivity on direct REC which suggested the presence of HBAb. The patterns of radiolabel percentage distribution produced by the 11 sera are shown in Table IX. The 10 sera which are grouped together (Nos. 245 through 221) were stated to contain HBAb on the basis of testing by passive hemagglutination (PHA). The mean percentage radiolabel distribution of 12 other sera (Nos. 203, 211, 212, 215, 216, 227, 230, 240, 241, 242, and 247) stated to lack HBAb detectable by PHA, and confirmed by REC, was taken as the negative control. In the first report of this data (Simons, 1973a) the approach adopted for the analysis of radiolabel distribution patterns was based on an index which expressed the degree of anodal migration of HBAg-I^{125}. The formula used for calculation is shown as footnote *b* of Table IX. By this approach all 10 sera positive for HBAb by PHA had an index less than 1 SD below the mean of the HBAb-negative sera. In retrospect it would have been more appropriate to use the reciprocal of this index so that high

Table VII. Techniques for Measuring Hepatitis B Antigen and Antibody (WHO, 1973a)

Technique	Relative sensitivity for detecting[a]		Ease of performance[b]	Relative cost	Time required for completion (hours)
	HBAg	HBAb			
Immunodiffusion[c]	1–5	1–10	simple	inexpensive	24–72
Counterimmunoelectrophoresis[d]	5–15	5–10	simple	moderate	2
Complement fixation[e]	15–20	5–10	moderate	inexpensive	2–24
Immune adherence[f]	20–2000	50–150	moderate	inexpensive	2
Latex particle agglutination[g] (antibody-coated)	15–100	–	simple	inexpensive	0.1–0.2
Passive hemagglutination and inhibition[h]	15–20	10,000	moderate	expensive	2
Radioimmunoassay[j]	2,000–10,000	10,000–1,000,000	complex	expensive	24–120
Immune electron microscopy[k]	1,000–2,000	–	complex	expensive	2–4

[a] The approximate reciprocal titer of an antigen or antibody was arbitrarily assigned a titer of 1 when tested by the two-dimensional micro-Ouchterlony immunodiffusion technique. Range of sensitivity values was obtained by various modifications of this basic technique.

[b] This includes the preparation of reagents.

c This is highly specific. Various modifications used to improve sensitivity were the use of templates, low concentration of agarose, radial diffusion, rheophoresis, and staining of precipitin lines.

d This is very useful for large-scale screening of sera, but sensitivity is markedly influenced by the quality of reagents and the skill of the technician in detecting faint precipitin lines.

e The usefulness of this method is limited by anticomplementary activity in a proportion of sera, but it is useful for quantifying antigen and antibody. Prozones occur with high-titer sera and can result in false negative results unless the sera are tested at several dilutions.

f Large prozones with high-titer antigen-positive sera can result in false negative results if the serum is not tested at several dilutions. However, this technique combines sensitivity with speed for detecting antigen.

g This is not fully evaluated, but simplicity and speed make it potentially useful. The relatively high frequency of nonspecific agglutination makes it necessary to include appropriate controls.

h This technique is comparable to complement fixation and counterimmunoelectrophoresis for detecting antigen. It is one of the most sensitive and useful techniques for detecting and quantifying antibody. The high frequency of nonspecific agglutination makes it necessary to include appropriate controls.

j Several types of radioimmunoassay method are in use, including double antibody and solid phase. This is one of the most expensive and elaborate of techniques, but the most sensitive for detecting antigen and antibody.

k This is not suitable for large-scale testing and requires special skills and expensive equipment, but this technique is very valuable for identifying morphological types of antigen and antibody specific to them.

TABLE VIII.   Distrubution Patterns of HBAg-I^{125}
when Migrated against Dilutions of HBAB
for 90 and 120 Minutes

EP time (min)	HBAb dilution	AbWZ-2	AbWZ-1	IWZ	AgWZ	Total cpm
90	2^0	3	5	19	73	754
	2^{-2}	9	12	46	33	743
	2^{-4}	11	23	52	14	711
	2^{-6}	26	43	24	7	699
	2^{-8}	43	37	14	6	689
	2^{-10}	48	34	11	7	745
	Control	51	32	10	7	765
120	2^0	3	4	17	76	821
	2^{-2}	11	15	55	19	754
	2^{-4}	14	26	50	10	865
	2^{-6}	44	43	9	4	868
	2^{-8}	65	25	6	4	817
	2^{-10}	70	21	6	3	843
	Control	73	17	5	5	863

values would correspond directly to levels of HBAb activity. A second approach is to directly compare corresponding zones and to express any difference in radiolabel distribution pattern between test and control reactions as the sum of the squares of differences by the formula given in footnote c of Table IX. Using both approaches for REC index determination, there was a clear trend in the values obtained for the 10 HBAb-positive sera with the 3 sera which were positive by CIE showing the highest HBAb activity by REC. Sera numbers 245, 246, and 229 had the lowest levels of HBAb by REC. In Table IX are shown results obtained by Dr. R. H. Purcell using radioimmunoprecipitation (RIP) (Purcell, 1972). The three sera (Nos. 245, 246, and 229) which had the lowest REC indices of the 10 HBAb-positive sera also produced the lowest binding of HBAg-I^{125} by RIP. There is a suggestion from the REC and RIP data that the testing of an undiluted sample by REC may provide semiquantitative information, in addition to enabling the presence or absence of HBAb to be determined. One additional serum (No. 225) consistently showed an HBAg-I^{125} binding pattern on REC indicative of the presence of HBAb, although HBAb was stated to be undetectable by PHA. This serum showed a mean binding of 18% by RIP and was interpreted as a doubtful positive.

Table IX. Distribution Patterns of HBAg-I^{125} when Migrated against Sera of the Reference Hepatitis B Antigen Panel No. 2

Panel serum No.	Radioelectrocomplexing						Radioimmunoprecipitation[d]	
	AbWZ	IWZ	AgWZ	Index[b]	Index[c]	Interpretation	% Binding[e]	Interpretation
HBAb negative (12 sera)	56	27	17[a]	0.126 ± 0.045(1 SD)	1	–	<10	–
225	37	44	19	0.044	654	+	18	±
245	49	30	21	0.077	74	+	41	+
246	49	28	23	0.076	86	+	62	+
229	47	35	18	0.074	146	+	66	+
248	46	31	23	0.064	152	+	78	+
257	45	29	26	0.059	206	+	85	+
258	45	29	26	0.059	206	+	77	+
259	39	26	35	0.042	614	+	80	+
224	27	46	27	0.021	1302	+	85	+
231	16	25	59	0.010	3368	+	81	+
221	17	18	65	0.014	3754	+	76	+

[a] Mean percent distribution of 12 sera.

[b] Index = X/% AgWZ, where X = % AbWZ/% IWZ.

[c] Index = $\Sigma(X-\bar{X})^2$, where X is the percent in each zone in the control reaction, and $\bar{X}$ is the percent in the corresponding zone in the test reaction.

[d] Performed by Dr. R. H. Purcell, NIAID, NIH, Bethesda, Maryland.

[e] Mean of triplicate determinations.

3. Comparison of the Sensitivity of REC and PHA for
HBAb Detection

Results obtained using the Reference Panel No. 2 indicated that REC had a sensitivity for HBAb detection which was at least comparable to that of PHA and RIP. Recent experiments have raised the possibility that REC may even be more sensitive than PHA. A panel of 15 sera was prepared for testing at a WHO-assisted Workshop on Hepatitis B Antigen held in Tokyo between October 29 and November 8, 1973. The HBAb content of the panel sera was designated by Dr. M. Mayumi, Department of Immunology, Jichi Medical School, Tochigi, Japan, on the basis of PHA testing, and in all samples the designation was confirmed by the results obtained by the nine Workshop participants (WHO, 1973b). One of the sera (J34) showed a reaction at dilutions of 1:2 and 1:4, but confirmatory testing for immunological specificity by the addition of excess HBAg did not result in the fourfold dilution difference conventionally adopted as a criterion of positivity. The results obtained by testing this serum and three others of the panel by REC are summarized in Table X. It is now realized that, by the gel-cutting approach to zone separation, the greatest sensitivity for detection of very low levels of antibody and antigen is achieved by subdivision of the AbWZ 2 mm anodal to the antibody well (Fig. 1). It is also now realized that to express the REC radiolabel patterns by an index based on summation of the squares of the differences between corresponding zones in the test and control reactions is the most suitable of the presently recognized approaches.

From Table X it can be seen that radiolabel distribution was similar in the triplicate test of each of the five sera. Two sera of the panel (J33 and J24), which had HBAb titers of 1:16 to 1:64 by PHA, had relatively high REC index values. The pattern of J34 was clearly different from that of the HBAb-negative control serum. J35, which was completely unreactive by PHA, gave a REC index value which was only minimally different from that of the negative control.

4. Effect of Inhibition by "Purified" HBAg on the Binding of
HBAg-I^{125} with Sera Suspected to Contain HBAb

The results of experiments such as that shown in Table X suggested that sera producing positive reactions on PHA but not fulfilling the criterion for HBAb positivity may, in fact, contain HBAb. This question was investigated by testing sera from a group of East Africans which were also tested by PHA at the WHO-assisted Workshop on Hepatitis B Antigen. In Table XI is shown the results obtained by testing four sera which produced minimum reactions when tested by PHA.

Each serum was tested in quadruplicate. In two of the reactions "purified" HBAg was reacted against the test samples by a brief period of electrophoresis.

Table X. Distribution Patterns of HBAg-I^{125}
when Migrated against Sera Previously Tested
for HBAb by PHA

Panel No.		AbWZ-2	AbWZ-1	(IWZ + AgWZ)	Total cpm	REC index	PHA
HBAb negative							
Control		33	55	11	365		
		35	54	11	343		
		34	56	11	338		
	average	34	55	11		1 (−)	(−)
J35		25	61	14	358		
		27	58	10	352		
		36	52	12	380		
	average	30	57	13		24 (−)	(−)
J34		30	47	23	365		
		36	50	14	348		
		36	47	17	390		
	average	34	48	18		98 (+)	(−)
J33		24	44	32	427		
		22	49	29	479		
		21	42	37	507		
	average	22	45	33		728 (+)	32 (+)
J24		21	32	47	411		
		20	33	47	352		
		16	31	53	413		
	average	19	32	49		2198 (+)	32 (+)

Veronal buffer was substituted for HBAg in the remaining two of the four reactions. After electrophoresis for 15 min, HBAg-I^{125} was added to all antigen wells and electrophoresis continued for two hours. This standard procedure for inhibition of REC has been described in the sections on HSA and AFP.

HBAg "inhibition" of the HBAb-negative control serum had very little effect on the pattern of radiolabel distribution. The REC index was calculated on the basis of the difference between the mean percentage of the reactions inhibited by HBAg, and uninhibited by HBAg for each of the three zones. For

Table XI. Effect of Inhibition by "Purified" HBAg on the Binding of HBAg-I^{125} with Sera Suspected to Contain HBAb

Serum	AbWZ-2	AbWZ-1	(IWZ + AgWZ)	Total cpm	REC index	PHA
HBAb negative control	24	48	28	696		
	25	46	29	682	8 (−)	(−)
HBAg inhibited	21	50	29	653		
	24	48	28	644		
Afr. 512						
	13	53	35	668		
	14	52	35	708	182 (+)	4/0 (+)
HBAg inhibited	24	43	34	724		
	23	44	34	704		
Afr. 538						
	10	57	33	671		
	13	57	30	623	72 (+)	8/2 (+)
HBAg inhibited	18	51	31	698		
	18	50	32	662		
Afr. 500						
	19	60	21	675		
	24	57	19	666	114 (+)	4/2 (−)
HBAg inhibited	23	46	31	682		
	22	53	25	683		
Afr. 511						
	16	52	32	642		
	17	51	32	615	56 (+)	4/4 (−)
HBAg inhibited	21	47	31	642		
	20	44	36	682		

the control serum the REC index was 8. The REC index values of sera Afr. 511 and Afr. 538, which were sevenfold and ninefold higher than that of the control, respectively, were interpreted as reflecting the presence of HBAb. These and other similar results support the suspicion that HBAb is present in at least some sera which produce equivocal reactions on testing by PHA. The results also suggest that the sensitivity of REC is sufficient for the detection of HBAb in amounts below the lower limit of detectability by PHA.

C. Hepatitis B Antigen

1. Detection of HBAg by Inhibition of the Binding of HBAg-I^{125} with HBAb

Detection of HBAg was attempted by the same approach as described in the previous section for demonstrating immunological specificity of the binding of HBAg-I^{125} with certain sera. Test sera were delivered into the antigen well, and a period of electrophoresis against reagent HBAb was initiated. After 15–20 min, HBAg-I^{125} was added to the antigen well and electrophoresis continued for 2 hours. Table XII shows the results obtained when a serum known to contain HBAg in high titer by CIE and a "purified" preparation of HBAg were assayed by the inhibition method. A dilution of HBAb was used which bound approximately 50% of the HBAg-I^{125}. It has been frequently observed that the proportion of radiolabel in the bound zones is slightly higher when HBAg-negative sera are tested undiluted as compared to when dilutions in a buffer of low protein content are used. Thus the reactivity of control and test sera should be compared at the same dilution. In this experiment the HBAg positive serum inhibited binding of HBAg-I^{125} with HBAb to a dilution greater than 2^{-12} Inhibition by the "purified" HBAg preparation occurred to a 2^{-8} dilution.

Table XII. Detection of HBAg by Inhibition of the Binding of HBAg-I^{125} with HBAb

Test sample	AbWZ-2	AbWZ-1	(IWZ + AgWZ)	Total cpm
HBAg negative control				
2^0	21	13	66	1615
2^{-2}	27	20	53	1577
2^{-4}	28	18	54	1552
HBAg positive serum				
2^0	67	19	14	1642
2^{-4}	62	17	21	1728
2^{-8}	63	21	16	1596
2^{-12}	45	31	24	1631
2^{-16}	30	17	53	1619
"Purified" HBAg				
2^0	59	21	20	1590
2^{-4}	49	19	32	1669
2^{-8}	31	26	43	1598
2^{-12}	25	15	60	1652

Evidence has been presented elsewhere (Simons, 1973b) that sera of the Reference Panel No. 2, which were positive for HBAg only by RIA, as well as those with levels of HBAg detectable by CIE and complement fixation, produced a pattern of radiolabel distribution distinguishable from those of sera stated to lack HBAg.

When the assay was applied to 102 sera from asymptomatic blood donors who were positive for HBAg by CIE, an inhibition pattern similar to that produced by "purified" HBAg was observed in 15. In the remaining 87, the proportion of radiolabel in the AgWZ was higher than in the "control" reactions of HBAg-negative sera. The difference persisted for varying electrophoretic times up to and including 2 hours.

2. Evidence for the Presence of HBAb in the Sera of HBAg-Positive Asymptomatic Blood Donors

Several types of experiments were undertaken to investigate the nature of the HBAg-binding serum factor(s). Following incubation of one of the sera with HBAg-I^{125} for 30 min at room temperature (22°C), the mixture was transferred to the antigen well and electrophoresis commenced immediately. At intervals of 5 min the agar on both sides of the antigen well was cut into sections of approximately 1 mm and counted. There was an initial rapid migration of radiolabel in a cathodal direction, followed by an apparent reversal of the direction of movement. This pattern was seen in each of 5 sera tested. The reagent HBAb serum produced the same initial cathodal migration of radiolabel but, in contrast to the HBAg-containing sera, a high proportion of the radiolabel persisted in the agar cathodal to the antigen well, even after electrophoresis for 2 hours. No cathodal migration occurred when HBAg-I^{125} was diluted in veronal buffer.

Inhibition of HBAg-I^{125} binding with HBAb can also be achieved by prefilling the antibody well rather than the antigen well. Figure 12 shows the percentage of radiolabel in the AgWZ and IWZ when HBAg-I^{125} was electrophoresed against dilutions of one of the five sera which showed the cathodal migration phenomenon, and against dilutions of the same "purified" HBAg which was tested by prefilling the antigen well (Table XII). The "purified" HBAg produced a dilution-dependent curve of HBAg-I^{125} binding inhibition to a titer similar to that obtained in the experiment summarized in Table XII. In marked contrast, the HBAg-positive serum required dilution to 2^{-5} (1:32) before maximum inhibition of binding occurred. The question arose as to whether the binding of HBAg-I^{125} with lower dilutions of this serum was immunologically specific. On theoretical grounds it can be assumed that the serum component binding with HBAg-I^{125} must migrate cathodally under the electrophoretic conditions employed and that, if the radiolabeled preparation contained proteins

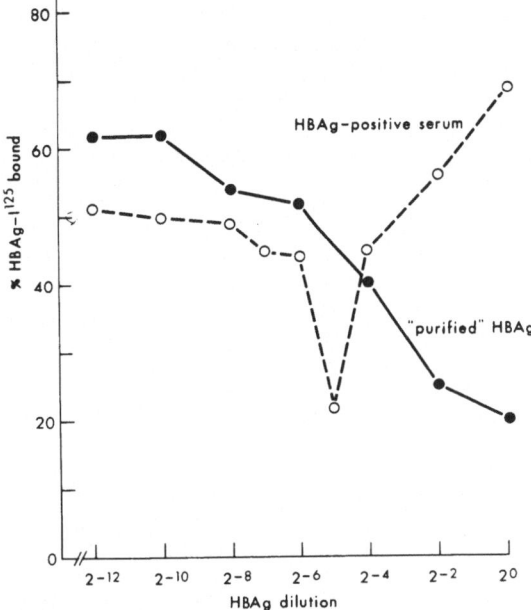

Figure 12. Inhibition of the binding of HBAg-I^{125} with HBAb by an HBAg-positive serum and by a "purified" HBAg solution.

other than HBAg in which substitution of I^{125} had also occurred, those molecules must have anodal migratory characteristics. These considerations would appear to exclude the possibility that the observations might be due to globulin–antiglobulin reactions since γ-globulins tend to migrate in the same direction on electrophoresis. It had been established that the HBAg solution which was radioiodinated contained no serum contaminants detectable by ID or by immunoelectrophoresis (Purcell, 1972). Furthermore, HBAg-I^{125} bound with sera known to contain HBAb (Table IX). It was therefore strongly suspected that the cathodally migrating component(s) of those HBAg-positive sera which bound HBAg-I^{125} was HBAb.

To test this hypothesis, 39 of the HBAg-containing sera were pipetted into the antibody well and electrophoresed against HBAg-I^{125}. In Table XIII the radiolabel distribution patterns of 14 sera tested on one slide of lantern-plate size are shown. The total radioactivity detected in the 4 zones of each reaction was comparable. In the first seven reactions a typical dilution-dependent response with the reagent HBAb serum was obtained. Dilutions were made in a serum lacking HBAb detectable by PHA or by REC. The last six reactions show the retardation of anodal migration of HBAg-I^{125} produced by 6 of

Table XIII. Evidence for the Presence of HBAb
in HBAg-Positive Sera from Asymptomatic Blood Donors:
Retardation of the Anodal Migration of HBAg-I^{125}

Serum		AbWZ-2	AbWZ-1	IWZ	AgWZ	Total cpm
Reagent HBAb	2^0	3	6	22	69	847
	2^{-2}	6	10	69	15	887
	2^{-4}	14	38	38	10	871
	2^{-6}	30	44	21	5	820
	2^{-8}	35	51	8	6	846
	2^{-10}	49	33	10	7	848
	2^{-12}	61	27	7	5	802
HBAb negative control		53	33	8	6	785
HBAg positive sera						
CIE/1		47	31	12	10	846
CIE/3		59	25	10	6	818
CIE/4		22	32	40	6	837
CIE/5		39	41	14	6	848
CIE/6		30	45	18	7	855
CIE/7		33	46	13	8	844

the first 7 HBAg-positive sera tested. Serum CIE/4 had a relatively high content of HBAg-I^{125} binding activity (REC Index of 1986). Sera numbers CIE/1, 3, 5, 6, and 7 had REC index values of 72, 104, 296, 774, and 598 respectively. The binding patterns of CIE/1, 5, 6, and 7 were significantly altered* by inhibition with purified HBAg as a confirmatory test for immunological specificity. Of 39 sera so far tested, 29 showed binding activity greater than that of the HBAb-negative control, and in 26 confirmation of the presence of HBAb by HBAg inhibition was obtained.

Five sera known to contain HBAg, and suspected to contain HBAb, have been tested for HBAg-I^{125} binding activity after absorption with various anti-immunoglobulin antisera. Table XIV shows the results of one experiment. It can be seen that absorption with anti-Ig serum resulted in a substantial reduction in binding activity. A similar although lesser effect resulted from absorption with anti-ϵ chain antiserum. Anti-μ chain antiserum had some effect, but anti-γ chain and anti-α chain did not appear to influence HBAg-I^{125} binding activity. All 5 sera were similarly affected by absorption with anti-Ig antiserum. In 2 of the 5

*A change in radiolabel distribution pattern by HBAg inhibition has been arbitrarily defined as significant if the REC index for inhibition of the test serum is ≥ 5 times that of the control HBAb-negative serum.

sera, binding activity was also substantially decreased following absorption with anti-ϵ chain antiserum. The remaining 3 of the 5 were affected by anti-γ chain antiserum but virtually uninfluenced by absorption with anti-ϵ chain absorption. Only a small number of sera have been tested. Nonetheless, absorption with anti-Ig antiserum had a consistent effect, and confidence in the interpretation of anti-heavy-chain absorption effects is strengthened by the finding that the effects were not observed with all 5 antisera in each test serum.

Based on the findings of experiments such as those reported in this section, it was concluded that a majority of HBAg-positive sera contain immunoglobulin with a specificity for binding HBAg-I^{125} . It must be clearly understood that the sera which have been studied are from asymptomatic blood donors living in a tropical country where the HB agent is endemic. All comments refer only to this category of subject. No information is presently available on patients with biochemically or clinically detectable hepatic dysfunction.

3. Approaches to the Simultaneous Detection of HBAg, HBAb, and HBAg/HBAb Complexes

It is likely that a proportion of HBAg and the putative HBAb exists as immune complexes. In relative antigen excess such complexes are most likely to be soluble. The postulate that HB antigenemia is often associated with specific immune complexemia has obvious relevance to the mechanism of induction and persistence of the antigenemic state. If immunological unresponsiveness is involved, the findings suggest that the immune defect is only partial. Other aspects of immune competence, particularly those mediated by lymphoid cells, remain

Table XIV. Absorption of a Serum Known to Contain HBAg, and Suspected to Contain HBAb, by Anti-immunoglobulin Sera; Effect on the Migration Pattern of HBAg-I^{125} in Direct REC

Reagent used for absorption	AbWZ	IWZ	AgWZ	REC index[a]
Nil	62	23	15	1
Anti-Ig	84	9	7	744
Anti-ϵ chain	79	12	9	446
Anti-μ chain	68	15	17	104
Anti-γ chain	66	23	11	32
Anti-α chain	62	23	15	0

[a] REC index = $\Sigma(X-\bar{X})^2$, where X is the percentage in each zone in the control reaction, and $\bar{X}$ is the percentage in the corresponding zone in the test reaction.

to be investigated. The contribution of the immune complexes to the total pathogenesis of HB agent infection also remains to be elucidated.

From the viewpoint of laboratory practice, an important objective is the development of a single approach to the detection of HBAg, HBAb, and specific immune complexes. One approach is to test sera for HBAb by direct REC, and for HBAg by inhibition of HBAg-I^{125} binding, in adjacent reactions using the two-well REC system. A three-well system, in which the third well, also of 3 mm diameter, is punched 4 mm to the cathodal side of the antigen well, is presently under investigation. When the test serum is introduced into the central well and subjected to electrophoresis, HBAg and HBAb move in opposite directions as in the CIE three-well method (Alter *et al.*, 1971). After a short period of electrophoresis a suitable dilution of reagent HBAb is dispensed into the antibody well and HBAg-I^{125} added to both the central and cathodal-end wells. Electrophoresis is then continued for 90–120 min. When HBAb is present, anodal migration of the cathodal-well HBAg-I^{125} is retarded between the cathodal-end well and the central well. When HBAg is present, inhibition of binding between central-well HBAg-I^{125} and reagent HBAb results in a higher proportion of radiolabel entering the AbWZ. When both HBAg and HBAb are present, radiolabel is increased in both the cathodal-end IWZ and the AbWZ. Problems of interpretation are still being encountered when the test serum contains neither HBAb nor HBAg because of the variable migration of cathodal-well HBAg-I^{125} into the anodal-end IWZ, and because of the migration of immune complexes of reagent HBAb and central-well HBAg-I^{125} cathodally into the cathodal-end IWZ. Reagent HBAb serum has been fractionated on starch block electrophoresis, and cathodally migrating fractions containing HBAb have been radioiodinated. Under investigation is the use of a three-well system for detection of both HBAg and HBAb by primary binding with the corresponding radiolabeled reagents.

V. SUMMARY AND CONCLUSIONS

In CIE, visible immune precipitation occurs in the zone between the wells. Thus in early REC studies the zone of bound Ag-I^{125} was taken as the interwell zone and the agar cathodal to it (IWZ and AgWZ, Fig. 1). Provided that care was taken to cut the agar in a constant position, binding curves of satisfactory reproducibility were obtained. This approach was adequate in those experiments in which "50% binding" was used as the end point. Where the objective was the detection of very small amounts of antibody or antigen, it became apparent that some sensitivity was lost when the agar was sectioned at the cathodal margin of the antibody well (junction of IWZ and AbWZ-1, Fig. 1), because bound Ag-I^{125} present around and anodal to the antibody well was not included in the zones of reaction. Detection sensitivity could be increased by extending the "bound zone" to include the AgWZ, IWZ, and AbWZ-1. The remainder of the gel was taken as the "free" or follow-through zone.

Division of the agar into "bound" and "free" zones has the advantages of simplicity and of minimizing the variation associated with multiple-zone cutting. The proportion of unbound Ag-I^{125} which does not migrate beyond the "bound" zone can easily be determined by the application of a formula (Section IIC). Semiquantitative information can be achieved by analysis of the distribution of Ag-I^{125} within the bound zone. This is a distinguishing feature of RIA electrophoretic methods. Theoretically, precise analysis of Ag-I^{125} distribution would be achieved by dividing the agar into extremely narrow zones. This ideal situation can be approached by scanning the gel for γ-ray emission, although problems of zone resolution and emission detection efficiency are encountered. When agar zones of approximately 1 mm width were examined, it was found that high-, medium-, and low-titer Ab solutions produced a localization of radiolabeled homologous antigen in the AgWZ, IWZ, and AbWZ-1, respectively. Correspondingly, the amount of Ag was reflected in the distribution of binding inhibition in the three zones; with low amounts, binding was inhibited only in AbWZ-1.

Several forms of REC index calculation for the expression of reaction positivity have been investigated (Simons, 1973a; Simons, 1973b; Table IX). Those based on the degree of Ag-I^{125} anodal migration are most suitable when changes in Ag-I^{125} distribution occur in all the zones being examined. When this is not the case, the proportion of Ag-I^{125} in corresponding zones of control and test reactions can be directly compared. When it is suspected that the Ag-I^{125} distribution produced by a test sample reflects a weak positive reaction, a confirmatory test of immunological specificity can be performed. The test and control reactions are then the Ag- or Ab-inhibited and uninhibited reactions, respectively.

The quantitative studies provided useful information on the sensitivity and reliability of REC. REC was capable of furnishing relative values for some reaction parameters which were in good agreement with values obtained by more definitive techniques. The relative binding constants of DNP derivatives and anti-DNP were of the same order as expected from measurements made by fluorescence quenching (Eisen and Siskind, 1964). The rate of dissociation of anti-DNP and DNP-conjugate was related to the binding constants, as had been determined by equilibrium dialysis. Also, on a molar basis, anti-DNP IgM antibody was about 4–5 times as effective as the IgG antibody for binding of antigen, in accordance with the valences of IgM and IgG antibodies. On the assumption that the molecular composition of complexes in extreme antigen excess approaches Ag_2Ab, then, at a constant level of antibody, there will be a concentration of antigen which saturates antibody. The limiting composition of Ag_2Ab seemed to have been reached; increasing concentrations of antigen added to a limited antibody concentration approached constant binding (Fig. 5B). Although sufficient data has not as yet been obtained to test the assumptions used to estimate the weight of antibody in an antiserum, as was done so elegantly by Osler (1971) and by Revoltella *et al.* (1971a) with a modified Farr technique (Farr, 1958), the results reported here suggest that such measurements are possible with REC. In this connection, estimation of the weight of anti-DNP antibodies in the low nanogram range by REC is of the same order of sensitivity as the modified Farr method (Revoltella *et al.*, 1971b). Thus, determination of standard curves and assay of antigens can be accomplished with a sensitivity similar to that which can be achieved by other RIA procedures (Hunter, 1967).

The quantitative studies also provided evidence that immune complexes which are formed during REC may subsequently dissociate. It was found that antibody avidity was probably a major factor in complex dissociability. With relatively high electrical current and prolonged electrophoresis some dissociation occurred even with antibody of high avidity. It is likely that some dissociation takes place at all dilutions, but at low dilutions there is sufficient Ab available for recomplexing to occur. At high dilutions, a greater proportion of Ag-I^{125} will escape recomplexing. For each Ag–Ab system, it is important to establish the conditions whereby association of reactants and separation of bound from free Ag-I^{125} is maximized while dissociation of bound Ag-I^{125} is minimized. Although immune complex dissociation is a complicating factor in the REC method, it may be possible to turn the phenomenon to advantage. Investigations are proceeding to determine whether complex dissociability can be used to measure Ab avidity.

Studies using HBAg-I^{125} suggested that immune complexes of HBAg/HBAb were present in the sera of some individuals with HB antigenemia. Since HBAg is in relative excess it is likely that some dissociation of immune complexes is necessary before HBAb is available to bind with HBAg-I^{125}. It therefore seems likely that the HBAb in HB antigenemic sera is of low avidity, and hence the complexes are relatively unstable. Although these studies are at an early stage, it is already apparent that REC can be used not only for detecting the presence of immune complexes, but also for identifying their immunological specificity. REC may therefore prove to be a useful technique in the investigation of the wide range of infectious diseases in man and experimental animals, in which immune complexemia and soluble-complex deposition pathology is known or suspected to occur (WHO, 1972).

The coexistence of HBAg and HBAb in certain sera is one reason the HBAg system is more complicated than that of the model system of DNP-HSA. Another is that the single term HBAg belies the antigenic complexity of the material. HBAg refers to multiple antigenic determinants at the surface of particulate material derived from the agent responsible for hepatitis type B (WHO, 1973a). There is at least one common antigenic determinant *a* and two groups of antigenic subspecificities (d and $y;$ w and r), the antigens of each of which behave in a mutually exclusive manner (Le Bouvier, 1971; Bancroft et al., 1972). Using antisera to a, d, and y, provided by Dr. G. Le Bouvier, and sera of the Reference Panel No. 2, evidence has been obtained that sera which contain HBAg detectable by REC can be subtyped by REC.

In the section of this review dealing with application of REC (Section IV), attention has been given to the HBAg system since it is the most complicated of those so far studied. By comparison, detection and estimation of serum levels of AFP and of hormones, such as insulin and growth hormone, is relatively simple. In the case of these latter three, purified antigenic preparations are available and can be radioiodinated. The antibody-containing solution need not be specifically purified; an antiserum raised against whole human serum was found to be adequate for the detection of HSA by REC. Antisera to low-molecular-weight molecules (<5000), such as angiotensin I, vasopressin, and oxytocin, can be produced by immunization with conjugates of the polypeptide and protein carrier. HSA is suitable for this purpose. Antisera have been raised to cortisone–HSA, testosterone–HSA, and estradiol–HSA conjugates (Erlanger et al., 1957; Jeffcoate, 1971). The conjugates have a fast anodal migration which can be exploited in REC.

REC is based on the principle of CIE (Lang, 1955; Watson and Whinfrey, 1958; Bussard, 1959; Culliford, 1964; Feinberg and Hill, 1968; Kohn, 1968; Lopez et al., 1969). CIE is in widest use for the identification of HBAg (Gocke and Howe, 1970; Pesendorfer et al., 1970; Prince and Burke, 1970; Alter et al., 1971; Yap et al., 1971). In addition, CIE methods have also been described for the detection of antibodies to a variety of antigens including diphtheria and tetanus toxins (Sgouris, 1972), treponemal antigens (Banffer, 1972), meningococcal antigens (Tobin and Jones, 1972; Edwards et al., 1972), Candida extracts (Hellwege et al., 1972), plasmodial extracts (Zaman et al., 1972), influenza virus (Berlin and Pirojboot, 1972), hepatitis B antigen (Alter et al., 1971), and seminal plasma antigens (Chen and Simons, 1973), and for the detection of antigenic components of serum such as α_1-antitrypsin (Manildi, 1973) and alpha-fetoprotein (Kohn, 1970; Sizaret et al., 1971). It is anticipated that REC will be adaptable to the investigation of these Ag–Ab systems. In principle, it should be possible to apply REC to the detection of all antigens which can be made to migrate either in a direction opposite to that of immunoglobulin, or in the same direction but at a differential migration rate.

REC has been found to have a sensitivity similar to that of other RIA methods. It is practicable in that the total process from preparation of agar slides to counting of agar zones takes 4–5 hours. One person can screen 30–40 sera per electrophoretic run, and make 3–4 runs per day. The limit of conservation of reagents is approached by REC; 5-μl volumes are sufficient. The method is relatively simple to perform; no washing or centrifugation is involved. It is also relatively safe. A low total radioactivity is required per electrophoretic run (20,000–30,000 cpm). There is no risk of spillage of radioisotope from the counting tubes, because both bound and free Ag-I^{125} are in the gel. Approaches to simplifying interpretation have been described. Undiluted sera can be used, since prozone phenomena do not appear to occur. Finally, REC appears to be more adaptable to automation than previously described RIA procedures (Knight *et al.*, 1971).

ACKNOWLEDGMENTS

These investigations were supported by the World Health Organization and the International Agency for Research on Cancer (MJS), and the United States Public Health Service (AAB) (Grant No. AI-05660). We thank Mr. Thomas Ee, Ms. Marianne Stella (WHO Immunology Research and Training Centre, University of Singapore), and Mr. Leonard Pollard (Department of Microbiology, University of Hawaii, Honolulu) for superb technical assistance. Dr. Yap Eu Hian (Department of Parasitology, University of Singapore), Mr. Tim Greenland (Service des Proteines, Institut Pasteur, Lyon, France), and Professor Gordon L. Ada (Department of Microbiology, Australian National University, Canberra) gave invaluable support and advice to MJS.

Radioisotope counting in Singapore was performed using a Panax Manual Well Crystal Counter lent by Dynatech Corporation, Cooke Engineering Division, Alexandria, Virginia.

REFERENCES

Aach, R. D., Grisham, J. W., and Parker, C. W., 1971, *Proc. Natl. Acad. Sci. U.S.* **68**:1056.
Abelev, G. I., Perova, S. D., Khramkova, N. I., Postnikova, Z. A., and Irlin, I. S., 1963, *Transplantation* **1**:174.
Abelev, G. I., Tsvetkov, V. S., Brvulina, T. I., Elgort, D. A., Olovnikov, A. M., Gusev, A. I., Yazova, A. K. Perova, S. D., Rubtsov, I. V., Shaborina, S. V., Kautorovich, B. A., Tur, V. M., Khazanev, A. I., and Levina, D. M., 1971, *Bul. Eksperim. Biol. i Med.* **4**:75.
Alter, H. J., Holland, P. V., and Purcell, R. H., 1971, *J. Lab. Clin. Med.* **77**:1000.
Ashman, R. F., and Metzger, H., 1969, *J. Biol. Chem.* **244**:3405.
Bancroft, W. H., Mundon, F. K., and Russell, P. K., 1972, *J. Immunol.* **109**:842.
Banffer, J. R. J., 1972, *Lancet* **1**:996.
Benedict, A. A., 1967, in Williams, C. A., and Chase, M. W. (eds.), *Methods in Immunology and Immunochemistry*, Vol. I, Academic Press, New York, p. 299.
Beng, C. G., Chan, G. L., Simons, M. J., and Lau, K. S., 1973, *Int. Arch. Allergy* **45**:352.
Berlin, B. S., and Pirojbott, N., 1972, *J. Infect. Diseases* **126**:345.
Berson, S. A., Yalow, R. S., Bauman, A., Rothschild, M. A., and Newerby, K., 1956, *J. Clin. Invest.* **35**:170.
Blumberg, B. S., 1964, *Bull. N.Y. Acad. Med.* **40**:377.
Bussard, A., 1959, *Biochim. Biophys. Acta.* **34**:258.
Caldwell, B. V., Burstein, S., Brock, W. A., and Speroff, L., 1971, *J. Clin. Endocrinol. Metab.* **33**:171.
Capalbo, E. E., 1972, *International Atomic Energy Agency*, Vienna, p. 41.

Chan, P., and Ti, T. K., 1973, Personal communication.
Chen, C. Y. H., and Simons, M. J., 1973, *Proc. 8th. Singapore-Malaysia Congress of Medicine*, Tan. N. C. (ed.), 8:295.
Coller, J. A., Millman, I., Halbherr, T. C., and Blumberg, B. S., 1971, *Proc. Soc. Exp. Biol. Med.* **138**:249.
Coller, J. A., Yin, L. K., and Crichlow, R. W., 1972, *Proc. Am. Assoc. Cancer Res.* **13**:95.
Coller, J. A., Crichlow, R. W., and Lo, K. Y., 1973, *Cancer Research* **33**:1684.
Cuatrecasas, P., Wilcheck, M., and Anfinsen, C. B., 1968, *Proc. Natl. Acad. Sci. U.S.* **61**:636.
Culliford, B. T., 1964, *Nature* **201**:1092.
Day, L. A., Sturtevant, J. M., and Singer, S. J., 1963, *Ann. N.Y. Acad. Sci.* **103**:611.
Edwards, E. A., Muehl, P. M., and Peckingpaugh, R. O., 1972, *J. Lab. Clin. Med.* **80**:449.
Eisen, H. N., and Siskind, G. W., 1964, *Biochemistry* **3**:996.
Eisen, H. N., 1964, in Eisen, H. N. (ed.) *Methods in Medical Research*, Vol. 10, Year Book Medical Publishers, Chicago, p. 94.
Erlanger, B. F., Borek, F., Beiser, S. M., and Lieberman, S., 1957, *J. Biol. Chem.* **228**:713.
Farr, R. S., 1958, *J. Infect. Diseases* **103**:239.
Feinberg, J. G., and Hill, C. W., 1968, *Arch. Allergy* **33**:120.
Froese, A., 1968, *Immunochemistry* **5**:253.
Gerloff, R. K., and Watson, R. O., 1967, *Am. J. Ophthalmol.* **63**:1492.
Ginsberg, A. L., Conrad, M. E., Bancroft, W. H., Ling, C. M., and Overby, L. R., 1972, *New Engl. J. Med.* **286**:562.
Gocke, D. J., and Howe, C., 1970, *Immunology* **104**:1031.
Hellwege, H. H., Fisher, K., and Blaker, F., 1972, *Lancet* **2**:386.
Hirai, H., Nishi, S., and Watabe, H., 1973, in Peeters, H. (ed.), *Protides of the Biological Fluids*, Vol. 20, Pergamon Press, Oxford, p. 579.
Hollinger, F. B., Vorndam, V., and Dreesman, G. R., 1971, *J. Immunol.* **107**:1099.
Hornick, C. L., and Karush, F., 1969, *Israel J. Med. Sci.* **5**:163.
Hornick, C. L., and Karush, F., 1972, *Immunochemistry* **9**:325.
Hunter, W. M., and Greenwood, F. C., 1962, *Nature (London)* **194**:495.
Hunter, W. M., 1967, Weir, D. M. (ed.), *Handbook of Experimental Immunology*, Blackwell Scientific Publications, Oxford, p. 608.
Ishii, M., 1973, *Monograph on Cancer Research* **14**:89.
Ishizaka, K., Ishizaka, T., and Campbell, D. H., 1959, *J. Exp. Med.* **109**:127.
Jeffcoate, S. L., 1971, in Kirkham, K. E., and Hunter, W. M. (eds.), *Radioimmunoassay Methods*, Churchill Livingstone, Edinburgh and London, p. 591.
Kirkham, K. E., and Hunter, W. M., 1971, *Radioimmunoassay Methods*, Churchill Livingstone, Edinburgh and London.
Kleczowski, A., 1959, *Immunology* **2**:97.
Knight, R. A., Caldwell, C., and Audhya, T. A., 1971, in Kirkham, K. E., and Hunter, W. M. (eds.), *Radioimmunoassay Methods*, Churchill Livingstone, Edinburgh and London, p. 598.
Kohn, J., 1968, in Smith, I. (ed.), *Chromatographic and Electrophoretic Techniques*, Heinemann, London, p. 137.
Kohn, J., 1970, *J. Clin. Pathol.* **23**:733.
Lang, N., 1955, *Klin. Wochschr.* **33**:29.
Landsteiner, K., 1945, *The Specificity of Serological Reactions*, Harvard University Press, reprinted 1962 by Dover Publications, Inc., New York.
Lander, J. J., Alter, H. J., and Purcell, R. H., 1971, *J. Immunol.* **106**:1166.
LeBouvier, G. L., 1971, *J. Infect. Diseases* **123**:671.
Levine, L., and van Vunakis, H., 1970, *Biochim. Biophys. Res. Commun.* **41**:1171.
Ling, C. M., and Overby, L. R., 1972, *J. Immunol.* **109**:834.
Little, J. R., and Donahue, H., 1968, in Williams, C. A., and Chase, M. W. (eds.), *Methods in Immunology and Immunochemistry*, Vol. II, Academic Press, New York, p. 344.
Lopez, M., Tsu, T., and Hyslop, N. E., 1969, *Immunochemistry* **6**:513.
Manildi, E. R., 1973, *Clin. Chem.* **18**:1019.
Masseyeff, R., Gilli, J., and Bonet, C., 1973, *Proceedings of the First International Meeting*

of the International Research Groups for Carcinoembryonic Proteins. Bull. Sapporo Med. College. Hirai, H., and Wada, T. (eds.) in press.

McConahey, P. S., and Dixon, F. J. 1966, *Intern. Arch. Allergy Appl. Immunol.* 29:185.

Minden, P., Anthony, B. F., and Farr, R. S., 1969, *J. Immunol.* 102:83.

Nishi, S., and Hirai, H., 1973, *Gann Monograph on Cancer Research* 14:79.

O'Conor, G. T., Tatarinov, Y. S., Abelev, G. I., and Uriel, J., 1970, *Cancer* 25:1091.

Onoue, K., Grossberg, A., Yagi, Y., and Pressman, D., 1968, *Science* 162:574.

Osler, A. G., 1971, in Williams, C. A., and Chase, M. W. (eds.), *Methods in Immunology and Immunochemistry,* Vol. 3, Academic Press, New York, p. 73.

Pauling, L., Pressman, D., and Grossberg, A. L., 1944, *J. Am. Chem. Soc.* 66:330.

Pesendorfer, F., Krassnitzky, O., and Wewalka, F., 1970, *Klin. Wochschr.* 48:58.

Prince, A. M., and Burke, K., 1970, *Science* 169:593.

Purcell, R. H., 1970, *Bull. World Health Organ.* 42:978.

Purcell, R. H., 1972, Personal communication.

Purves, L. R., Macnab, M., Gedes, E. W., and Bersohn, I., 1968, *Lancet.* 1:921.

Purves, L. R., and Geddes, E. W., 1972, *Lancet* 1:47.

Purves, L. R., and Purves, M., 1972, *S. Africa Med. J.* 46:1290.

Revoltella, R., Adler, L. T., and Osler, A. G., 1971a, *J. Immunol.* 106:1507.

Revoltella, R., Adler, L. T., and Osler, A. G., 1971b, *J. Immunol.* 106:1519.

Ruoslahti, E., and Seppala, M., 1971, *Int. J. Cancer* 8:374.

Simons, M. J., 1972, *Proc. Aust. Soc. Immunol.* (Abst.) p. 60.

Simons, M. J., 1973a, *Bull. World Health Organ.,* 48:499.

Simons, M. J., 1973b, *Bull. World Health Organ.,* in press.

Simons, M. J., and Hosking, C. S., 1973, unpublished observations.

Simons, M. J., Yu, M., and Shanmugaratnam, K., 1973, *Proceedings of the First International Meetings of the International Research Groups for Carcinoembryonic Proteins.* Bull. Sapporo Med. College (Edited by H. Hirai), in press.

Singer, S. J., and Campbell, D. H., 1955, *J. Am. Chem. Soc.* 77:4851.

Sizaret, P. P., McIntyre, R. K., and Princler, G. L., 1971, *Cancer Research* 31:1899.

Sgouris, T. J., 1972, *Vox Sanguinis* 22:359.

Tabert, G. C., and Lachman, D. B., 1965, *J. Immunol.* 94:959.

Tatarinov, Y. S., 1964, *Vopr. Med. Khim.* 10:90.

Thomson, D. M. P., Krupey, J., Freedman, S. O., and Gold, P., 1969, *Proc. Natl. Acad. Sci. U.S.* 64:161.

Tilden, R. L., and DeLand, F. H., 1972, *J. Nucl. Med.* 13:599.

Tobin, B. M., and Jones, D. M., 1972, *J. Clin. Pathol.* 25:583.

Waldmann, T. A., and McIntire, K. R., 1972, *Lancet* 2: 1112.

Walsh, J. H., Yalow, R., and Berson, S. A., 1970, *J. Infect. Diseases* 121:550.

Watson, D., and Whinfrey, H., 1958, *Lancet* 2:1375.

Weigle, W. O., and Deichmuller, M. P., 1960, *J. Immunol.* 84:434.

Werblin, T. P., and Siskind, G. W., 1972, *Immunochemistry* 9:987.

WHO, 1972, *Bull. World Health Organ.* 47:257.

WHO, 1973a, *Viral hepatitis. World Health Organ. Technical Report Series,* No. 512.

WHO, 1973b, *Proceedings of the WHO-assisted Workshop on Hepatitis B Antigen.* Tokyo, Japan, in preparation.

Wofsy, L., and Burr, B., 1969, *J. Immunol.* 103:380.

Yalow, R. S., and Berson, S. A., 1960, *J. Clin. Invest.* 39:1157.

Yalow, R. S., and Berson, S. A., 1964, *Methods Biochem. Analy.* 12:69.

Yap, E. H., Ee, T. I., and Simons, M. J., 1971, *Southeast Asian J. Trop. Med. Public Health* 2:486.

Zaman, V., Ascheim, L., Yap, E. H., and Simons, M. J., 1972, *Singapore Med. J.* 13:6.

Index